Pediatric Disorders of Feeding, Nutrition, and Metabolism

Pediatric Disorders of Feeding, Nutrition, and Metabolism

INGEBORG KRIEGER, M.D.
Professor of Pediatrics
School of Medicine
Wayne State University
Director, Nutrition and Metabolism Service
Children's Hospital of Michigan
Detroit, Michigan

1807 175 YEARS OF PUBLISHING 1982

A WILEY MEDICAL PUBLICATION
JOHN WILEY & SONS
New York • Chichester • Brisbane • Toronto • Singapore

Library of Congress Cataloging in Publication Data:

Krieger, Ingeborg.
Pediatric disorders of feeding, nutrition, and metabolism.

(A Wiley medical publication)
Includes index.
1. Nutrition disorders—in children.
2. Metabolic disorders in children. 3. Children—Diseases—Nutritional aspects. I. Title.
II. Series: Wiley medical publication. [DNLM:
1. Nutrition disorders—In infancy and childhood.
2. Metabolism, Inborn errors. WS 115 K92p]
RJ390.K74 618.92′39 81-21923
ISBN 0-471-08730-0 AACR2

Printed in the United States of America

10 9 8 7 6 5 4 3 2 1

To JACQUELINE and SUZANNE

Preface

The need for education in nutrition is now well recognized by the medical community, especially as it relates to nutrition of the fetus and infant as a determinant of health throughout life. As a result of this insight, nutrition education has been integrated into the curriculum of many medical schools, and a number of excellent books and symposia dealing with normal nutrition or different aspects of clinical nutrition have been published in recent years. There has not yet been, however, a comprehensive book of pediatric clinical nutrition that presents in a single volume clinically relevant nutrition information essential for normal child care and the management of diseases.

This book introduces medical students, pediatric house staff, and practitioners caring for children to the full range of normal and abnormal conditions that require consideration of nutrition—either as a cause of disease, as a tool in the diagnosis of metabolic disorders, or in therapy. Whereas the major emphasis is on nutritional deficiencies and diseases of overnutrition, the book also covers genetic disorders that resemble nutritional deficiencies and diseases that respond to nutritional therapy although they themselves are not caused by abnormal nutrition. Thus the book includes sections on select inborn errors of metabolism, gastrointestinal disorders, and allergic or immunodeficiency diseases.

Normal nutrition is presented as a function of age in an introductory chapter, together with a brief presentation on infant foods and an overview of nutritional assessment methods. Chapters dealing with infant feeding disorders, emotional deprivation syndromes, obesity, and anorexia nervosa include in-depth discussions of psychological factors that make the book relevant to the entire health care team, including nurses and social workers. The clinical approach to diagnosis is stressed in the presentation of disorders that share a common disease expression—for example, hypoglycemia, failure to thrive, and chronic diarrhea. Practical therapeutic guidelines are given for each condition or disease, stressing health maintenance and including the latest therapeutic approaches to the nutritional treatment of genetic metabolic diseases. The biochemical or physiologic aspects of disease are covered only to the extent necessary for an understanding of disease processes or the approach to therapy.

The proper use of references has been a most difficult task, since it is impossible to give due credit to all the workers in the field who have made contributions in the many areas of nutrition discussed in this book. Consequently, historically important references are mentioned only infrequently, and no attempt is made to cite original contributions that have become part of common knowledge. The book is not intended to be a reference source, although attempts are made to quote at least a few references on all recent advances, which consequently may be used by the student as a starting point for further literature research. The choice does not represent bias in instances where a determination of priority or importance of a contribution was not possible for the author. Occasionally, single observations are cited, because they were too recent to have been confirmed but seem to contribute to basic nutrition knowledge—for instance, in the case of rare single-nutrient deficiencies. When only one reference seemed appropriate, as in other rare disorders—like inborn errors of vitamin metabolism—a specific reference may have been chosen not because of it's originality, but because it covered the most recent studies of enzyme function. Quotations of the author's own research are intended as a means of giving added credibility to those discussions where the author can claim expertise.

Finally, I would like to acknowledge the help of my secretary, Fran Blaske, and co-workers Qamar Taqi and Mike Fracassa.

I.K.

Contents

Pediatric Disorders of Feeding, Nutrition, and Metabolism

1 Nutritional Requirements as a Function of Age

INTRAUTERINE NUTRITION
Basic Principles
Fetal Growth Retardation
Recommendations

THE FULL TERM (FT) AND LOW BIRTH WEIGHT (LBW) NEONATE
Nutrition as a Function of Gastrointestinal Maturation
Effects of Food Introduction on Gastrointestinal Function
Protein Digestion and Absorption
Fat Digestion and Absorption
Carbohydrate Digestion and Absorption
Recommendations
Nutritional Goals
Choice of Nutrients
Quantity of Nutrients

INFANCY
Nutrition as a Function of Neuromuscular Maturation
Recommendations
Semisolid Foods: Time and Sequence of Introduction
Meal Schedule

PRESCHOOL YEARS, SCHOOL AGE, AND ADOLESCENCE
Nutrition as a Function of Growth and Sexual Maturation
Growth
Nutrient Requirements
Assessment of Nutrient Intake
Special Considerations for the Teenage Athlete

RECOMMENDED DIETARY ALLOWANCES (RDA)

INTRAUTERINE NUTRITION

A wealth of data has appeared in the literature over the past decades dealing with the effect of calorie and protein restriction during pregnancy on fetal growth and postnatal development. Most of these investigations have shown that nutrient restriction causes retardation of statural growth and organ size, hormone deficiencies, and an increase in mortality.

Basic Principles

Improved understanding of the mechanisms that are responsible for the profound and potentially lasting influence of maternal nutrition on the fetus comes mainly from rat experiments. Enesco and Leblond (1) first recognized that intrauterine growth occurs either through cell proliferation or cell enlargement. In the early months following conception, when organs like the heart and kidney develop and differentiate, growth is primarily due to rapid cell multiplication. This *hyperplastic* phase is followed by an intermediate phase, in which cell proliferation continues but is associated with an increase in cell size. During the final, *hypertrophic* phase, body and organ mass increase mainly by cell enlargement.

Nutritional insults have a different effect during each of these growth phases. The earlier the insult, the more likely it is to result in irreversible damage. Undernutrition during the proliferative phase slows the rate of cell division. If realimentation is delayed until the time that is programmed for cell proliferation has passed, cell number will be permanently reduced. By contrast, fetal growth retardation that develops during the hypertrophic phase is reversible.

The effect of a nutritional insult varies in different species and organs because the timing of these growth sequences is not the same in each. Growth of the human brain through cell proliferation continues after birth but slows down at around 1 to 2 months of age; it reaches a plateau toward the end of the first year (2). A reduction in the total number of brain cells of up to 20% has been recorded in infants who died of undernutrition during early infancy (3). The cell number of infants who had a low birth weight and died of undernutrition was reduced to 60%. This represents a comparatively large reduction in brain cell number, which may have been the combined result of pre- and postnatal deprivation. The same group of investigators had observed that the effect of undernutrition in rats throughout two proliferative phases was more pronounced than the sum of the effects seen in each single phase (4). The reduction in total brain cell number of infants who were undernourished beyond 8 months of age is accompanied by a reduction in total cholesterol and phospholipids. In view of a normal lipid concentration, this finding was interpreted to be caused by a decrease in the number and length of myelin sheaths.

Fetal growth retardation in humans is manifested by a low birth weight

(LBW) for length of gestation. This group of LBW infants should be distinguished from infants who are small because of prematurity. Premature infants may sustain injury due to undernutrition if the rate of weight gain, which can be accomplished after birth, is significantly below that in utero. By contrast, if the small for gestational age (SGA) infant has suffered an earlier insult, it may be irreversible. Major differences between the two groups are evidenced by the fact that the typical neonatal complications of premature infants are respiratory distress and hyperbilirubinemia, whereas SGA infants are prone to become hypoglycemic and a larger percentage seems to have irreversible growth failure.

Fetal Growth Retardation

The incidence of fetal growth retardation is high, according to Lubchenco (5), who estimates that 30% of all LBW infants are SGA. In underdeveloped countries the incidence is considerably higher (6).

Causes of low birth weight for length of gestation are (*1*) a decrease in the inherent growth potential of the fetus or (*2*) deficient growth support by the mother. Chromosomal abnormalities and other genetic dwarfing syndromes are examples of the former. Growth support may be deficient because of decreased nutrient concentration in the maternal blood, deficient transfer of nutrients across the placenta, or a decreased rate of placental blood flow. Although circulatory abnormalities may seem equivalent to undernutrition, there is evidence from rat experiments to indicate that the effects of these two insults are different (7). Rats with a compromised fetal blood supply due to uterine artery ligation had offspring with "asymmetrical" growth failure, where the brain was almost completely spared. Analogous differences have been observed in SGA human infants (8).

When a pregnancy is carried to term or longer and the placenta becomes infarcted, or when the blood supply is compromised toward the end of gestation for other reasons, the neonate will be wasted; length will be normal or only slightly decreased, and the head will be normal for height but large relative to body size. The "postmature" infant is thus as long as the full term infant, but birth weight is decreased due to consumption of nutrients, including glycogen stores in the liver. SGA infants with normal length should be distinguished from those with a significantly decreased length and a small head for height because the prognosis appears to be different.

Malnutrition is one cause of fetal growth retardation in humans, as suggested by observations made during the Dutch famine of World War II and by the high incidence of SGA births to women on reducing diets. It has been estimated that maternal nutrition contributes about 45% to birth weight; genetic factors, 25%, and all others, including maternal height, prepregnant weight, age, and smoking, the rest. Several studies in underdeveloped countries have shown that the incidence of LBW infants can be reduced significantly by giving dietary supplements to pregnant women. A similar beneficial effect was observed in a poor black urban population in the United States (9). Balanced protein-calorie supplements increased length of gestation and reduced the proportion of LBW infants, but raised the mean birth weight of the total group by only 41 g, which was not significant. A noteworthy observation was the adverse effect of high-protein supplements. They were associated with significant growth retardation up to 37 weeks' gestation and with an excess of very early premature births and neonatal deaths.

Other causes of SGA are chromosomal abnormalities, viral infections, hypertension, smoking, and alcohol ingestion by the mother, extremes of age and parity, toxemia, twinning, and placental abnormalities. Only in some of these instances can the mechanism be linked to a form of malnutrition—which is present, for example, in twinning—because it may lead to competition for blood and nutrient supply. Infants of toxemic mothers most resemble the offspring of rats with a ligated uterine artery because their length and brain, heart, and lung weight are not severely affected while body weight and weight of liver, spleen, and adrenals are disproportionately small (8).

The prognosis for later growth and intellectual development varies in different SGA infants, although precise data that might allow prediction based on growth parameters at birth are not yet available. By and large, it can be stated that the prognosis for growth is better in infants with a normal or only slightly decreased height for length of gestation. Regardless of height, prognosis for intellectual development is poor in infants with a head circumference at or below the third percentile. There is still doubt whether maternal malnutrition throughout gestation can irreversibly affect the brain and cause permanent stunting. Primate studies support the contention that rat data cannot be applied to humans. For instance, protein and calorie restrictions on pregnant monkeys cause fetal growth retardation only if the deficit is so severe that the mother has used up all her body stores. Since proliferation of brain growth in humans, in contrast to rats, continues throughout the first 2 years, one can expect that a prenatal nutritional insult can be compensated for after birth. The disproportionately large reduction in brain cell number observed by Winick and coworkers (3,4) in LBW infants who died of malnutrition during infancy was not proven to be due to intrauterine malnutrition. Infection or teratogenic insults may have played a role. Reductions in the number of cells in the brain and other parenchymal organs have been observed following intrauterine viral infections (10).

Recommendations

In the past, women were encouraged to keep their weight gain during pregnancy to between 7 and 8 kg. This practice stemmed from the erroneous belief that the limitation would decrease the incidence of eclampsia. There is now sufficient evidence that inadequate weight gain increases the incidence of LBW infants. A weight gain of 11 to 12 kg is currently considered desirable. The RDA for pregnant women is 300 kcal/day more than the basic caloric requirement of mature nonpregnant women. Protein intake is also an important consideration, since the pregnant woman must synthesize complex new tissues. An additional 30 g/day over the basic allowance is therefore recommended.

The rate of maternal weight gain should roughly parallel fetal growth, with little gain in the first trimester (approximately 500 g/month) and a rapid increase in the second trimester, when weight gains usually amount to about 500 g/week. If the mother gains slightly more but at a regular rate, criticism of her dietary habits is not warranted. A gain, however, in excess of 3,000 g/month should be cause for concern. Women tend to add to their own body fat stores approximately 20% of the recommended total weight gain, or about 5 lb. This amount can be lost easily after delivery. Fifty percent of the total gain is for the products of conception and 30% for an increase in blood volume, excess body water, and tissues added to the reproductive organs. Considering that demands on nutritional support are minimal during the first trimester, one may assume that malnutrition during the first trimester has little effect on the fetus because the demand can be supplied by maternal stores of fat and muscle.

THE FULL TERM (FT) AND LOW BIRTH WEIGHT (LBW) NEONATE

Gastrointestinal digestive and absorptive function of the full term (FT) infant appear adequate for growth and development, if judged only by the fact that mankind has survived and developed and used the species' intellectual potential. This was accomplished by raising infants on breast milk, which is ideal, for reasons we are only now beginning to understand. Breast feeding is being done with increasing frequency again today. However, since artificial feeding will inevitably continue, it is important to examine whether commercial formulas and supplemental solid foods impose a burden on the digestive system, with the possible risk of causing illness and unnecessary loss of nutrients.

Adequacy of gastrointestinal function is even more important in premature infants, especially since there now are many formulas on the market that are not all equally suitable for premature infants. Since 10% of infants in the United States and up to 40% in underdeveloped countries are born prematurely, feeding these infants and assuring adequate catch-up growth and development are important tasks.

Nutrition as a Function of Gastrointestinal Maturation

The neonate, who has received nutrients throughout gestation from the mother in a readily usable form by way of the placenta, is suddenly faced with the digestion and absorption of food in amounts that are much greater relative to body weight than in the adult. This task must be accomplished at a time when the turnover rate of the intestinal brush border is slow and when—in addition to digestion and absorption—many other functions, like sucking and swallowing, esophageal and intestinal motility, gastroesophageal sphincter control and gastric emptying, are immature.

Effects of Food Introduction on Gastrointestinal Function

Animal experiments indicate that the development of gastrointestinal function follows in an intrinsic ontogenetic sequence that is only to a degree modified by food. For instance, the lactase activity of rats drops around weaning time, while sucrase activity rises. This drop is not related to the diet change at weaning, because lactase activity declines even when weaning is delayed. However, the introduction of food is not without effects on gastrointestinal function; intestinal weight increases after exposure to food because of an increase in mucosal mass, which is accompanied by an increase in enzyme activity. Although this appears to be an induction phenomenon, it is not specific for individual foods. Examples are the stimulation of lipase activity by protein, disaccharidase by glucose, and tryptic activity by elemental diets composed of amino acids.

These programmed changes in gastrointestinal enzyme activity may be related to changes in endocrine function. Although knowledge is incomplete to date, there is evidence from animal data indicating that certain hormones have a stimulatory effect. For instance, cortisone given to pregnant rats induces sucrase activity, and thyroidectomy delays and dampens the increase in enzyme activity that occurs normally after birth. While these observations suggest a therapeutic role for hormones, such therapy is not advisable at this time because of the possibility of undesirable side effects.

Protein Digestion and Absorption

The proteolytic activity of newborn infants is low compared to that of older infants. This applies to the tryptic activity of duodenal juices as well as the gastric secretion of pepsin and hydrochloric acid. An abrupt, nearly threefold rise occurs during the latter two-thirds of the first year. After reaching a peak between 1 and 2 years, tryptic activity levels off and at 4 years is only about double what it is at birth. Since the rise is roughly proportional to body weight and calorie intake (11), we have assumed that the low activity after birth does not reflect deficiency. Indeed, nitrogen balance studies of young infants indicate that protein absorption is adequate, even on intakes of up to 4.5 g/kg/day. Fecal nitrogen is in the normal range.

Trypsin and enterokinase activity can be demonstrated between 26 and 28 weeks of gestation. The amount at this time represents only one-third the activity of FT infants. By contrast, intestinal mucosal peptidase and absorptive capacity for amino acids are well developed in LBW infants. Moreover, a high-protein diet stimulates trypsin production, which, according to Zoppi et al. (12), is higher in LBW infants at 10 days of age than in the FT infant at birth. Differences between premature and FT infants have been reported by some investigators, but they appear to be of little practical significance. The past practice of giving high-protein diets to LBW infants has not caused gastrointestinal problems.

Fat Digestion and Absorption

Fat digestion begins with exposure of food to the gastric juice. Gastric lipolytic activity is induced after birth by the introduction of food (13). Gastric lipolysis plays a greater role in the fat digestion of newborns than of older infants because their pancreatic lipolytic capacity is limited by low bile salt concentration; bile acids are not essential for gastric hydrolysis.

The contribution of gastric juice to fat digestion is even greater in LBW than in FT infants, because pancreatic lipase is poorly developed between 30 and 34 weeks' gestation. Monoglycerides and fatty acids, which are products of gastric digestion, promote the solubilization of nonpolar lipids (triglycerides, diglycerides, and cholesterol) and prepare them for digestion by pancreatic lipase (14). A study that compared two groups of infants at 30 weeks' gestation indeed showed lower fat excretion in a group fed by nasogastric tube (14.9%) than in one fed by nasojejunal tube (23.0%), thereby proving that gastric digestion is important (15).

Pancreatic lipase activity in FT infants is low, according to Norman et al. (16). By contrast, Widdowson (17) reported only a minor decrease in digestive and absorptive capacity. Pancreatic lipase is decreased in LBW infants, but by 1 week of age, lipase activity surpasses that of the full term infant at birth (12). Feeding a high-protein diet stimulates the production of lipase, while high fat alone does not have a stimulatory effect.

The molecular structure of fat is a factor in fat utilization, according to studies by Holt et al. (18) and Filer et al. (19). These investigators found that the absorption of free palmitic acid is low and that the absorbability of the ester is 84% if the fatty acid is in the 1-position, compared to 92% in the 2-position. Holt observed that vegetable oils containing unsaturated fatty acids are better absorbed than butter fat. Both findings agree with subsequent reports showing that fat absorption is better from human milk than from cow's milk, which has less unsaturated fatty acids and higher esterification in the 1-position (20). Fat losses ranging from 30 to 55% have been observed in LBW infants after ingestion of cow's milk (21), an observation that is similar to that reported for full term infants by Fomon (22). Infants less than 10 days of age absorb only about 60% of butter fat, while they demonstrate acceptable absorption rates (in excess of 80%) of oils from coconuts, corn, safflower, and peanuts. These oils are better absorbed from milk-based formulas than from formulas whose protein source is a soy isolate, a finding that should concern pediatricians prophylactically treating newborns with an atopic constitution with a low-allergenic formula. Absorption of soybean oil is also affected by the protein source.

Morales et al. (23) showed that the percentage of fat absorption remains the same whether a diet of high or low fat content is offered. They suggest that energy retention can be increased by offering a high-fat diet. Whether or not increased fat excretion is harmful when absolute fat absorption is adequate remains unknown.

Inadequate bile acid concentrations of less than 2 mmoles/l in duodenal aspirates of 3- to 15-day-old infants are probably a major cause of steathorrhea in the newborn period (16,24). Whereas their values are variable in full term infants, bile concentrations in LBW infants are uniformly low. The bile acid pool increases with age, although the synthesis of bile acids remains the same, an observation that can be explained by improved enterohepatic circulation. Bile acids are the limiting factor in fat absorption because they facilitate the action of pancreatic lipase and solubilize the end products of lipolysis.

Since exocrine pancreatic function of the LBW infant is adequate after enzyme induction through feeding, steathorrhea of prematurity appears to be caused mainly by inadequate bile acid excretion. The bile acid pool of the premature infant is approximately half that of the full term infant. The concentration in duodenal juice has ranged in most studies below the 2 mmoles/l required for formation of micellar solutions (25). Excessive losses of bile acids in the stools have been reported (26).

Studies of fat absorption in newborns by Snyderman et al. and subsequently by other investigators have shown that triglycerides containing medium chain fatty acids are well absorbed by both premature and FT infants (27). Utilization of medium chain triglycerides (MCT) is not lipase dependent and does not require bile acids for micelle formation. Gastric hydrolysis liberates medium chain fatty acids, which are then able to short-circuit the lymphatic system. Resynthesis of triglycerides in the intestinal epithelium is not required. Medium chain fatty acids are absorbed directly into the venous system, where they complex readily with serum albumin and are transported to the liver.

Carbohydrate Digestion and Absorption

There is no convincing evidence that healthy FT infants have a problem with disaccharide digestion. Tests for fecal reducing substances are, by and large, negative. Moreover, lactase activity is greater during infancy than in later life. Glucose, galactose, and fructose, the split products of disaccharide digestion, are well absorbed, according to in vitro accumulation studies using human intestine. Some perfusion experiments, on the other hand, have been indicative of deficiency, but these results were probably a function of the methodology, which does not reflect physiologic intestinal conditions. That the rate of glucose absorption is decreased after a large load is suggested by the fact that neonates often do not achieve peak plasma glucose levels until 60 minutes after an oral glucose tolerance test.

The capacity of the LBW infant may be limited for disaccharidase digestion, mainly lactase, which appears to be low prior to 8 months' gestation. During the last month of gestation, lactase rises sharply to birth levels, which are subsequently maintained throughout infancy (28). It has been estimated that the premature infant can hydrolyze only about one-third the amount hydrolyzed by the FT infant. In contrast to the development of lactase activity, maltase and sucrase appear earlier, rising sharply at around 6 months' gestation and reaching levels during the eighth month that are comparable to those of full term infants (28).

The capacity for starch digestion has not been questioned until recently. Data are now appearing that suggest that starch digestion may be limited in newborn infants. At birth, amylase is about one-tenth the adult value, and tolerance tests by and large show only minimal increases in blood glucose concentration following oral ingestion of starches. By 4 months of age, all infants have generally adequate starch digestion (29). The concentration appears to be crucial because feedings containing 3.5% starch are well tolerated in young infants, but higher concentrations of about 6% may cause fermentative diarrhea due to fecal excretion of dextrins and glucose (30).

Recommendations

Nutritional Goals

Good nutrition should be aimed at accomplishing a normal rate of growth. The weight gain that must be achieved after birth is greater than at any other time in life. It amounts to 30 to 40 g/day, or 7.5 g/kg/day at 2 weeks of age, 5.7 g/kg/day at 1 month, and 2.8 g/kg/day at 5 months of age.

Determination of the nutritional goal for LBW infants is more difficult than for full term infants. Some neonatologists believe that one should strive to imitate the rate of weight gain that would have taken place in utero if the infant had been carried to term. During the last trimester, the gain amounts to more than 30 g/day, or 15 g/kg/day for infants of 33 weeks' gestation. On a per kilogram basis, this is twice the rate of a FT infant. To accomplish this rate of growth, calorie requirements are higher—130 cal/kg/day or more. Infants recovering from malnutrition, who gain 15 g/kg/day or more, generally tolerate that much food. However, in view of their immaturity and changed environment after birth, growth rates of a similar magnitude may not be physiologic for all LBW infants.

Weight gains of about 4 oz/week or 15 g/kg/day are possible and have been reported in premature infants of 1.12 kg after they regained their birth weight at 3 weeks of age (31,32). By 3 months of age, which would have been the normal time of birth for these infants, weight gains were comparable to those of FT infants (i.e., almost 2 lb/month). However, catch-up growth cannot occur unless postnatal growth exceeds that of normal infants. Studies from the United States and abroad show that height and weight usually remain below standard curves during the first year and even up to 4 years of age (31,33,5). Head circumference deviated least from the norm.

Choice of Nutrients

The selection of food in early infancy should be determined by the digestive and absorptive capacity of the newborn infant. Three limiting factors must be taken into consideration: (*1*) fat digestion and absorption are deficient in some FT and most LBW infants; (*2*) digestion of lactose may be limited in LBW infants; and (*3*) both FT and LBW infants are deficient in starch digestion.

A certain degree of fat malabsorption may not present a problem for the healthy FT infant who has a good appetite and an adequate volume capacity. LBW infants, on the other hand, who require formulas with high caloric density, may be affected by the fecal loss of fat since it represents a significant energy drain and thus increases calorie requirements per body weight even more. The use of formulas that supply a percentage of fat as medium chain triglycerides is therefore recommended for LBW infants. FT infant formulas are best made up of blends of vegetable oils and animal fats.

The need for elimination of lactose from the diet of LBW infants is debatable. This currently requires the use of hypoallergenic formulas because they are the only ones on the market without lactose. Protein hydrolysate formulas that are also lactose free are not necessary in LBW infants since their protein digestion is not decreased. Special formulas have been introduced in recent years that address the nutritional problem of LBW infants by providing (*1*) a portion of the carbohydrate as polycose, (*2*) part of the fat as MCT, and (*3*) increased caloric density without increased osmolality. They are Similac 24 LBW (Ross) and Enfamil premature formula (Mead Johnson).

Recommendations regarding the use of cereals present no difficulty because cereals offer no advantage to the neonate that cannot be obtained from milk. Thus, they need not be introduced until the LBW infant is about 4 months old.

Quantity of Nutrients

The amount of food required by the neonate is a function of body composition and the desired rate of growth (see Table 1-1 to 1-3). Feeding should commence on the second day of life because the infant is born with reserves of glycogen and water that are not adequate for a longer period of time. The practice of feeding only water during the first few days in order to avoid aspiration has been abandoned. LBW infants and infants

Table 1-1. Recommended Dietary Allowances (Revised 1980)

	Age (years)	Weight (kg)	Weight (lb)	Height (cm)	Height (in)	Protein (g/kg)	Protein (g/day)	*Fat-Soluble Vitamins:* Vitamin A (μg Retinol Equiv)[a]	Vitamin D (μg)	Vitamin E (mg Tocopherol Equiv)	*Water-Soluble Vitamins:* Vitamin C (mg)	Thiamin (mg)	Riboflavin (mg)	Niacin (mg Niacin Equiv)	Vitamin B_6 (mg)	Folacin (μg)	Vitamin B_{12} (μg)	*Minerals:* Calcium (mg)	Phosphorus (mg)	Magnesium (mg)	Iron (mg)	Zinc (mg)	Iodine (μg)
Infants	0.0–0.5	6	13	60	24	2.2	13	420	10	3	35	0.3	0.4	6	0.3	30	0.5[g]	360	240	50	10	3	40
	0.5–1.0	9	20	71	28	2.0	18	400	10	4	35	0.5	0.6	8	0.6	45	1.5	540	360	70	15	5	50
Children	1–3	13	29	90	35	1.8	23	400	10	5	45	0.7	0.8	9	0.9	100	2.0	800	800	150	15	10	70
	4–6	20	44	112	44	1.5	30	500	10	6	45	0.9	1.0	11	1.3	200	2.5	800	800	200	10	10	90
	7–10	28	62	132	52	1.2	34	700	10	7	45	1.2	1.4	16	1.6	300	3.0	800	800	250	10	10	120
Males	11–14	45	99	157	62	1.0	45	1000	10	8	50	1.4	1.6	18	1.8	400	3.0	1200	1200	350	18	15	150
	15–18	66	145	176	69	0.9	56	1000	10	10	60	1.4	1.7	18	2.0	400	3.0	1200	1200	400	18	15	150
	19–22	70	154	177	70	0.8	56	1000	7.5	10	60	1.5	1.7	19	2.2	400	3.0	800	800	350	10	15	150
	23–50	70	154	178	70	0.8	56	1000	5	10	60	1.4	1.6	18	2.2	400	3.0	800	800	350	10	15	150
	51+	70	154	178	70	0.8	56	1000	5	10	60	1.2	1.4	16	2.2	400	3.0	800	800	350	10	15	150
Females	11–14	46	101	157	62	1.0	46	800	10	8	50	1.1	1.3	15	1.8	400	3.0	1200	1200	300	18	15	150
	15–18	55	120	163	64	0.9	46	800	10	8	60	1.1	1.3	14	2.0	400	3.0	1200	1200	300	18	15	150
	19–22	55	120	163	64	0.8	44	800	7.5	8	60	1.1	1.3	14	2.0	400	3.0	800	800	300	18	15	150
	23–50	55	120	163	64	0.8	44	800	5	8	60	1.0	1.2	13	2.0	400	3.0	800	800	300	18	15	150
	51+	55	120	163	64	0.8	44	800	5		60	1.0	1.2	13	2.0	400	3.0	800	800	300	10	15	150
Pregnancy							+30	+200	+5	+2	+20	+0.4	+0.3	+2	+0.6	+400	+1.0	+400	+400	+150	[b]	+5	+25
Lactation							+20	+400	+5	+3	+40	+0.5	+0.5	+5	+0.5	+100	+1.0	+400	+400	+150	[b]	+10	+50

[a] One Retinol Equivalent equals 3.33 IU Vitamin A from retinal.

[b] Increased iron requirements during pregnancy are not met by the habitual American diet nor by the existing iron stores of most women. Therefore, the use of 30–60 mg of supplemental iron is recommended. Iron needs during lactation are not different from those of nonpregnant women, but continued supplementation for 2–3 months after parturition is advised in order to replenish stores depleted during pregnancy and blood lost during delivery.

Table 1-2. Recommended Dietary Allowances (Revised 1980)—Mean Heights and Weights and Recommended Energy Intake[a]

Category	Age (years)	Weight (kg)	Weight (lb)	Height (cm)	Height (in)	Energy Needs (with range) (kcal)	Energy Needs (with range) (per body weight)
Infants	0.0–0.5	6	13	60	24	kg × 115(95–145)	kg × 115
	0.5–1.0	9	20	71	28	kg × 105(80–135)	kg × 105
Children	1–3	13	29	90	35	1300 (900–1800)	kg × 100
	4–6	20	44	112	44	1700 (1300–2300)	kg × 85
	7–10	28	62	132	52	2400 (1650–3300)	kg × 85
Males	11–14	45	99	157	62	2700 (2000–3700)	kg × 60
	15–18	66	145	176	69	2800 (2100–3900)	kg × 42
	19–22	70	154	177	70	2900 (2500–3300)	kg × 42
Females	11–14	46	101	157	62	2200 (1500–3000)	kg × 48
	15–18	55	120	163	64	2100 (1200–3000)	kg × 38
	19–22	55	120	163	64	2100 (1700–2500)	kg × 38
Pregnancy						+300	
Lactation						+500	

[a] The energy allowances for young adults are for doing light work. Values for adults, listed in parentheses, are ranges based on a variation in energy needs of ± 400 kcal. Values for children, listed in parentheses, are 10th and 90th percentiles of energy intake.

who do not take adequate amounts orally should be fed by gavage or intravenously.

Calorie requirements can be partitioned into calories to cover basal expenditures (55 kcal/kg), activity, environmental stress, fecal losses and calories for growth (5 kcal/g weight gain). An allotment for postprandial heat production ("specific dynamic action") is omitted since it reflects the work of growth (35,36). Total requirements of the young infant, who is gaining 7 g/kg/day, consequently add up to 115 kcal/kg/day. Although weight gain per unit of body weight decreases during the first year, calorie requirements remain fairly constant. This can be explained by the reallocation of consumed energy from growth to activity.

The resting metabolic rate is low in the first 12 hours after birth, rises during the ensuing days, and reaches by the seventh day a value similar to that of older infants. Although body composition is different in preterm, small-for-date, and large-for-date infants, resting metabolic rate per body weight is not measurably different according to current techniques (34). The higher requirements of LBW infants (>120 kcal/kg) are attributable to their greater rate of growth (>7.5 g/kg). Cold stress may contribute unnecessarily to the energy burden if LBW infants are not kept in a controlled environment, because extreme conditions of cold stress increase the resting rate of heat production by as much as two and a half times due to their lack of insulation by fat.

Table 1-3. Safe and Adequate Intakes for 12 Nutrients Not Listed in the RDA

		Vitamins			*Trace Minerals*						*Electrolytes*		
	Age (years)	*Vitamin K(μg)*	*Biotin(μg)*	*Pantothenate (mg)*	*Copper (mg)*	*Manganese (mg)*	*Fluoride (mg)*	*Chromium (mg)*	*Selenium (mg)*	*Molybdenum (mg)*	*Sodium (mg)*	*Potassium (mg)*	*Chloride (mg)*
Infants	0–0.5	12	35	2	0.5–0.7	0.5–0.7	0.1–0.5	0.01–0.04	0.01–0.04	0.03–0.06	115–350	350–925	275–700
	0.5–1	10–20	50	3	0.7–1.0	0.7–1.0	0.2–1.0	0.02–0.06	0.02–0.06	0.04–0.08	250–750	425–1275	400–1200
Children	1–3	15–30	65	3	1.0–1.5	1.0–1.5	0.5–1.5	0.02–0.08	0.02–0.08	0.05–0.1	325–975	550–1650	500–1500
and	4–6	20–40	85	3–4	1.5–2.0	1.5–2.0	1.0–2.5	0.03–0.12	0.03–0.12	0.06–0.15	450–1350	775–2325	700–2100
Adolescents	7–10	30–60	120	4–5	2.0–2.5	2.0–3.0	1.5–2.5	0.05–0.2	0.05–0.2	0.1 –0.3	600–1800	1000–3000	925–2775
	11+	50–100	100–200	4–7	2.0–3.0	2.5–5.0	1.5–2.5	0.05–0.2	0.05–0.2	0.15–0.5	900–2700	1525–4575	1400–4200
Adults		70–140	100–200	4–7	2.0–3.0	2.5–5.0	1.5–4.0	0.05–0.2	0.05–0.2	0.15–0.5	1100–3300	1875–5625	1700–5100

The recommended protein intake of newborn infants is 2.2 g/kg (Table 1-1). A higher amino acid load in the neonatal period may exceed the metabolizing capacity of the infant and result in metabolic acidosis or hyperammoniemia, especially in LBW infants. Commercially prepared infant formulas, which are used during the first 6 months of life, usually contain about 1.5 g/dl of protein, which supplies the recommended amount if the infant drinks 150 ml/kg. The protein content of human milk is less, and there is increasing concern that it is insufficient for small premature infants. Several studies failed to demonstrate a superiority of cow's milk over human milk, but these studies did not prove that LBW infants fed human milk can maintain on human milk a rate of growth comparable to intrauterine growth. While this may not be a prudent goal, protein deficiency should be considered when a LBW infant on human milk does not gain at least 7.5 g/kg/day. Protein supplementation of pooled human milk or mother's own milk may become routine practice before too long.

Fat is the vehicle for essential fatty acids (linoleic and arachidonic) and fat-soluble vitamins and supplies a major portion of the infant's caloric requirements. A minimum of 30% fat calories is recommended. Formulas that provide 40 to 50% of total calories from fat are recommended for LBW infants. Breast milk provides 50% fat. The recommended intake of linoleic acid is 300 mg/100 kcal or 3% of total calories. Higher amounts of linoleic acid are not advised unless they are covered by an appropriate amount of vitamin E (Chapter 11).

Carbohydrate calories should not exceed 50% of the total because of the risk of inducing diarrhea and acidosis. When lactose is the sole carbohydrate, this risk is greater than with sucrose (37).

The osmolality of most mammalian milks and commercial formulas in regular dilution (67 kcal/dl) is approximately 300 mOsm/kg water. Concentrations in excess of 400 mOsm/kg water are potentially harmful, as they may cause enterocolitis. Recently, formation of lactobezoars has been linked with feeding concentrated formulas to very immature or stressed infants whose gastric emptying time may be delayed, thus causing formation of the milk-containing semisolid mass in the stomach. Most high-caloric formulas supplying 90 kcal/dl have a caloric density of about 420 mOsm/kg/water and are contraindicated; special low-sodium preparations are an exception.

Fluid requirements, which are highest during the first 3 months of life, are a function of the solute load. This, in turn, is related to the infant's ability to consume nutrients and to grow. A 3-kg infant who consumes 100 kcal/kg in the form of a regular 67 kcal/dl formula maintains, under normal environmental conditions, a urine specific gravity below 1.015. On an 80 kcal/dl formula, urine specific gravity tends to be around 1.015. This translates into a fluid intake of about 120 to 150 ml/kg body weight. Consequently, no extra water is needed if the formulas have an acceptable osmolality. However, since the oxidation of food in a mixed diet yields about 12 ml of water per 100 kcal, water must be offered when formulas and solid foods provide 100 kcal with less than 100 ml water.

Commercial infant formulas contain ample vitamin supplementation. Breast milk, by contrast, provides only marginal levels for most vitamins, including B_{12}, and is deficient in vitamin D (Table 2-2). However, since colostrum and early postpartum milk have a high B_{12} concentration, B_{12} acquired from this source and stored may protect the breast-fed infant (38). A multiple-vitamin preparation including vitamin D is recommended for breast-fed infants, especially in cases where the mother's vitamin nutriture is questionable (Vi-Daylin drops [Ross], 1 ml/day).

Calcium and phosphorus requirements are high during infancy. Evidence has been presented indicating that human milk does not contain enough calcium and phosphorus to sustain a postnatal rate of growth corresponding to that of the intrauterine period from 28 to 36 weeks' gestation. Both Fomon et al. (39) and Forbes (40) came to a similar conclusion, based on literature data on fetal content of these elements at various stages of gestation, percent retention from food, and growth and maintenance needs. Actual measurements are needed. Supplementation is not recommended until this issue has been adequately studied. The ratio of calcium to phosphorus intake should be no less than 1.1 and no more than 2.0.

Infants receive adequate amounts of sodium, chloride and potassium in human or cow's milk and in most commercial infant formulas, including those for LBW infants. The Committee of Nutrition recommends that the ratio of sodium to potassium (in mEq) should not exceed 1.0, and the ratio of sodium plus potassium to chlorine should be at least 1.5 (41). Very low birth weight infants excrete sodium readily and may be at risk of developing metabolic acidosis. Rather than altering the formula in these cases, alkaline supplementation may be tried, providing other metabolic causes of acidosis have been ruled out. Attention should also be paid to the ratio between anions and cations in commercial formulas. A low chloride intake over 3 to 5 months caused by a deficient formula, has been shown to result in hypokalemic metabolic alkalosis with failure to thrive, deficient head growth and muscle weakness.

Commercial formulas contain adequate amounts of trace minerals, while breast and cow's milk are insufficient in iron. The recommended intake of 10 mg/day for term infants and 2 mg/kg for LBW infants should be supplied by a formula that provides at least 1 mg/l, but these milks contain only 0.5 mg/l (Table 2-2). Nevertheless, breast-fed infants rarely develop anemia, apparently because of improved iron absorption (49%). After 6 months some breast-fed infants will deplete their iron stores even if absorption is optimal (42). Supplemental iron is therefore recommended in all infants on cow's milk and after 6 months in breast-fed infants. Iron may be administered as a combination vitamin-iron preparation (Vi-Daylin

Plus Iron Drops). This drug and many other similar preparations provide 10 mg of iron per milliliter. Most iron-supplemented commercial formulas provide more iron than is necessary for the prevention of deficiency (i.e., 6–10 mg/l).

INFANCY

Nutrition as a Function of Neuromuscular Maturation

The development of feeding skills occurs in an orderly fashion, influenced by maturation of the nervous system, which controls the acquisition of gross and fine motor functions, including the oral motor skills necessary for sucking, chewing, swallowing, and so on. The newborn infant is endowed with a number of primitive reflexes that probably developed as a survival mechanism (43,44). They are adaptive reflexes; in the case of suckling, swallowing, and rooting reflex, they promote the acquisition of liquid foods. The rooting reflex directs the infant's head toward the side where the cheek is stimulated by stroking, as though this reflex were conditioned by the touch of the breast. Since satiety influences the rooting and suckling reflex, it is hard to elicit them when the infant is full. They are consequently not useful for testing maturation. The coordination of rhythmic sucking and swallowing, which allows the alimentary and respiratory pathways to cross over in the pharynx, requires considerable nervous system maturation (45,46). The complexity of this process is often not recognized until one has the opportunity to observe a very immature infant or one with central nervous system disease who is unable to perform this vital function.

The manner is which the infant obtains milk during the first 3 to 4 months of life is called *suckling,* This is distinct from mature *sucking,* an acquired function of the orofacial muscles that must be learned. In the absence of central nervous system dysfunction, the neonate is born with the ability to suckle. A suckling motion is initiated by lowering the mandible with the mouth closed, thus creating a negative pressure. The tip of the tongue moves forward and, as the mandible is raised, compresses the nipple. The vigorous up-and-down movement can be painful and may be perceived as biting. The liquid is milked out as the curled tongue draws back and moves the nipple compression from the front of the mouth toward the back. During sucking, the mouth is more pursed, and the tongue moves back and forth, in contrast to the mandibular up-and-down movement of suckling. Backward movement of the tongue creates smacking noises that the infant makes spontaneously at about the time sucking is learned.

A forward motion of the tongue on dropping the lower jaw is typical of the first 3 months. Some infants move the tongue out and in spontaneously in a monotonous, repetitive fashion, as if they were using the tongue as a pacifier. During this phase semisolid foods are not accepted readily. Attempts to overcome the tongue protrusion are equivalent to forced feeding. Parents not infrequently misinterpret tongue protrusion as a conscious act of food rejection, motivated by a discriminating taste. Although they may correctly refrain from further attempts to introduce semisolid food, they may not reintroduce the specific item for an unnecessarily long period of time, thinking that it is disliked.

Oral anatomical structures are also adapted for sucking. The tongue is disproportionately large, the maxilla protrudes over the mandible, and the tip of the tongue lies between. There is a prominent fat pad in the cheeks, which seems to act like a prop for the buccinator muscle, keeping the cheeks rigid during sucking. A mucosal fold on the free edge of the gum seals the curvature of the jaw in the region of the canine teeth. The fold disappears by 3 to 4 months, around the time when the infant learns to seal the oral cavity more effectively with the lips alone. Up to that time the lateral corners of the lips tend to gape, allowing milk to flow out when the nipple is withdrawn. As the infant grows, the oral cavity becomes larger, and the tongue no longer fills the mouth, although it is by that time longer. These changes afford, at about 8 months of age, increased mobility of the tongue, which by then can protrude, receive food, and pass it between the gum pads or erupting teeth for chewing.

Like most other primitive reflexes, the rooting and suckling reflex has disappeared by 3 to 4 months of age. Sucking becomes volitional, and the infant recognizes the breast or bottle as a source of food. By 4 months, the infant opens the mouth for the spoon and closes the lips over it, but sucks the food from the spoon rather than shoving it back with the lips. Tongue projection may still occur when the spoon is removed. The ability to draw in the lower lip as the spoon is removed and to shift semisolid food in the mouth and swallow it is necessary for coordinated eating of semisolid food. This function is generally well developed by 6 months. The normal bite begins around that time. The up-and-down movement for chewing is well developed by 7 to 8 months, together with the ability to move the tongue laterally. The infant licks the spoon and enjoys biting it, as well as other objects, such as the rim of a cup or the nipple—a fact that makes breast feeding increasingly painful in the second half of the first year.

Also at about 6 months of age, the infant can sit without support and move the body freely. The control of head, neck, and body allows the infant to withdraw and reject food more effectively, thus avoiding overfeeding. The infant is able to grasp objects in a direct fashion with the radius upward, but still uses only thumb and four-finger apposition. At about 9 months, the pincer movement of the thumb and forefinger develops, allowing the infant to handle finger foods and pick up bite-sized pieces. Table foods are easily chewed, and the infant can now drink from the bottle independently in a sitting posture and can even tip the bottle

.t empties. As the first year ends and the "terrible twos" tend to use food to express all their newfound motor skills. ,oy mashing a cracker or poking a finger into the food dish, cup and watching the fluid spill out. They like to mash food ands as they become more interested in the feel of things. ıobility allows the infant to spit, and blowing, with noisy vibratıng ..ıovements of the lips, is a favorite pastime of some. Tongue projection may occur again, now as a voluntary action, because the tongue is freer and the infant likes to explore with it.

Recommendations

Semisolid Foods: Time and Sequence of Introduction

When and how semisolid foods are introduced are guided by nervous system maturation; the need for additional nutrients should not be a motivating factor. Thus, an infant may be raised solely on breast milk up to 1 year of age, providing vitamin D and iron supplements are given. A parent who insists on "natural" vitamin and trace mineral sources must offer meats and egg as an iron source by 6 months of age and must provide vitamin D through sun exposure. Commercial infant cereals that are fortified with iron are a popular supplement that should be started by 4 to 6 months. Infants fed commercial formulas that provide additional vitamins and minerals do not need supplemental semisolid foods until their calorie requirements exceed those supplied by a quart of milk, which is usually at about 6 months of age, when the infant weighs approximately 7 kg.

At six months, the infant is also neurologically ready to handle semisolid foods. Readiness may be measured by loss of tongue protrusion, ability to swallow solid food and sit with support. Early introduction of semisolid foods often leads to infantile obesity, since the infant is not able to express satiety and overcome the force of the spoon, which may be pushed into the mouth by an eager parent.

Earlier introduction is often done for the wrong reasons. They include the belief that solid foods given before bedtime will encourage the infant to sleep through the night. This is not true, because foods given at that time do not have a significantly higher caloric density than milk. Whereas protein foods may help an infant to sleep longer through the night, the foods usually given as bedtime snacks do not provide more protein than milk. Some parents introduce cereal because they think the infant is hungry. However, infants usually adjust their total calorie intake when calorie density is high by decreasing the amount per feeding. Other parents may push for early introduction because they think this represents a developmental landmark, not realizing that forced feeding semisolids can be done even in infants with central nervous system dysfunction.

Breast milk and iron-fortified commercial infant formulas generally provide all the nutritional needs of full term infants during the first 6 months of life. When the infant weighs 6 to 7 kg and consumes 1 qt of milk, which provides about 100 kcal/kg/day, it is time to add more calories in the form of semisolid food. Too early introduction not only encourages overfeeding but an emotional reaction toward feeding may also develop because semisolids are introduced before neuromuscular function has sufficiently matured. Single-ingredient food items should be introduced first, one at a time, to allow the detection of food sensitivities. It is also advisable to start with a small amount, like 1 teaspoon, and to offer increasingly more until 9 teaspoons (i.e., 3 tablespoons) are taken by the ninth day, at which time a new food item may be tried.

Juices can be offered much earlier and are generally already accepted during the first month of life. They are a means of letting the infant get accustomed to a different taste sensation. They are not a crucial part of the diet of infants on commercial formulas that are fortified with vitamins, including vitamin C.

Cereal is usually the first semisolid food offered. It trains the infant to accept a new food texture. By 4 to 6 months, a nutritional need for iron-fortified cereal arises, especially in infants on breast milk or prepared formulas that are not iron-fortified. Earlier introduction is not desirable in breast-fed infants, because the admixture of other foods to human milk changes the intestinal flora. The improved bioavailability of iron in human milk provides enough for growth during the first half-year of life to obviate the need for other iron sources. If cereals are introduced by 6 weeks, as was the practice in the past, the intended calorie enrichment may not be accomplished, because starch digestion may be incomplete before 4 months of age.

Fruits and vegetables are usually introduced next. This is recommendable after 6 months since at that time most infants are switched from formulas to homogenized milk, which has twice the protein concentration. Consequently, low-protein solids such as fruits and vegetables are a suitable energy supplement. Infants who remain on breast milk longer than 6 months will benefit from protein-rich semisolid foods after the age of 6 months. High-protein cereals and high-protein dinners are recommended in this case rather than fruits and pure vegetables.

Meats are added at about 8 or 9 months because the infant has grown; energy needs have increased further; and the addition of cereal, fruit, and vegetables has diluted the protein content of the daily diet, making protein-rich supplements, such as meat and egg, desirable.

By 9 months motor function has matured, and the mouth has developed into a sensory organ that can handle solids. Foods that do not crumble into pieces, which may be aspirated, should be chosen. Commercially prepared cookies for infants satisfy this special need, but other foods like animal crackers, soft cheese, white bread, and so on are equally satisfactory. Such foods train infants to use their hands for eating; by 1 year they should start using the spoon for feeding and learn to drink from a cup.

Meal Schedule

Feeding times can be arranged to satisfy the infant's demand without imposing an unnecessary burden on the mother. *Demand feeding* of the newborn is advisable. However, it must be remembered that infants with decreased vitality—for instance, those with congenital heart disease or deprivation syndrome—may not cry when hungry. Usually, a pattern develops spontaneously, consisting of six meals per day, spaced roughly 4 hours apart. The infant will sleep through one of the six meals by 2 to 3 months; by 6 months, when solids are introduced, the infant will be able to get along on four meals—three coinciding with the traditional adult schedule of breakfast, lunch, and dinner and one additional nighttime "snack." It must not be assumed that parents are aware of the limited volume capacity of small infants and will space the three meals evenly over 16 hours of daytime activities.

It is customary, although without specific reason, to feed cereal for breakfast and for the last meal before bedtime. The remaining food items can be given for lunch or dinner in any pattern the parent wishes to use. Semisolids and solids should be given before the milk. The amount offered should be guided by the infant's willingness to accept solids, leaving enough appetite so that 750 ml milk will be accepted readily in four meals per day. Together with the milk used in cereals, total milk intake should not exceed 1 l/day.

PRESCHOOL YEARS, SCHOOL AGE, AND ADOLESCENCE

Nutrition as a Function of Growth and Sexual Maturation

Growth

At no other time in life is the relation between growth and energy requirements more apparent than in the first 3 years, when calorie intake drops from 115 to 85 kcal/kg as growth decelerates. The decreasing appetite is often disturbing to parents, who tend to complain that their child "doesn't eat anymore." Weight gain decelerates somewhat earlier than linear growth, causing the 3-year-old to look thin relative to the 2-year-old, thus heightening parental concern. It is important to recognize the causal relationship between growth and energy requirements and not to encourage unnecessary worry by the parents, who should direct their energies into creating a happy home atmosphere.

During the negativistic period of the "terrible twos," the child may use food to express resistance to the socialization process. Later, during the early school years, children often refuse to eat breakfast because they are tense and anxious in the morning before school. However, this habit does not have serious consequences providing the total intake per day is adequate. On the whole, the period of steady growth, which overlaps with an emotionally quiet, "latent" period, is not characterized by special nutritional problems.

Following the fourth year of life, growth is fairly constant until puberty, with growth rates ranging from 7 cm down to about 5 cm/year until midpuberty. Calorie requirements are also fairly constant and are similar for boys and girls, averaging 85 kcal/day. Linear growth then begins to accelerate and reaches a maximum at the end of puberty, at 13 years in girls and 15 years in boys, averaging 8–9 cm/year (Figs. 1-1, 1-2).

During the teens, growth in body mass and stature is related to sexual

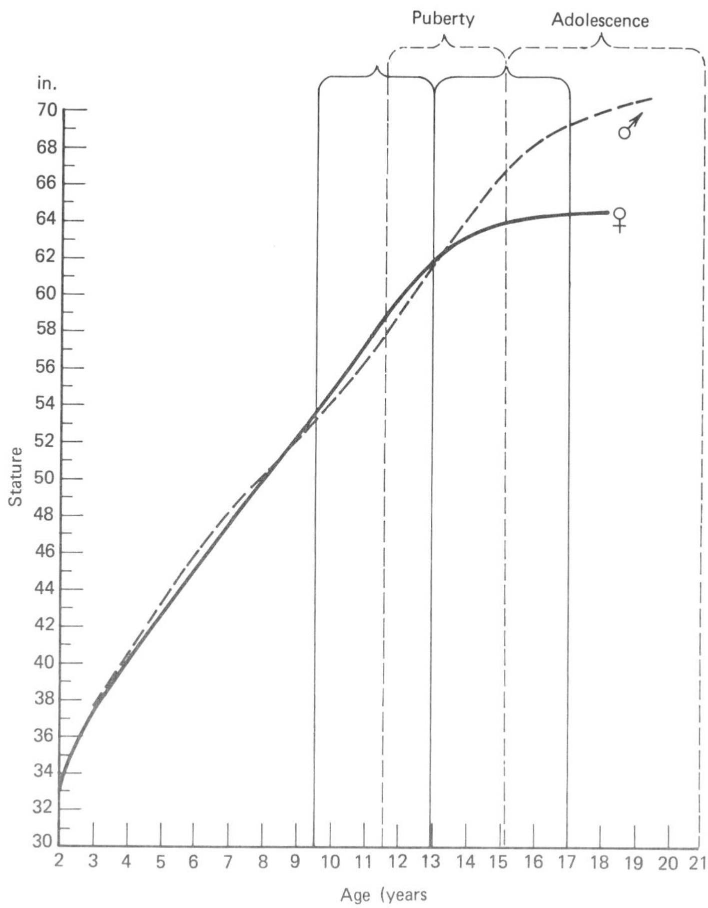

Figure 1-1. MEAN STATURE FOR AGE IN BOYS AND GIRLS

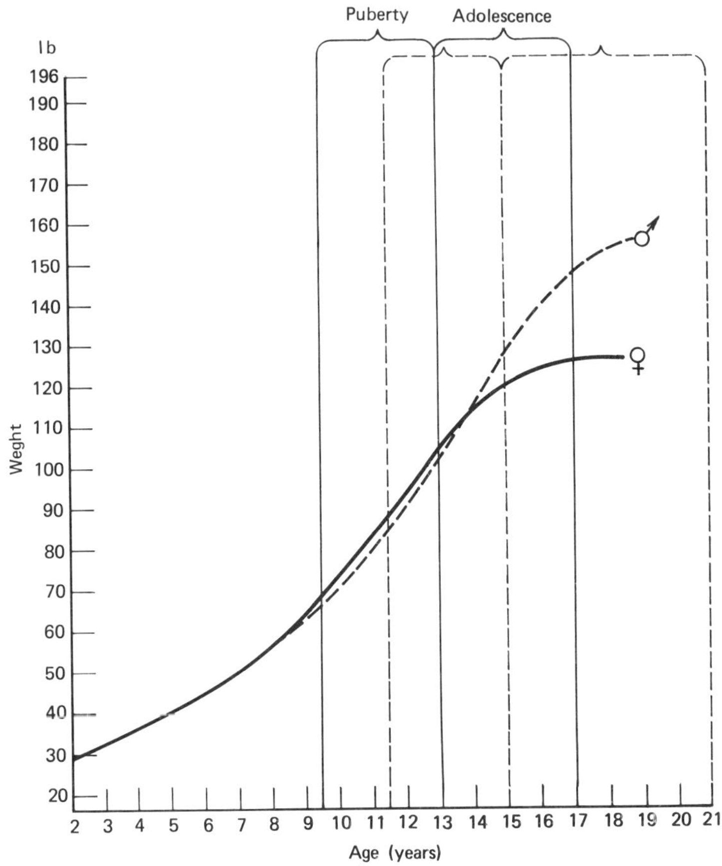

Figure 1-2. MEAN WEIGHT FOR AGE IN BOYS AND GIRLS

maturation. *Pubescence,* the beginning of sexual maturation, starts in boys at about 11.5 years and in girls 1 to 2 years earlier. Puberty ends with the emergence of the capacity for sexual reproduction. Linear growth decelerates sharply with the onset of adolescence to only about 2 cm/year within the time span of 1 year. Deceleration is more gradual in some, especially children with a delayed pubertal growth spurt. *Adolescence* is the term for the period of growth that starts with the end of puberty and lasts until linear growth comes to a complete halt at about 17 years in girls and 21 years in boys. Since linear growth lasts altogether 2 years longer in boys than in girls, boys' final stature tends to be greater.

Weight gain accelerates at the beginning of puberty and decelerates during early adolescence. Since the weight increase begins at a time when the linear growth rate is still very low, especially in girls, they tend to be chubby between 9 and 11 years of age. Fat mass increases steadily in girls throughout puberty and adolescence. Boys, on the other hand, show a sharp increase during puberty, which is followed by a marked decline in fat accumulation after 15 years of age (47). Muscle mass increases at a comparable rate in both sexes until 13 years of age, at which time increments begin to be greater in boys than in girls. Moreover, growth in muscle mass continues for a longer period of time in boys.

Nutrient Requirements

The energy need of boys are highest between 15 and 18 years of age (2,100 to 3,900 kcal/day) when growth in muscle mass is greatest. Calorie recommendations for girls are highest toward the end of puberty and in early adolescence (1,500 to 3,000 kcal/day) because increments in height, weight, fat, and muscle mass are high. When calorie recommendations or actual measurements of healthy adolescents do not reflect the rate of growth, it is usually due to the higher energy needs imposed by activity. Thus, calorie requirements of boys 11 to 14 years old exceed those for girls by 500 kcal/day, although height and weight are similar and growth rates even somewhat higher in girls. The wide range of energy needs, listed in the RDA, are intended to cover normal variations due to activity. The adequacy of a patient's calorie intake consequently cannot be evaluated solely from intake records. Rather, if a person has a normal weight for height and a normal height for stage of sexual maturation, caloric adequacy may be assumed.

Racial differences in height and weight exist and may be nutrition related. The Ten-State Nutrition Survey (48,49), which assessed the food intake of lower-income families in the United States, showed that the energy intakes of black adolescents of both sexes were well below the recommended levels. This was supported by earlier studies conducted during the 1960s that showed white boys to be taller and heavier after 14 years than black boys. On the other hand, the Ten-State Nutrition Survey showed the intake of white female adolescents to be below that recommended for their age. This is probably a consequence of current cultural trends, which equate attractiveness with having a slender, boyish figure. The fact that intakes tend to be marginal in teenage girls must be kept in mind during periods of added stress, such as illness, pregnancy, or competitive sports events.

Growth during puberty and adolescence imposes additional requirements for specific nutrients, like iron. The RDA for other minerals, like calcium, phosphorus, and magnesium, is also higher between 11 and 18 years of age than it is later. The recommendations for iron in girls provide a safe margin to compensate for menstrual losses. The higher requirements for adolescent boys are intended to cover the expanded blood volume associated with their marked increase in lean body mass and the rise in hemoglobin secondary to the androgenic stimulation of erythropoiesis. The greater demand for iron can be correlated with a higher incidence of anemia in pubescent males than in females from lower-income groups.

The RDA of iron in teenagers (18 mg/day) is just barely met by the average American diet, which contains about 9 to 18 mg of iron daily. Deficiency develops in adolescents because dairy products, which are low in iron, make up a large percentage of their calorie intake. Moreover, many teenagers are currently vegetarians or limit meat intake severely, thus eliminating a source of easily absorbed iron. Vitamin B_{12} deficiency, which causes anemia, also tends to develop on vegetarian diets. Many foods popular among teenagers (ice cream, french fries, carbonated beverages, etc.) are low in vitamin C. Consequently, borderline deficiencies may be anticipated.

Certain occurrences common to adolescence, including anorexia nervosa, obesity, bowel disorders such as ulcerative colitis, and competitive sports activities, make unusual demands on nutrition that may require careful assessment of food intake. Teenagers are susceptible because of the emotional stress inherent in "growing up." They have to develop career goals, come to grips with their sexuality, separate from their families, and find their own identity. Competitive sports, jogging, and other exercises are a positive way of dealing with the task, but these activities may be overdone and are occasionally not supported by adequate nutrition, especially by girls who use sports as a means of weight reduction. The teenager with a poor body image may withdraw from social contact, lead a sedentary life, and find compensatory pleasure in eating, thus setting the stage for a lifelong habit that results in obesity. There is also evidence that some bowel disorders are stress related. The way teenage girls tend to cope with these disorders poses unique problems, because they often hide the diarrhea, which is embarrassing to them, thus delaying treatment and compounding nutrient deficiency. Such a patient may deny or successfully hide the symptom, even in the hospital or doctor's office, causing a misdiagnosis of anorexia nervosa. (These disorders are discussed in more detail in later sections.)

Assessment of Nutrient Intake

Evaluating the adequacy of nutrient intake in teenagers is extremely difficult for several reasons. The foregoing discussion indicates that an assessment must include consideration of psychological makeup and evaluation of environmental factors, in addition to growth and sexual maturation.

The practical approach of assessing nutrient adequacy by comparing the patient's growth with standards for age, sex, and race may not adequately reflect deficiencies of single nutrients. Evaluation is further complicated in adolescents because minimum requirements have not been defined and because quantitatively accurate diet records are difficult to obtain. Moreover, reconstruction of past food intakes is bound to be inaccurate in teenagers because, nearly one-third of 12-year-old schoolchildren and half the 17-year-olds in the United States take only one meal with the family. School lunches, although scientifically constituted, are often not taken by the young teenager who has the money to buy food at a popular "fast-food" restaurant. It therefore is often not feasible to insist on an accurate account of nutrient intake. Diet histories should be aimed at the detection of nutritional imbalances that are common in teenagers because of diet fads and habits peculiar to their culture. To rule out the more common disturbances of this age group, appropriate tests—such as serum iron; vitamin A or carotene levels; calcium, phosphorus, and alkaline phosphatase; vitamin B_{12} and folate—should be performed.

Special Considerations for the Teenage Athlete

Pediatricians and nutritionists are frequently asked about the particular needs of the athlete, either in an official capacity as team physician or as the family doctor. For example, it is not uncommon for a parent to be concerned about a son "stuffing" himself after a sports events with carbohydrate-rich, so-called junk foods. Some insight into the specific requirements of athletes is therefore useful.

The objectives of nutrition modification are variable and should be discussed first, since they determine the type of nutritional care and prophylaxis that is necessary prior to an athletic event. The competitiveness of the young athlete should also be considered. In sports such as weight lifting and football, the athlete may want to build muscle mass and gain weight, whereas weight loss may be the major goal prior to events like small-boat racing or featherweight boxing, which match competitors on the basis of body weight. The objective is different again in high-energy-expending athletic events or sports in which the ratio between strength and weight is crucial, such as figure skating or gymnastics.

For muscle building or the maintenance of an efficient ratio between muscle strength and body weight, a balanced diet with a normal nutrient density is important. Regular meals and a varied diet, using the four food groups, will satisfy the athlete who avoids drastic weight changes during training. Meatless fruit and vegetable diets are also adequate providing they include milk and eggs. Supplements, such as vitamins and minerals, are not needed when a balanced diet is offered, especially since athletes consume larger amounts. A balanced diet, which is based on meat protein, tends to be costly and may present problems for low-income families. However, since protein in excess of 8 to 10% of total calories is not necessary, this amount can be supplied by less expensive milk products, because they contain high-quality protein.

An intake of about 800 to 1,000 kcal/day beyond normal requirements for age and weight will cause an approximate weight gain of 1 kg/week. There is a tendency to consume this extra energy in the form of fat, especially when meat intake is high, because the so-called lean meats, like high-quality steak, are high in fat content. Fat calories should be limited to 30 to 35% of total intake. Fat of vegetable origin is preferred. It is desirable to distribute this high intake fairly equally over the waking hours. Occasionally, it may be necessary to monitor weight gain through measuring skinfold thickness in order to avoid obesity. The athlete who wishes to increase lean body mass should realize that this requires muscle work. Consequently, while attempting to reduce skinfold thickness, it is necessary that the athlete decrease intake of calories and increase muscle-building exercises at the same time.

Weight reduction should never exceed more than 1 kg/week except in severely obese people. Weight loss should be accomplished while athletic activities are continued at a high level, balancing energy intake and output in such a way that the deficit does not amount to more than 1,000 kcal/day, equivalent to 1 kg of fat loss per week.

A sudden, brief energy output, required for such events as the shot put or high jump, requires little extra nutritional preparation because it can be accomplished with existing adenosine triphosphate (ATP) as a ready energy source and some glycogen. Sports that require energy expenditure for prolonged periods of time call for more calories than are ordinarily stored as glycogen in muscle. A high intake of starchy foods, taken in regular intervals on the day of competition, is advised. Moreover, sufficient time should be allowed between events, and high-carbohydrate, low-fat liquids should be given to replenish glycogen stores.

Dietary manipulations have been devised that increase the muscle glycogen content several-fold in hopes of prolonging high energy output by long-distance runners, cross-country skiers, and so on. For this purpose carbohydrate intake should be limited during training before the event. If this regimen results in depletion of muscle glycogen and is followed by a regimen that provides, for several days just prior to the event, a bolus of 1500 kcal as low-residue carbohydrates, muscle stores of glycogen increase (50).

Hydration and electrolyte balance should be of concern to the nutritionist who takes care of the athlete during training or before and during the main event. Ordinarily, on a varied diet no special need exists for extra electrolytes. Indeed, excess intake of electrolyte-containing beverages designed for athletes may cause fluid retention. Salt tablets are rarely needed and may be dangerous, since it is difficult to match precisely the intake of a pure salt with an appropriate fluid intake. It should be remembered that sweat has the lowest sodium concentration of all extracellular body fluids (5 to 40 mg/l). Scheduled fluid intakes are advised during an athletic competition that is expected to cause fluid loss. About 500 ml should be taken 15 minutes before the event. During training, fluid loss may be monitored by measuring daily changes in body weight prior to the event. Assuming that food intake does not vary immediately before a competition, weight changes of more than of 2.5% of body weight from one day to the next signals water imbalance, which must be avoided.

It is advisable to be aware of the fact that an athlete may occasionally try to reduce to reach a mandatory weight for a given event by forced dehydration.

RECOMMENDED DIETARY ALLOWANCES (RDA)

Initial publication of the "Recommended Dietary Allowances (RDA) (Tables 1-1, 1-2, 1-3) by the Food and Nutrition Board, National Academy of Sciences–National Research Council, came in 1942. Since then, the RDA have been updated approximately at 5-year intervals on the basis of new nutritional knowledge or different interpretations of existing data. These allowances are intended to provide for individual variations that exist among most normal people living in the United States under usual environmental stresses. They are directed toward nutritionists, physicians, dietitians, and other health care personnel as a guide for diet therapy, nutrition education, nutrition labeling of foods, planning of public assistance programs, and so on. They are not for use directly by the consumer. With the exception of allowances for energy (Table 1-2), the RDA are generally higher than the requirements of most people and far exceed minimum requirements. For instance, the RDA for most nutrients are higher than the amount that can be obtained by breast feeding an infant. In the case of iron, RDA is based on a 10% absorption rate, although the absorption of heme iron is at least double that amount. The RDA provide this margin of safety because absorption of nonheme iron is lower, and because individual variations in absorption must be expected. Similar considerations have gone into the establishment of other values.

Important changes in the revision of the RDA in 1980 included the addition of two new tables; one lists recommended energy intakes, and the other gives safe and adequate intakes for 12 additional nutrients, including trace elements for which there is insufficient information about human requirements. The upper limit for trace elements in the new table should not be habitually exceeded, because toxic levels may be only several times the usual intake.

REFERENCES

1. Enesco M, Leblond CP: Increase in cell number as a factor in the growth of the organs of the young male rat. *J Embryol Exp Morphol* 10:530, 1962.
2. Winick M: Changes in nucleic acid and protein content of the human brain during growth. *Pediatr Res* 2:352, 1968.
3. Winick M: Malnutrition and brain development. *J Pediatr* 74:667, 1969.
4. Winick M: Cellular growth during early malnutrition. *Pediatrics* 47:6, 1971.

5. Lubchenco LO: *The High Risk Infant.* Philadelphia, WB Saunders Co, 1976.
6. Mata L, Urrutia JJ, Mohs E: Implicaciones de baja peso al nacer pare la salud publica. Arch Latinoam Nutr (Suppl. 1) 27:198, 1977
7. Wiggelsworth J: Experimental growth retardation in the fetal rat. *J Pathol Bact* 88:1, 1964.
8. Naeye RL: Abnormalities in infants of mothers with toxemia of pregnancy. *Am J Obstet Gynecol* 95:276, 1966.
9. Rush D, Stein Z, Susser M: A randomized controlled trial of prenatal nutritional supplements in New York City. *Pediatrics* 65:683, 1980.
10. Naeye RL, Blanc W: Pathogenesis of congenital rubella. *JAMA* 194:1277, 1965.
11. Delachaume Salem E, Sarles H: Evolution en fonction de l'age de la sécrétion-pancréatique humaine normale. *Biol Gastroenterol* 2:135, 1970.
12. Zoppi G, Androetti G, Pajno-Ferrara DM, et al: Exocrine pancreas function in premature and full term neonates. *Pediatr Res* 6:880, 1972.
13. Fredrikzon B, Hernell O: Role of feeding on lipase activity in gastric contents. *Acta Paediatr Scand* 66:479, 1977.
14. Hamosh M, Sivasubramanian KN, Salzman-Mann C, et al: Fat digestion in the stomach of premature infants: I. Characteristics of lipase activity. *J Pediatr* 93:674, 1978.
15. Roy RN, Pollnitz RP, Hamilton JR, et al: Impaired assimilation of nasojejunal feeds in healthy low-birth-weight newborn infants. *J Pediatr* 90:431, 1977.
16. Norman A, Strandvik B, Ojamäe O: Bile acids and pancreatic enzymes during absorption in the newborn. *Acta Paediatr Scand* 61:571, 1972.
17. Widdowson EM: Absorption and excretion of fat, nitrogen and minerals from "filled" milks by babies one week old. *Lancet* 2:1099, 1965
18. Holt LE Jr, Tidwell HC, Kirk CM, et al: Studies in fat metabolism I. Fat absorption in normal infants. *J Pediatr* 6:427, 1935.
19. Filer LJ Jr, Mattson FM, Fomon SJ: Triglyceride configuration and fat absorption by the human infant. *J Nutr* 99:293, 1970.
20. VandeKamer JH, Weijers HA: Malabsorption syndrome. *Fed Proc* (Suppl.) 20:335, 1961.
21. Davidson M, Bauer CH: Patterns of fat excretion in feces of premature infants fed various preparations of milk. *Pediatrics* 25:375, 1960.
22. Fomon SJ, Ziegler EE, Thomas LN, et al: Excretion of fat by normal full-term infants fed various milks and formulas. *Am J Clin Nutr* 23:1299, 1970.
23. Morales S, Chung AW, Lewis JM, et al: Absorption of fat and vitamin A in premature infants: I. Effect of different levels of fat intake on the retention of fat and vitamin A. *Pediatrics* 6:86, 1950.
24. Poley JR, Dower JC, Owen CA Jr, et al: Bile acids in infants and children. *J Lab Clin Med* 63:838, 1964.
25. Watkins JB, Ingall D, Szczepanik P, et al: Bile salt metabolism in the newborn: Measurement of pool size and synthesis by Stable Isotope technique. *N Engl J Med* 288:431, 1973.
26. Signer E, Murphy GM, Edkins S, et al: Role of bile salts in fat malabsorption of premature infants. *Arch Dis Child* 49:174, 1974.
27. Snyderman SE, Morales S, Holt LE Jr: The absorption of short chain fats by premature infants. *Arch Dis Child* 30:83, 1955.
28. Auricchio S, Rubino A, Murset G: Intestinal glycosidase activities in the human embryo, fetus and newborn. *Pediatrics* 35:944, 1965.
29. DeVizia B, Ciccimarra F, DeCicco N, et al: Digestibility of starches in infants and children. *J Pediatr* 86:50, 1975.

30. Lilibridge CB, Townes PL: Physiologic deficiency of pancreatic amylase in infancy: A factor in iatrogenic diarrhea. *J Pediatr* 82:279, 1973.
31. Babson SG: Growth of low birth weight infants. *J Pediatr* 77:11, 1970.
32. Levin B, Mackay HM, Neill CA, et al: Weight gains, serum protein levels and health of breast fed and artificially fed infants, full term and premature. *Med Res Counc Mem (Lond.)* 296:1, 1959.
33. Clarkson JE, Silva PA, Buckfield PM, et al: The later growth of children who were preterm and small for gestational age. *NZ Med J* 81:279, 1975.
34. Hills JR, Robinson DC: Oxygen consumption in normally grown small for dates and large for dates newborn infants. *J Physiol* 199:685, 1968.
35. Ashworth A: Metabolic rates during recovery from malnutrition: The need for a new concept of specific dynamic action. *Nature* 223:407, 1969.
36. Krieger I, Whitten CF: Energy metabolism in infants with growth failure due to maternal deprivation, undernutrition or causes unknown: II. Relation between nitrogen balance, weight gain and postprandial excess heat production. *J Pediatr* 75:374, 1969.
37. Fosbrooke AS, Wharton BA: "Added Lactose" and "Added Sucrose" cow's milk formulas in nutrition of low birth weight babies. *Arch Dis Child* 50:409, 1975.
38. Samson RR, McClelland DB: Vitamin B_{12} in human colostrum and milk: Quantitation of the vitamin and its binder and the uptake of bound vitamin B_{12} by intestinal bacteria. *Acta Paediatr Scand* 69:93, 1980.
39. Fomon SJ, Zeigler EE, Vasquez HD: Human milk for small premature infants. *Am J Dis Child* 131:463, 1977.
40. Forbes GB: Is human milk best for low birth weight infants, abstracted. *Pediatr Res* 12:433, 1978.
41. Committee on Nutrition: Commentary on breast-feeding and infant formulas, including proposed standards for formulas. *Pediatrics* 57:278, 1976.
42. Gary PJ, Owen GM, Hooper EM, Gilbert BA: Iron absorption from human milk and formulas with and without iron supplementation. *Pediatr Res* 15:822, 1981.
43. Ingram TTS: Clinical significance of the infantile feeding reflexes. *Dev Med Child Neurol* 4:159, 1962.
44. Peiper A: The neurology in food intake, in Peiper A: *Cerebral Function in Infancy and Childhood,* New York Consultants Bureau, 1963, p 396.
45. Ardran GM, Kemp FH, Lind JA: Cineradiographic study of bottle feeding. *Br. J Radiol* 31:11, 1958.
46. Ardran GM, Kemp FH, Lind JA: Cineradiographic study of breast feeding. *Br. J Radiol* 31:156, 1958.
47. Reynolds EL: The distribution of subcutaneous fat in childhood and adolescence. *Soc Res Child Dev* 15:1, 1950.
48. Ad Hoc Committee to Review the Ten-State Nutrition Survey: Nutrition, growth, development and maturation: Findings from the Ten-State Nutrition Survey of 1968–1970. *Pediatrics* 56:306, 1975.
49. Ad Hoc Committee to Review The Ten-State Nutrition Survey: The Ten-State Nutrition Survey. *Pediatrics* 51:1095, 1973.
50. Smith NJ: *Food for Sport,* Palo Alto, Calif, Bull Publ Co, 1976.

2
Foodstuffs for Infant Feeding

HUMAN MILK COMPARED TO COW'S MILK

Traditionally, human milk has been considered superior to cow's milk because it is the physiological food that has permitted survival of the species. With the advent of industrialization, affluent women began to use formulas made from cow's milk, because wet nurses were no longer readily available. The popularity of this practice spread when it could be demonstrated that bottle-fed infants were thriving and that their weight gain was better than that of breast-fed infants. In time, working mothers discovered the convenience of bottle feeding. Although preparation initially required measuring a variety of ingredients, mixing, and terminal sterilization, most women considered formulas superior to breast feeding. As the demand increased, industry developed formulas that imitate the relative concentration of the major nutrients in human milk and later introduced ready-to-use bottles that obviate sterilization measures.

The recognition in recent years of the anti-infectious properties of human milk once again renewed the controversy over what constitutes the best milk for young infants. Reexamination of the entire issue brought to light many other advantages of breast feeding. As a result, the practice of breast feeding has doubled over the past 8 years.

Nutritional Characteristics

Protein

Twenty percent of the calories in cow's milk and 7% of the calories in human milk are supplied by protein. Values reported for human milk range from 0.9 to 1.2 g/dl. This variability is related to a number of factors, including the time after conception. Thus, breast milk from the early postpartum days has a higher concentration of protein than mature milk, and the milk of mothers giving birth to premature infants has a higher protein content than the milk produced after a full 9 months gestation. Moreover, values based on Kjeldahl analysis overestimate protein content by about 25%, since they include nonprotein nitrogen.

An infant's weight gain after birth is frequently used as a measure of protein adequacy when comparing human with cow's milk, because the two are calorie equivalent and protein concentration constitutes a major difference. Although breast-fed infants seem to be satisfied, they do not regain their birth weight as fast as bottle-fed infants. This difference may be related to difficulties in establishing an adequate milk supply rather than to the lower protein concentration of human milk. However, after the second week of life, when birth weight has been regained, breast-fed infants continue to gain at a slightly lower rate, with differences between breast- and bottle-fed infants ranging as high as 12% in some studies. Only part of the greater initial weight gain of bottle-fed infants can be attributed to water retention. However, these differences in weight gain do not appear to have long-range implications for the health of full term infants.

Controversy is more acute with regard to premature infants, because they may require a higher protein intake than that provided by human milk. A group of Finnish investigators (1), who fed either pooled human milk or cow's milk yielding 114 to 118 kcal/kg/day to premature infants, found no difference between the rates of growth in weight, length, and head circumference from when birth weight was regained until a weight of 2.4 kg was reached. In another study of infants (33 to 36 weeks' gestation) who were given equivalent amounts, no difference was observed between those on mature pooled breast milk and others on milk formulas providing 2.7 g protein per 100 ml. However, weight gain was slower in infants on breast milk who were more premature—28 to 32 weeks' gestation (2).

The higher protein content of cow's milk is responsible for higher plasma amino acid, total serum protein, and blood urea nitrogen (BUN) values. By and large, these BUN values are not high enough to be considered injurious to the infant. It is not known whether the higher serum protein and amino acid values represent an advantage.

High-protein formulas carry a risk of causing hyperammonemia in the newborn period. The mechanism is not clear. Although the phenomenon is transient, it may be so severe as to cause letheragy, coma, and convulsions. Azotemia, metabolic acidosis, and hyperammonemia have been observed in newborns fed casein-predominant formulas supplying 4.5 g/kg/day (1). High-protein diets are especially dangerous to infants with inborn errors of amino acid metabolism because they may develop catastrophic illness when the protein load is high because of intake or catabolic protein breakdown.

The protein in cow's milk differs qualitatively from that in human milk in that casein makes up 80% and whey protein, only 20%. Casein precipitates in the acid environment of the stomach to form a tough, rubbery curd that is hard to digest if the milk is not treated before ingestion by heating, homogenization, or acidification. Human milk, which contains less casein but comparable amounts of whey, has a casein/whey protein ratio of 40/60. Alpha-lactalbumin and lactoferrin are the main whey protein constituents in human milk. Beta-lactoglobulin is not present. Some superiority has been attributed to these differences, based mainly on animal data, which show whey protein to be more effective in the promotion of growth and albumin synthesis. Human data lead to different conclusions. Thus, full-sized infants receiving 7% of protein calories from either human or cow's milk have consistently demonstrated comparable rates of growth (3). In another study, Barness et al. (4) showed that premature infants fed artificial formulas with the casein/whey protein ratios similar to either human or cow's milk had comparable growth rates.

However, the higher cystine content of whey (see later) and the absence of lactoglobulin in human milk may constitute an advantage, since this protein inhibits pancreatic lipase by competing at the oil–water interface of the emulsified triglyceride substrate (5). In view of the neonate's poor fat tolerance, even a minor contribution to the improvement of fat absorption can be important.

Amino Acids

Newborn infants must consume an adequate amount of essential amino acids to promote growth. Although the protein content of milk is below that which is considered the minimum requirement, it is sufficient to promote growth. This fact alone suggests that certain features of human milk protein are unique and particularly suited to the needs of the newborn infant.

In comparing the amino acid composition of the two milks, one recognizes that the higher content of most amino acids in cow's milk is due to the higher total protein concentration, which amounts to about 300%. Cystine is an exception, because it is only 50% higher in cow's milk. The relatively high cystine concentration of human milk thus may constitute a significant advantage, since this is an essential amino acid to the neonate, whose capacity to form cysteine is limited due to transient deficiency of cystathionase (6). The taurine content of human milk also exceeds that of cow's milk. The significance of this difference is still not known, but there is evidence that taurine is important in central nervous system and neuromuscular function. This amino acid is unique in that it is not a component of brain proteins. Its presence in the free form suggests that it has a specific functional role. In most species, including humans, taurine concentrations are higher in the developing brain than the mature brain. Since relatively little is synthesized by adults and less by the neonate, who is deficient in the enzyme cysteine sulfinic acid decarboxylase, provision of taurine in the diet may be important. There is evidence that this amino acid is an inhibitory neurotransmitter. It is therefore understandable that teleological meaning has been attributed to the high taurine concentration in human milk.

Hyperphenylalaninemia occurs as a transient phenomenon in approximately 2 of every 100 live births. It is often associated with tryosinemia. Both disorders are more common in premature infants, probably as the result of functional immaturity of the enzymes that regulate phenylalanine hydroxylation and tyrosine oxidation. The high protein content of cow's milk, which leads to a correspondingly higher intake of phenylalanine and tyrosine, represents an unnecessary burden to the newborn infant. The plasma phenylalanine concentration of infants on milk-based formulas may approach levels considered harmful in phenylketonuria. Whether or not transient neonatal hyperphenylalaninemia is benign remains an unsettled question. The condition is less frequent in infants fed human milk (7). Premature infants on a high protein intake may develop transient hypermethioninemia. Adverse effects are not known.

Nonprotein Nitrogen

Urea, creatine, creatinine, uric acid, peptides, and free amino acids provide nonprotein nitrogen. Concentrations are equal in the two milks. However, if expressed as a percentage of total protein nitrogen, the value is higher for human milk—25% compared to 6% for cow's milk. Although peptides are absorbed and may be utilized more efficiently than proteins, the nutritional significance of nonprotein nitrogen remains unknown.

Solute

Because of the greater protein and mineral content of cow's milk, solute concentration is high. Thus, sodium, potassium, and calcium concentrations in cow's milk are three times higher than in human milk. This characteristic constitutes a definite disadvantage, because the newborn's renal capacity for solute excretion is limited and the obligatory water loss for the excretion of solutes is high. Since the surplus of free water is small in newborn infants, they are at risk of developing hypernatremia, which may cause irreversible CNS damage.

The ratios of sodium to potassium (0.6) and of sodium plus potassium to chlorinc (2.0) are similar in the two milks. An important difference exists with regard to the calcium/phosphorus ratio. It is 2.0 to 2.4 in human milk and only 1.2 in cow's milk, since cow's milk contains three times as much calcium but six times as much phosphorus as human milk. This relatively high phosphorus content has been implicated as an etiologic factor in neonatal tetany, which develops toward the end of the first week of life or later if infants are suddenly switched from human to cow's milk. Whereas the higher Ca/P ratio represents an advantage, the low absolute amount of calcium and phosphorus in human milk may constitute a disadvantage (see later).

Fat

The concentration of fat in human milk is variable, though roughly comparable to cow's milk. Hytten (8) observed a rise in fat content, both during feeding and throughout the day. The speculation that the rise during the course of feeding is a signal for the baby to stop sucking and that it represents a protection against overfeeding has not been tested. Another cause of variability in fat content is the duration after delivery. The concentration decreases after birth, especially in the reflex milk. Whereas mean fat concentration in human milk is similar to that in cow's milk, the molecular structure of triglycerides is dissimilar. A high percentage of the total palmitic acid content of human milk is esterified in the 2-position of the triglyceride molecule. By contrast, in cow's milk palmitic acid is predominantly in the 1- or 3-position. Pancreatic lipase hydrolyzes fatty acids from the 1- and 3-positions. Since palmitate is poorly absorbed, it may be precipitated by calcium and excreted as calcium palmitate, causing a loss of both fat and calcium. By contrast, human milk offers the advantage that palmitic acid in the 2-position is absorbed as the monoglyceride.

Fat provides 50% of the calories in human milk, which includes 4% as essential fatty acids (EFA), principally linoleic acid. By contrast, EFA in cow's milk make up only 1% of total calories. This is less than the minimum recommended for infant formulas by the Committee on Nutrition (9)—300 mg/100 cal, or approximately 2.7% of total calories.

Much significance has been attached to differences in the cholesterol content of human and cow's milk because of a rat study showing that pups fed a high-cholesterol diet after birth subsequently had lower levels of serum cholesterol than control subjects. The suggestion has been made that the high cholesterol concentrations in human milk are necessary to induce enzyme systems for the regulation of cholesterol metabolism, thus resulting in lower cholesterol levels in later life. Retrospective studies of individuals who as infants received either breast or bottle feedings have not shown differences in plasma cholesterol concentration or incidence of arteriosclerosis.

Carbohydrate

Lactose is the disaccharide in human and cow's milk that provides a ready source of energy. Lactose (6.8 g/dl) supplies approximately 42% of the calories in human milk. In cow's milk, lactose supplies 30% of the calories, or 4.9 g/dl. The higher carbohydrate content of human milk compensates for a lower protein concentration so that total energy concentration is similar.

Bifidus Factor

N-containing oligo- and polysaccharides, including bifidus factor, which are essential for the growth of certain species of lactobacilli, are prevalent in human milk. An intestinal flora consisting mainly of *Lactobacillus acidophilus*, *L. casei*, and *L. bifidus* is therefore characteristic of breast-fed infants and is responsible for the acid pH of their stools. By contrast, the stool pH of infants on cow's milk is shifted toward the neutral or alkaline range. Strains of lactobacillus have been found to possess inhibitory properties against intestinal pathogens and food spoilage organisms. This action of lactobacilli in human milk has been attributed to the acid pH and the production of peroxide and natural antibiotics, such as nisin, acidolin, and lactocidin. Within a day after onset of breast feeding, there is a preponderance of lactobacilli, whereas artificially fed infants harbor Gram-negative organisms. It must be recognized, however, that actual benefits of a breast milk-induced flora have not been proven.

Fat Absorption

Fecal fat losses are considerably higher in newborns fed cow's milk than in breast-fed infants (10). This represents a decisive advantage of human over cow's milk, which can be attributed to two specific properties. One is the molecular structure of triglycerides in human milk, which facilitates the absorption of palmitate as the monoglyceride esterified at the 2-position. The other property (11) is a higher content of bile salt-stimulated lipase (BSSL). This enzyme has characteristics that make it particularly suitable for lipolytic action in newborns. Thus, it is stable at a low pH and able to pass the stomach; it is not affected by proteolytic enzymes and does not require a high bile acid concentration for its activation. The contribution of BSSL to the digestion of milk triglycerides is important in view of the rather low levels of pancreatic lipase and bile acids in the intestines of newborn infants. The products of hydrolysis by BSSL are different from the ones resulting from pancreatic lipase activity inasmuch as BSSL hydrolyzes all three ester bonds. BSSL activity thus complements that of pancreatic lipase and seems to assure sufficient digestive capacity. Following a feeding of fresh human milk, the BSSL concentration in duodenal contents is similar to that in the milk itself (12). Heating and homogenization destroy BSSL activity, a fact that has implications for the treatment of milk from human milk banks.

Anti-Infectious Properties

The superiority of human milk over cow's milk with regard to its anti-infectious properties has been recognized for some time, but the reasons for this have become better understood during the past decade (Table 2-1).

Table 2-1. Anti-Infectious Factors in Breast Milk

Factor	*Function*
Immunoglobulins secretory IgA	Protection against invading bacteria
Lactoferrin and transferrin	Inhibition of bacterial multiplication
Lysozyme	Lysis of bacteria
Lactoperoxidase	Bactericidal (streptococci and enteropathogens)
Complement (C3 and C4)	Opsonization
Interferon	Antiviral
Cellular components	
B cells	Synthesis of immunoglobulin
T cells	Surveillance and response to histoincompatible cells and proteins
Monocytic phagocytes	Synthesis of lysozymes

Vulnerability of the Newborn

The newborn infant is vulnerable to infection because of decreased B-cell proliferation, decreased complement, and decreased opsonic and chemotactic activity. In addition, the small intestine of the newborn is deficient in IgA-producing cells within the lamina propria. Both feces and saliva have low IgA levels. This deficiency constitutes a risk because secretory IgA plays an important role as part of a complex barrier mechanism that protects the intestinal epithelium from bacterial and viral penetration and absorption of antigenic macromolecules. Breast milk and colostrum contain some of the immunological factors that are missing in the young infant. The protective property of breast milk is most crucial in developing countries. Only a few studies from the United States have shown a lesser incidence of gastrointestinal and respiratory infections, otitis media, sepsis, and meningitis in breast-fed infants as compared to matched control subjects on cow's milk. Studies from other affluent societies also have shown no difference.

Soluble Components

The mammary gland has the capacity for synthesis and storage of immunoglobins. Thus, breast milk contains secretory IgA (S-IgA) and a number of other soluble components of the immune defense system, including intact IgM, IgG, lysozyme, lactoperoxidase, and interferon. The origin of immunoglobulins is not the blood because changes in concentration occur after birth that are not parallel in the two body fluids. IgA and IgM levels in breast milk are high during the first week and drop subsequently, while IgG levels remain relatively constant. Titers of specific S-IgA in milk correlate with the concentration in feces (13). Neutralizing antibodies against enteroviruses as well as immunoglobulins with activity against rotaviruses have been found in colostrum and breast milk. Human milk also contains lactoferrin and transferrin, two iron-binding proteins that have bacteriostatic properties providing they are not saturated by iron (14). The presence of trypsin inhibitor in human milk may play a role in that it prevents the digestion of antibodies that consequently retain immunological activity.

Cellular Components and Their Products

Protection is also conferred by cellular components that reflect the mother's infectious experience. Pregnant women, immunized by mouth against such bacteria as strains of *Escherichia coli*, have cells in their colostrum that produce antibodies against the antigen given by mouth. These antibody-producing cells are seen in colostrum even when there are no such cells in the peripheral blood. Specific antibodies are synthesized by colostral cells within a few days of oral immunization. Colostrum, which is more potent in antibody production than mature milk, thus is important for the protection of infants during the first few days of life. Gut lymphoid cells, stimulated by oral immunization, apparently travel to distant sites like the mammary glands, where they can transfer the immunological experience to other cells. The possibility exists that protection can be conferred in this manner against viral diarrhea, an important cause of morbidity in infancy. Some cellular elements in colostrum and breast milk possess antimicrobial activity by virtue of their capacity to phagocytose such pathogenic organisms as *E. coli* and *Candida albicans.*

Infectious agents, such as *E. coli,* rubella, CMV, and herpesvirus, have been recovered from human milk. While they are potentially harmful, low quantities may have a beneficial effect if the infection produces immunity without causing disease.

Anti-Allergic Properties

Infants with a family history of allergy may benefit from breast feeding because human milk is less allergenic because of the absence of lactoglobulin, and because the presence of immunologically active cells may prevent the adherence of foreign protein to the intestinal mucosa. These cells are thereby able to prevent entry of antigen and subsequent sensitization of the atopic individual. The small infant is at risk of being sensitized because the intestinal mucosa is more permeable to macromolecules in early infancy than later on. Within a few days following the ingestion of cow's milk, antibodies can be found in serum. Chronic, occult gastrointestinal blood loss, which has only been reported in infants receiving cow's milk, may be due to milk allergy. Eczema and allergic rhinitis are also more common in infants from allergic families fed cow's milk than in those who are fed breast milk.

Ligands Promoting Mineral Absorption

The concentration of iron is the same in human and cow's milk, yet infants receiving cow's milk without iron supplementation have a higher incidence of iron-deficiency anemia. The greater bioavailability of iron from human milk is the reason for this. Thus, newborns absorb approximately 50% of the iron from human milk but only 10% from cow's milk. It is therefore possible for a breast-fed infant to remain iron sufficient for up to 1 year, providing the diet is composed solely of breast milk. The responsible ligand has not been identified, nor is it known what mechanism is responsible for the decrease in bioavailability that occurs if breast feeding is supplemented by other foods (15).

Human milk also improves the bioavailability of other trace metals. The first indication of such a mechanism came when it was recognized that acrodermatitis enteropathica (AE), a disorder cured by breast milk, is caused by insufficient absorption and/or retention of zinc. Breast milk seems to supply a ligand that may be deficient in AE. Picolinic acid was recently identified as a zinc-binding ligand in human milk and was shown capable of improving zinc absorption in rats (16) and patients with AE (17). Its concentration in human milk is higher than in cow's milk.

Emotional Aspects of Infant Feeding

Breast feeding can be a major factor in the development of mother–infant bonding, providing the conditions are optimal. A number of studies in recent years have shown that the quality of the mother–infant relationship is not the same in breast- and bottle-fed infants. It has not been proven that the process of breast feeding itself is the deciding factor. It is possible therefore that the type of mother who chooses to breast feed is a more important influence, since the desire to breast feed may be an expression of her "mothering" personality. Infants therefore can be emotionally satisfied equally well through bottle feeding and mothers who want to breast feed but are unable to do so should be assured that bottle feeding represents an equally good opportunity for mother–infant bonding. Certainly, nothing can be gained by pressing a mother to breast feed if she has an aversion toward the process.

Disadvantages of Breast Milk

Enthusiasm over breast feeding should be accompanied by an awareness of its negative effects. Among these are deficient vitamin D and marginal levels of most other vitamins (Table 2-2). This should not be a deterrent, however, since the deficit can be compensated for. It appears that human milk is also inadequate for maximal growth of premature infants, as it provides only about half the estimated protein needs, three-fourths the sodium, and a quarter of the calculated calcium requirements (18).

The decision on nursing may be a difficult one for mothers who must receive medication, because only a few drugs have been evaluated for use by nursing mothers. Some are definitely contraindicated; others may cause problems but may be used if the nursing infant is watched closely. As more knowledge is accumulated, drugs now considered safe may be revealed as being otherwise (Table 2-3). Tolerance by the infant depends upon the drug's mechanism of excretion and degree of transmission into breast milk, as well as on absorption by the infant, who in turn may have variable tolerance, depending on genetic makeup, maturity of metabolizing enzyme systems, and rate of excretion. For some drugs, including tetrahydrocannabinol (contained in marijuana), milk is the only medium of excretion for that portion of the drug that has entered the breast. Other drugs, like isoniazid, may be concentrated in breast milk (19).

Environmental pollutants, such as polychlorinated or polybrominated biphenyls (PCP, PBP), DDT, and organophosphate insecticides, are ex-

Table 2-2. Nutrients in Human and Cow's Milk[a]

Composition	*RDA/day Infants 0.0-0.5 Years*	*Recommendations CON (1976)[b] (Minimum)*	*Human Milk*	*Cow's Milk*
Energy (kcal/dl)			71	79
Solute (Osm/100 kcal)			10	40
Protein (g/dl)(g/100 kcal)		1.25(1.8)	1.1(1.5)	3.3(5.3)
Casein (% of total)			40	82
Whey (% of total)			60	18
Albumin (mg/dl)[a]			50	30
α-Lactoalbumin (mg/dl)[a]			260	110
β-Lactoglobulin (mg/dl)[a]			0	360
Lysozyme (mg/dl)[a]			50	trace
Lactoferrin (mg/dl)[a]			170	trace
Lactose (g/dl)			6.8	4.9
Fat (g/dl)		2.3	3.1–4.6	3.7
Cholesterol (mg/dl)			26–29	14
Essential fatty acids (% kcal)(mg/100 kcal)		3(300)	4	1
Palmitate (% of total)			23	43
Polyunsaturated/Saturated fatty acids			0.2/1	0.08/1
Vitamin E / Polyunsaturated fatty acids		0.7/1	0.7/1	0.1–2.0/1
Amino Acids, essential (mg/dl)				
Histidine			22	95
Isoleucine			68	228
Leucine			100	350
Lysine			73	277
Methionine			25	88
Phenylalanine			48	172
Threonine			50	164
Tryptophan			18	49
Valine			70	245
Major Minerals				
Calcium (mg/l)	360 mg	340	340	1170
Phosphorus (mg/l)	240 mg	170	140	920
Sodium (mEq/l) (mg/l)	(>115 mg)	6(140)	7	22
Potassium (mEq/l) (mg/l)	(>350 mg)	14(560)	13	35
Chloride (mEq/l) (mg/l)	(>275 mg)	11(385)	11	29
Magnesium (mg/l)	50 mg	40	40	120
Trace Minerals				
Iron (mg/l)	10 mg	1.0	0.5	0.5
Zinc (mg/l)	3 mg	3.4	3–5	3–5
Copper (μg/l)	500 μg	400	400	300

Table 2-2. (Continued)

Composition	*RDA/day Infants 0.0-0.5 Years*	*Recommendations CON (1976)[b] (Minimum)*	*Human Milk*	*Cow's Milk*
Vitamins				
Vitamin A (IU/l)	1400/μ	1700	1900	1025–1690[d]
B-carotene (μg/1)			610[c]	trace
Thiamine (μg/l)	300 μg	270	160	440
Riboflavin (μg/l)	400 μg	400	360	1750
Niacin (mg/l)	6.0 mg[e]	1.70	1.47(4.4)[e]	0.94(8.9)[e]
Pyridoxine (μg/l)	300 μg	238	100	640
Panthothenate (mg/l)	2 mg	2	1.85	3.46
Folacin (μg/l)	30 μg	27	52	55
B_{12} (μg/l)	0.5 μg	1	0.3	4
Vitamin C (mg/l)	35 mg	56	43	11–21[f]
Vitamin D (IU/l)	400 IU	270	22	14–33[d]
Vitamin E (mg/l)	3 mg	2	1.8	0.4
Vitamin K (μg/l)	12 μg	27	15	60

[a] Values adapted from Fomon SJ: Infant Nutrition. Philadelphia, WB Saunders Co, 1974, p 362, except for protein values; see Hambraeus L: *Pediatr Clin North Am* 24:17, 1977.

[b] CON = Committee on Nutrition; their original recommendations are for 100 kcal (9). For the purpose of this comparison, their values are recalculated for 68 kcal/dl milk.

[c] Higher in colostrum.

[d] Winter and summer milk.

[e] Includes preformed vitamin plus 1 mg nicotinamide equivalent for each 60 mg of tryptophan.

[f] Higher values are for fresh milk.

creted in milk. To date, adverse effects have not been demonstrated in infants fed milk contaminated with PCP. However, it is too soon after the original exposure to rule out long-term effects. Given the current state of knowledge, advising exposed mothers against breast feeding is not warranted, although the unknown risk should be pointed out. Fat-soluble pollutants, like PCP, are not present in skim milk. Since these chemicals concentrate with the ascent in the food chain, their concentration in vegetable oils is low, and formulas made with vegetable oils are consequently safer in this regard.

Another negative effect is the possible transmission of infective organisms, notably cytomegalovirus and hepatitis virus B. While they may have an immunizing effect in very small amounts, sufficient quantities may be transferred to the infant and thus cause disease.

Breast milk contains a number of hormones. Some mothers have high concentrations of pregnanediol. This may be the cause of the prolongation

Table 2-3. Acceptability of Drugs in Nursing Mothers

Contraindicated	*Reason ("Infant" indicates actual observation)*
Chloramphenicol	Infant: bone marrow depression
Metronidazole (Flagyl)	Blood dyscrasia, neurological effects, possibly carcinogenic
Tetracycline	Infant: enamel hypoplasia, discoloration
Reserpine	Infant: lethargy, nasal congestion, diarrhea
Quinine	Infant: thrombocytopenia
Pyrimethamine	Bone marrow depression, convulsions
Meprobamate	(Up to four times higher in milk than plasma)
Lithium	(Plasma concentration is up to half that of mother)
Primidone (Mysoline)	Contraindicated on manufacturer's advice
Ergot alkaloids	Infant: ergotism
Cascara and most laxatives	Infant: diarrhea
Propylthiouracil	(Up to 12 times higher in milk than plasma)
Tetrahydrocannabinol	Infant: drowsiness
Phenytoin, Trimethadione	
Iodides	Infant: goiter
	Judicious Use Allowed
Valium	Infant: sedation with high doses
Theophyllin	Infant: thrombocytopenia, 1 case
Sulfonamide	Hemolytic anemia in G-6PD-deficiency
Nalidixic acid	Hemolytic anemia and kernicterus possible
Nicotine	Infant: nicotine intoxication
Isoniazid	Hepatitis, neuropathy
Phenobarbital and Morphine	Infant: sedation with hypnotic doses
Atropine	
Alcohol	Infant: sedation, congenital anomalies
	Unknown Effects
Large doses of Salicylate, Caffeine, Methyldopa, Imipramine, Phenothiazine, Thorazine, Prochlorperazine, Trifluoperazine, Phenolphthalein (Ex-Lax)	
	Acceptable
Dicumerol, Warferin, Guanethidine, Propranolol, Penicillins, Chloralhydrate, Antihistamines, Occasional Use of Aspirin, Acetaminophen	

and exacerbation of "physiologic" jaundice in certain newborns, because pregnanediol seems to inhibit hepatic glucoronyl transferase. Recently, evidence has been presented which suggests that breast milk jaundice is due to the inhibitory effect of non-esterified fatty acids which are increased as a result of BSSL activity (20). Other hormones in breast milk are thyroxine and triiodothyronine. Whether they have a protective effect in infants with hypothyroidism is an unsettled question. They are probably not harmful.

Finally, allergens consumed by the mother may affect the infant even though breast milk has some protective effect against the entry of antigens. It is not necessary to discontinue breast feeding in these cases, since the omission of cow's milk and other allergens from the mother's diet may be sufficient.

Leiner's disease, a dermatitis suggestive of seborrhea complicated by staphylococcal infection, occurs predominantly in breast-fed infants and improves after discontinuation. The reason why is unclear.

Summary and Recommendations

The question of whether to recommend breast feeding (Table 2-4)—possibly with some "arm twisting"—became a hotly debated issue in the late 1970s. The American Academy of Pediatrics selected human lactation as one of its priorities for emphasis during 1979, the International Year of the Child. The emotionalism with which the crusade for breast feeding was carried out was unusual. It occurred during the decade when the women's liberation movement gained momentum and persisted during the time that consumer rights and patient rights to informed consent were successfully championed. There is no need for controversy; the pros and cons of breast feeding are easily summarized to the mother, who can make up her own mind. Unbiased pamphlets in lay language are available. Only the mother, who has to be comfortable with breast feeding, knows her own feelings and her capacity to manage a 4-hourly feeding schedule around the clock within her time constraints. The physician might point out to the mother who cannot commit herself for a long period that even a few weeks of breast feeding have advantages, especially where anti-infective and anti-allergic protection is concerned. A trial may give the mother who hesitates the opportunity to test the emotional experience of breast feeding. At no time should a mother be coerced and made to feel guilty for not nursing or for discontinuing after a trial period. There is currently controversy over the advantages of pooled mother's milk for the feeding of small premature infants. While these infants would benefit from the anti-infectious and anti-allergic qualities of human milk and its ability to promote fat absorption, there is justifiable concern over low protein content and the low marginal concentration of several minerals, mainly calcium and phosphorus. Evidence in support of the contention that human milk prevents enterocolitis in LBW infants is not as strong as it was originally thought to be. Hopefully, new information concerning ways to improve on human milk will soon become available.

A mother who wishes to breast feed but is unable to nurse should be

Table 2-4. Advantages and Disadvantages of Breast Feeding

Advantages
Low but adequate content of protein and specific amino acids, which prevents toxicity
Relatively high content of cystine and taurine
Low solute load
Physiologic calcium/phosphorus ratio
Improved fat absorption due to molecular structure of triglycerides and content of bile salt stimulated lipase
Bifidus factor
Anti-infectious properties conferred by content of:
immunoglobins
lactoferrin and transferrin
lysozyme
lactoperoxidase
complement (C3 and C4)
interferon
monocytic phagocytes
B and T cells
Anti-allergic properties
High concentration of ligands for trace metal absorption
Opportunity for mother–infant bonding
Disadvantages
Low vitamin D and marginal content of vitamin C, E, K, and B-complex
Protein content too low for maximal growth of LBW infants
Calcium and phosphorus content too low, sodium content marginal for maximal growth of LBW infants
Iron content insufficient after age 4–6 months
Carrier of environmental pollutants
Potential content of drugs, including nicotine, alcohol, etc.
Transmission of infective organisms
Transmission of allergens ingested by the mother

instructed in the pumping and proper care of the breast and the handling of milk in order to avoid contamination and destruction of immunologic factors and BSSL by heating. Terminal sterilization is not advisable. Pasteurization also destroys some factors, such as IgA. Fresh mother's milk can be used safely if the mother is healthy, if she washes hands and breasts, discards the first 6 ml of pumped-off milk, and collects the milk in clean containers, such as used baby food jars that are rinsed in boiling water. Refrigeration is satisfactory if the milk is used within 1 day. Otherwise, milk should be frozen. Addition of warm milk to the frozen milk should be avoided.

PREPARED FORMULAS

A variety of commercially prepared formulas are available in the United States. The food industry has been very responsive to new knowledge about the nutritional needs of infants and has made appropriate changes where needed. Some of the more popular formulas are listed in Table 2-5. Formulas are available for those with specific nutritional needs, such as LBW infants, atopic individuals, or infants with gastrointestinal dysfunction and metabolic diseases (Table 2-6).

Standard formulas are based on nonfat cow's milk for protein and lactose but use vegetable oils instead of butter fat. Their protein and electrolyte content is higher than that of human milk but lower than that of cow's milk. Three products are currently marketed that have the whey protein to casein ratio of human milk (Similac PM 60/40, Enfamil Premature Formula, and SMA S-26).

Hypoallergenic formulas are prepared mainly from soy protein isolates; some use meat base and others, casein hydrolysate. Since soy protein is low in sulfur amino acids, methionine was added. Heat processing diminishes the known goitrogenic effect of soy products. Soy formulas are lower in carnitine than either human or cow's milk, which may be a disadvantage in some cases. The high phytate content affects absorption of some minerals, but no adverse effects have been demonstrated to date. Lactose is not a component of any of the hypoallergenic formulas. Aside from its protein source, this constitutes a major difference that must be borne in mind when improvement of diarrhea is observed after switching a patient from a milk base to a hypoallergenic formula. The carbohydrate in hypoallergenic formulas is usually a mixture of sucrose, maltose, dextrins, and starch, which is therapeutic in lactase deficiency as well as milk allergy. Only one product (Prosobee) currently does not contain sucrose. The absence of lactose and sucrose makes this product suitable in the treatment of glycogen storage disease, type I, where fructose, which is contained in sucrose, and galactose cannot be utilized.

LBW formulas have a higher caloric density (81 instead of 67 kcal/dl), an adequate mineral concentration, yet relatively low osmolality. This is accomplished by using, in addition to lactose, either polycose (Similac 24 LBW) or glucose polymers (corn syrup). The fat source is a mixture of vegetable oil and MCT oil.

An easily digestible formula is Pregestimil, because it offers all three major foodstuffs in readily absorbable form—that is, protein as casein hydrolysate, fat as MCT oil, glucose polymers as the glucose source, and no other carbohydrates that may be difficult to digest except modified starch. Nutramigen also contains casein hydrolysate as the sole protein source, but fat and carbohydrate are not as easily digestible. Carbohydrate-free formulas, which are usually made from soy protein isolate and

Table 2-5. Nutritive Value of Commercial Infant Formulas

Name	*Company*	*Classification*	*Source of Protein, CHO and Fat*	*kcal oz*	*Protein (g/dl) (g/100 kcal)*	*Fat (g/dl) (g/100 kcal)*	*CHO (g/dl) (g/100 kcal)*	*Osmolality*
Enfamil	Mead-Johnson	Standard infant food	Nonfat milk Lactose Soy-coconut oil	20	1.5 (2.3)	3.7 (5.6)	7.0 (10.2)	278
Similac	Ross	Standard infant food	Nonfat milk Lactose Coconut oil	20	1.5 (2.3)	3.6 (5.3)	7.0 (10.2)	290
SMA 20	Wyeth	Infant food: 60/40 lactalbumin/casein	Nonfat Milk Lactose Corn-coconut-soy-oleo	20	1.5 (2.3)	3.6 (5.3)	7.2 (10.3)	300
SMA 24	Wyeth	High caloric infant food: 60/40 lactalbumin/casein	(See SMA 20)	24	1.8 (2.3)	4.3 (5.4)	8.6 (10.7)	364
Enfamil-24	Mead-Johnson	High caloric infant food	(See Enfamil)	24	1.8 (2.3)	4.5 (5.6)	8.3 (10.2)	340
Similac-24	Ross	High caloric infant food	(See Similac)	24	2.2 (2.7)	4.2 (5.3)	8.4 (10.5)	360
Similac-27	Ross	High caloric infant food	(See Similac)	27	2.4 (2.7)	4.8 (5.3)	9.5 (10.5)	420
SMA 27	Wyeth	High caloric infant food: 60/40 lactalbumin/casein	(See SMA 20)	27	2.5 (2.8)	4.8 (5.3)	9.5 (10.5)	—
Similac 24 LBW	Ross	LBW infant food: MCT-rich low osmolar	Nonfat milk Lactose, polycose MCT-coconut-soy oil	24	2.2 (2.7)	4.4 (5.5)	7.1 (10.5)	290
Enfamil Premature Formula	Mead-Johnson	LBW infant food: 60/40 lactalbumin/casein, MCT-rich, low osmolar	Nonfat milk Corn syrup, lactose MCT-corn-coconut oil	24	2.4 (3.0)	4.1 (5.0)	8.9 (11.0)	300

Similac PM 60/40	Ross	Infant food: 60/40 lactalbumin/casein low electrolyte	(See Similac)	20	1.5 (2.3)	3.7 (5.6)	6.9 (10.1)	260
ProSobee	Mead-Johnson	Hypoallergenic infant food	Soy protein Corn syrup Soy oil	20	2.0 (2.9)	3.6 (5.3)	6.9 (10.1)	200
Isomil	Ross	Hypoallergenic infant food	Soy protein Corn syrup, sucrose Coconut-soy oil	20	2.0 (2.9)	3.6 (5.3)	6.8 (10.0)	250
Soyalac	Loma Linda	Hypoallergenic infant food	Soy protein Corn syrup, sucrose Soy-corn oil	20	2.1 (3.1)	4.0 (6.0)	6.0 (9.0)	190
Neomullsoy	Syntex	Hypoallergenic infant food	Soy protein Sucrose Soy oil	20	1.9 (2.8)	3.6 (5.3)	6.6 (9.7)	273
MBF (Meat-Base Formula)	Gerber	Hypoallergenic infant food	Beef heart protein Sucrose, tapioca Sesame oil	20	2.7 (4.0)	3.2 (4.8)	6.0 (8.9)	—
Nutramigen	Mead-Johnson	Hypoallergenic infant food	Casein hydrolysate Sucrose, tapioca Corn oil	20	2.2 (3.2)	2.6 (3.9)	8.8 (13.0)	479
Portagen	Mead-Johnson	MCT–rich infant food	Sodium caseinate Corn syrup, sucrose MCT, Corn oil	20	2.4 (3.5)	3.2 (4.8)	7.8 (11.5)	236
Pregestimil	Mead-Johnson	Easy digestible, hypoallergenic infant food	Casein hydrolysate + cys + tyr + tryp Corn syrup, tapioca Corn oil, MCT	20	1.9 (2.8)	2.7 (4.0)	9.1 (13.5)	348

soybean oil, allow the addition of single sugars, either for diagnostic purposes or for treatment of gastrointestinal and metabolic diseases. A number of formulas for inborn errors of amino acid metabolism are on the market that are also composed of amino acid mixtures, but one or more amino acid is removed, either completely or partially. They are discussed in Chapter 13.

Home-prepared formulas are rarely used in the United States except for economic reasons. This practice need not be discouraged (Table 2-7) providing the infant is full term and healthy. Since the protein and electrolyte contents of cow's milk and of reconstituted evaporated milk are

Table 2-6. Indications for Special Formulas

Soy-protein formulas	Milk allergy
(Isomil, Mullsoy, Soyalac)	Lactose intolerance (lactase deficiency)
	Galactosemia
(Prosobee)	Same, plus glycogen storage disease
Casein hydrolysate formulas	Sensitivity to intact proteins
(Nutramigen)	Postgastroenteritis syndrome
(Pregestimil)	Fat malabsorption syndromes
	Transition after parenteral feeding
	(Not necessary for disaccharidase deficiencies)[a]
CHO-free formulas	Test diet (carbohydrate malabsorption)
with fructose[b]	Glucose-galactose malabsorption
	Severe intractable diarrhea
Special formulas for LBW infants	LBW infants
(Similac 24 LBW, Enfamil Premature Formula)	Protein-calorie malnutrition
	Biliary atresia, fat malabsorption
Low-electrolyte formulas	Renal failure
(Similac PM 60/40, SMA 20)	Heart failure
in < standard dilution	Severe malnutrition
Low phenylalanine	Phenylketonuria
(Lofenalac)	
Low branched chain amino acids (MSUD Diet Powder)	Maple sugar urine disease
Low tyrosine, low phenylalanine (Product 3200AB)	Hereditary tyrosinemia
Low methionine (Product 3200K)	Homocystinuria, unresponsive to vitamins
High MCT content	Fat malabsorption syndromes
40%: Enfamil Premature Formula	Exudative protein-losing gastroenteropathy
50%: Similac 24 LBW	
80%: Portagen (lactose free)	
40%: Pregestimil	

[a] Cheaper formulas are available: soy formulas for lactase deficiency and milk-base formulas for sucrase-isomaltase deficiency.

[b] RCF: Ross Carbohydrate Free Soy Protein Formula.

Table 2-7. Home Preparation of Infant Formulas[a,b]

Formula	*Milk* (ml)	*Water* (ml)	*Karo Syrup* (tablesp/ml)	*Calories* (per dl)
Evaporated	90	180	1/15	67
Evaporated	90	130	1/15	81
Homogenized	180	90	1/15	67

[a] Preparation of a single feeding is preferable to preparation of the daily formula at one time in order to prevent bacterial growth.
[b] *Supplements of vitamin C and iron* (7 mg/day) are necessary.

above the recommended maximum concentration for infants, it is necessary to make proper dilutions. Moreover, evaporated milk and homogenized milk formulas are inadequate sources of vitamin C and therefore require supplementation. There is also biochemical evidence that evaporated milk formulas are deficient in essential fatty acids and vitamin E, because blood levels of these two nutrients have been low during the first 3 to 6 months of life. As soon as fruits, vegetables, and cereals are added to the diet, these substances are usually supplied in adequate amounts. Skim milk formulas provide insufficient energy and therefore promote overeating by volume, which may lead to the development of unsound eating habits. In addition, they are an insufficient source of essential fatty acids and have an excessive protein and mineral content. Home-prepared formulas should be heated (terminal sterilization) both to reduce contaminants and allergenicity.

SEMISOLID AND SOLID INFANT FOODS

Serving Size

Commercially prepared infant foods are available in finely pureed form for small infants ("strained" baby foods) and in slightly chunkier consistency for older infants ("junior" foods). Texture and serving size are appropriate for two age groups—4 to 10 months and 10 months and older. Jars with strained food generally contain 128 to 135 g and junior foods, 213 to 220 g. The exceptions are strained and junior meats (99 g) and toddler meals (170 to 177 g). By the time the infant is ready for these foods, capacity is about ½ to 1 jar per meal. Jars are convenient for the measurement of nutrient intake.

Types of Food

Cereals

There is a nearly endless variety of infant food on the market (Table 2-8). Cereals are available as single-grain infant cereals (rice, oatmeal, and

Table 2-8. Nutritive Values of Commercial Infant Foods

Foods	*Jar (g)*	*Calories (per jar)*	*Calories (per 100 g)*	*Protein (per 100 g)*	*Specific Nutrient Content (% RDA)*
Dry cereals (per serving, with milk[a])					
Regular, barley, oat, rice, mixed		100[a]		2.0[a]	Vit. B, (45) Fe
High protein		110[a]		5.0[a]	" " "
High protein with fruit		100[a]		4.0[a]	" " "
Cereals with fruit					
Strained	135	100–120	70–86	0.4–1.4	Vit. C B, (45) Fe
Junior	220	170–200	76–81	1.2–1.5	" , " " "
High protein with banana	135	120	86	5.1	" " " "
Desserts					
Strained	128–135	100–130	71–100	0.1–2.0	
Junior	220	170–220	71–100	0.1–2.0	
Desserts with cottage cheese					
Strained	128	120	92	3.0	
Junior	220	220	99	3.0	
Vegetables: beets, carrots, spinach, vegetables, green beans, squash, peas					
Strained	128	30–60	26–44	0.7–3.3	Vit. A (100)
Junior	213	60–100	27–45	0.7–2.7	" "
Creamed corn, sweet potatoes					
Strained	128	90	67–72	1.2–1.4	Vit. A (100)
Junior	213	130–150	69–72	1.2–1.4	" "
Fruits: applesauce with pineapple pears with pineapple					
Strained	128	60	43–51	0.2–0.4	Vit. C (45)
Junior	213	90–110	42–52	0.3–0.4	" "

Apple with blueberry, with raspberry, apricotts or bananas with tapioca					
Strained	135	90–120	68–76	0.2–0.5	Vit. C (45)
Junior	220	140–160	68–76	0.2–0.5	″ ″
Applesauce with apricots, peaches, prunes (junior), plums (strained or junior)					
Strained	135	140	91	0.3	Vit. C (45)
Junior	220	170–200	78–91	0.3–0.6	″ ″
Egg yolk: Strained	94	180	195	9.7	Vit. A, B_2, B_6 (25–45), Fe (15)
Meats (excluding chicken) Strained	99	90–120	87–117	12.6–14.8	Vit. B (20–40), Fe (10)
(excluding sticks) Junior	99	100–120	94–120	14.3–15.7	
Chicken, strained/junior	99	130/150	132/153	13.6–14.6	
Sticks of chicken, turkey, etc., junior	71	130	178–195	12.9–14.4	
Toddler meals	177	110–150	57–86	4.6–5.2	Vit. A (50), Fe (15)
High-meat dinners					
Strained	128	90–120	74–92	6.0–6.3	
Junior	128	100–130	76–98	6.2–7.8	
Cottage cheese with pineapple	135	160	131	6.6	
Vegetable–meat dinners (excluding those listed below)					
Strained	128	60–70	41–57	1.6–2.7	Vit. A (40–80)
Junior	213	90–120	47–58	1.7–2.8	″ ″
Cream of chicken, grits with eggs, macaroni and cheese, vegetable and bacon					
Strained	128	80–100	63–75	1.6–2.7	
Macaroni and cheese, split peas with ham, vegetable and bacon, spaghetti and beef					
Junior	213	130–170	63–73	2.2–3.1	
Cookies, Zwieback (2)		60		1–2	
Pretzels (2) *teething biscuit* (1)		45		1	

[a] Mix 6 tablespoons with 70 ml milk.

barley) and as combination cereals—either "mixed" (oat, corn, wheat, and soy) or "high-protein" cereals (soy, oat, and wheat). Cereal and fruit combinations are on the market that appeal to the flavor preferences of older children. They may instead eat home-prepared cooked farinas and cereal–fruit combinations, which are cheaper. Cereals are valuable for their supply of energy; fortified cereals also provide iron, 45% of the U.S. RDA for thiamine and niacin, and 30% for riboflavin. The iron in cereal is electrically reduced and therefore readily absorbed. Five tablespoons supply 5.5 mg, which is an adequate daily intake because of the improved absorption of electrically reduced iron. Preparation of commercial infant cereals consists of precooking, partial hydrolysis by diastase, and drying. Rice is polished, but the external layers are re-added.

Fruits

Although fruits are usually introduced a month or so after cereals, they may be given at the same age—one item at a time. They mainly provide energy because of their high carbohydrate content, fructose and glucose. The majority have sugar added, which increases the natural calorie content per jar from about 60 kcal to 90 or 120 kcal. Most fruit products are enriched with vitamin C to compensate for the loss that occurs during processing and storage. Pureed and junior fruits are an ideal energy source for malnourished infants.

Vegetables

With the exception of sweet potatoes, corn, and peas, vegetables are by and large a low-calorie food. They supply minerals, fiber, and vitamins, especially vitamin A. Creamed vegetables, which contain milk solids and modified food starches, have a higher calorie content (about 60 kcal/jar) than such noncreamed vegetables as carrots, beets, green beans, and squash (30–40 kcal/jar).

Vegetable–Meat Combinations

Since vegetable–meat combinations are readily confused with other dinners, it should be noted that the vegetable is listed before the meat. They do not contain as many calories as high-protein dinners, and their protein concentration is only slightly higher than that of pure vegetable preparations. By contrast, meat–vegetable combinations that list the meat first are "high-protein" dinners, with a protein concentration about half that of pure meats.

Meats

Meat preparations are a source of high-quality protein, have a high protein concentration, are rich in iron, and have a high caloric density. However, they should not be used to increase calorie intake because of the potentially very high protein load. Pure meats have a lower fat content than most table meats, but as a result have a dry, grainy texture. They are not well accepted by many infants. Consequently, parents often mix them with other foods, including fruits.

Desserts

Desserts include fruit custards and puddings with a high caloric density because of their sugar content. They are ideal for use in high-caloric diets, especially for infants recovering from malnutrition. Vanilla and chocolate custard have the highest calorie density. Homemade custards serve the same purpose.

Toddler Meals

Toddler meals are meat–vegetable preparations or pasta mixtures with a chunkier consistency than most junior foods. They have a relatively high caloric density, 76 to 86 kcal/100 g (excluding beef stew, which is lower). Their calorie density is thus comparable to that of creamed vegetables, sweetened fruits, high-meat dinners, and a few vegetable–meat combinations.

A number of significant changes in the preparation of commercial infant foods occurred during the late seventies: (*1*) the reduction or elimination of added sugar in fruits and some desserts; (*2*) the elimination of added monosodium glutamate; and (*3*) the reduction or elimination of added salt. These changes were apparently made as a matter of good policy, since adverse effects of their prior use had not been demonstrated conclusively.

Pureed infant foods can be prepared at home in a blender. Cooked cereals and farinas may be used by young infants. Other table foods, like apple sauce, mashed potatoes, creamed spinach, mashed cooked carrots, and puddings are soft enough to be used in place of junior foods. The 1-year-old may accept such table foods as liverwurst, ground meat, minced tuna, and mashed chicken livers. If home-prepared foods are not consumed soon after preparation, care must be taken to avoid contamination. Single portions may be frozen. Another cause for caution is the high salt content of table foods, which was shown to be 64% higher in one study (21) than the maximum acceptable sodium level for commercially prepared foods recommended by the Food and Nutrition Board of the National Academy of Sciences.

REFERENCES

1. Räihä NCR, Heinonen K, Rassin DK, et al: Milk protein quantity and quality in low birth weight infants: I. Metabolic responses and effects on growth. *Pediatrics* 57:659, 1976.
2. Davies DP: Adequacy of expressed breast milk for early growth of preterm infants. *Arch Dis Child* 52:296, 1977.

3. Fomon SJ, Filer LJ Jr, Thomas LN, et al: Relationship between formula concentration and rate of growth of normal infants. *J Nutr* 98:241, 1969.
4. Barness LA, Omans WB, Rose SC, et al: Progress of premature infants fed a formula containing determined whey. *Pediatrics* 32:52, 1963.
5. Borgström B, Erlanson C: Interactions of serum albumin and other proteins with porcine pancreatic lipase. *Gastroenterology* 75:382, 1978.
6. Gaull, G, Sturman JA, Räihä NCR: Development of mammalian sulfur metabolism. Absence of cystathionase in human fetal tissues. *Pediatr Res* 6:538, 1972.
7. Hambraeus L, Ranne L: The plasma phenylalanine level in newborn infants of normal and low birth weights fed on human milk. *Biol Neonate* 13:315, 1968.
8. Hytten FE: Clinical and chemical studies in human lactation. *Br Med J* 1:175, 1954.
9. Committee on Nutrition, American Academy of Pediatrics: Commentary on breast feeding and infant formulas including proposed standards for formulas. *Pediatrics* 57:278, 1976.
10. Fomon SJ, Ziegler EE, Thomas LN, et al: Excretion of fat by normal full term infants fed various milks and formulas. *Am J Clin Nutr* 23:1299, 1970.
11. Hernell O: Human milk lipases. III. Physiological implications of the bile salt stimulated lipase. *Eur J Clin Invest* 5:267, 1975.
12. Fredrikzon B, Hernell O, Blackberg L, et al: Bile salt stimulated lipase in human milk: Evidence of activity in vivo and of a role in the digestion of milk retinol esters. *Pediatr Res* 12:1048, 1978.
13. Gindrat JJ, Gotherfors L, Hanson LA, et al: Antibodies in human milk against E. Coli of the sero groups most commonly found in neonatal infections. *Acta Paediatr Scand* 61:587, 1972.
14 Bullen JJ, Rogers HJ, Leigh L: Iron binding proteins in milk and resistance to escherichia coli infection in infants. *Br Med J* 1:69, 1972.
15. Saarinen UM, Siimes MA: Iron absorption from breast milk, cow's milk and iron supplemented formula: An opportunistic use of changes in total body iron determined by hemoglobin, ferritin and body weight in 132 infants. *Pediatr Res* 13:143, 1979.
16. Evans GW and Johnson PE: Characterization and quantitation of a zinc binding ligand in human milk. *Pediatr Res* 14:876, 1980.
17. Krieger I: Picolinic acid in the treatment of disorders requiring zinc supplementation. *Nutr Rev* 38:148, 1980.
18. Forbes GB: Is human milk best food for low birth weight infants, abstracted. *Pediatr Res* 12:433, 1978.
19. Wilson JT: Drugs in breast milk. ADIS Press, New York 1981.
20. Poland RL: Breast milk jaundice. *J Pediatr* 99:86, 1981.
21. Kerr CM Jr, Reisinger KS, Plankey FW: Sodium concentration of homemade baby foods. *Pediatrics* 62:331, 1978.

3 Nutritional Assessment

The approaches most commonly used in nutritional assessment of infants and children are (*1*) clinical evaluation, including anthropometric measurements; (*2*) assessment of past and current nutrient intake; and (*3*) biochemical measurements. Since each of these tools has serious limitations, diagnosis should never rest on just one of them.

CLINICAL EVALUATION

History and Physical Examination

Historical data, which are extremely important because they influence the interpretation of nutritional information, are birth weight and length of gestation, anthropometric measurements recorded in the past, time of development of secondary sex characteristics and menarche, past illnesses, chronically used medications that retard growth, a family history of short stature, metabolic diseases, and siblings born small for length of gestation. Developmental assessment by history is useful and can be done with the help of the parent, who may fill out a questionnaire in advance of the physical exam (Table 3-1). Development is slow in patients with environmental deprivation and in central nervous system disease. Because of weakness, gross motor development may be slower than fine motor and language development in cases of debilitating chronic disease and undernutrition.

The physical examination may show signs of specific nutrient deficiencies or evidence of diseases that cause nutritional disorders. Manifestations that commonly reveal single-nutrient deficiency states are listed in Table 3-2. Unfortunately, these signs and symptoms are not characteristic, as they may be seen in diseases of an entirely different nature. Moreover, certain clinical signs, such as angular stomatitis, may be caused by a deficiency of more than one nutrient. It is obvious, therefore, that interpretation of such findings must be supported by other clinical and laboratory data.

Determination of the developmental age is important in many nutritional disorders. Assessment by history, using the parents' report of developmental landmarks, should be combined with an examination of psychomotor function, feeding skills, developmental reflexes, and so forth. The infant and preschool child may be tested by the pediatrician through the use of the Denver Developmental Test (1). School records and formal intelligence tests are necessary for the evaluation of older children.

In low birth weight (LBW) infants assessment of gestational age (Fig. 3-1) should be done during the first 24 hours. This is necessary to determine whether the newborn is premature and has an appropriate weight for gestational age (AGA) or has been carried to term and is small for gestational age (SGA) because of intrauterine growth failure. This evaluation is extremely important in the nutritional management of LBW

Table 3-1. Developmental Landmarks[a]

Activity	*Mean*	*Range (Months)*[b]
Lifts up head while lying on belly	1 month	0–2
While held in sitting position, infant keeps head erect and steady	2 months	1–3
Turns over from back to stomach or vice versa	3 months	2–4
Sits alone for 5 seconds after support is released	6 months	5–6
Stands holding onto solid object	7 months	5–8
Pulls self to standing position	8 months	6–9
Stands alone 2 to 3 seconds if outside support is removed	10 months	9–12
Picks up small object (raisin or button) with two fingers	11 months	10–12
Walks with support	1 year	11–13
Says first words	1 year	9–15
Walks upstairs without help	$1\frac{1}{2}$ years	14–21
Points to named body parts	$1\frac{1}{2}$ years	15–22
Pedals a tricycle	2 years	21–30
Uses plurals	2 years	20–32
Pulls shirt overhead	2 years	30–30
Three-word sentences	$2\frac{1}{2}$years	24–36
Identifies primary colors	3 years	33–45
Copies a circle	$2\frac{1}{2}$ years	24–36
Copies a cross	3 years	33–45
Buttons	3 years	30–42
Hops on one foot	$3\frac{1}{2}$ years	38–48
Dresses without support	$3\frac{1}{2}$ years	30–48

[a] This or a similar list may be used as a questionnaire to be filled out by the infant's parents before the examination.
[b] 25th to 75th percentiles, according to Denver Developmental chart (1).

infants, because the prognoses for postnatal growth are different for premature AGA infants and mature SGA infants. The clinical assessment by the method of Dubowitz (2) has proven its value over the past decade. It is based on 10 neurological and 11 external signs that can be objectively scored from 0 to 5, where the lowest score reflects the more immature infant. The sum of the scores is plotted on a graph for determination of gestational age (Fig. 3-2). By relating gestational age to the patient's birth weight, one is able to determine whether the LBW infant has an appropriate weight (is AGA) (Fig. 3-1).

Anthropometric Measurements

In growth failure, anthropometric measurements achieve two goals: (*1*) the determination of present size relative to normal standards and (*2*) the

Table 3-2. Physical Signs Suggestive of Specific Nutrient Malnutrition[a]

Skin
- Dry and scaly (vitamins B_3 and A)
- Seborrhea (vitamins B_2 and B_6, biotin, and hypervitaminosis A)
- Follicular hyperkeratosis (vitamin A)
- Peripheral erythematous rash (vitamin B_3)
- Xerosis (vitamin A)
- Pallor (iron, folate, vitamin B_{12}, copper)
- Edema (protein)
- Petechii (vitamin C)

Hair
- Dry and brittle (kwashiorkor, thyroxin)
- Pulls out easily (protein)
- Depigmentation (kwashiorkor)
- Alopecia (vitamins B_6 and biotin, zinc)

Lips and mouth
- Cheilosis (vitamins B_2 and B_6)
- Marginal gum redness and swelling (vitamin B_3)
- Bleeding gums (vitamin C)
- Glossitis (vitamin B_3, B_6, B_{12}, and folic acid)
- Tongue papillae atrophic (iron, vitamin B_2)

Eyes
- Conjunctivitis (vitamin B_2)
- Corneal dryness, xerosis (vitamin A)
- Corneal vascularization (vitamin B_2)
- Corneal opacities (vitamin B_2)
- Angular conjunctival vascularities (vitamin A)
- Bitot's spots, yellow, over bulbar conjunctiva (vitamin A)

Head, face and neck
- Frontal bossing (vitamin D)
- Thyroid enlargement (iodine)

Skeleton
- Leg bowing (vitamin D)
- Broad epiphyses (vitamin D)
- Beading of the ribs (vitamin D)

[a] Nutrients listed in parentheses are deficient except where otherwise specified.

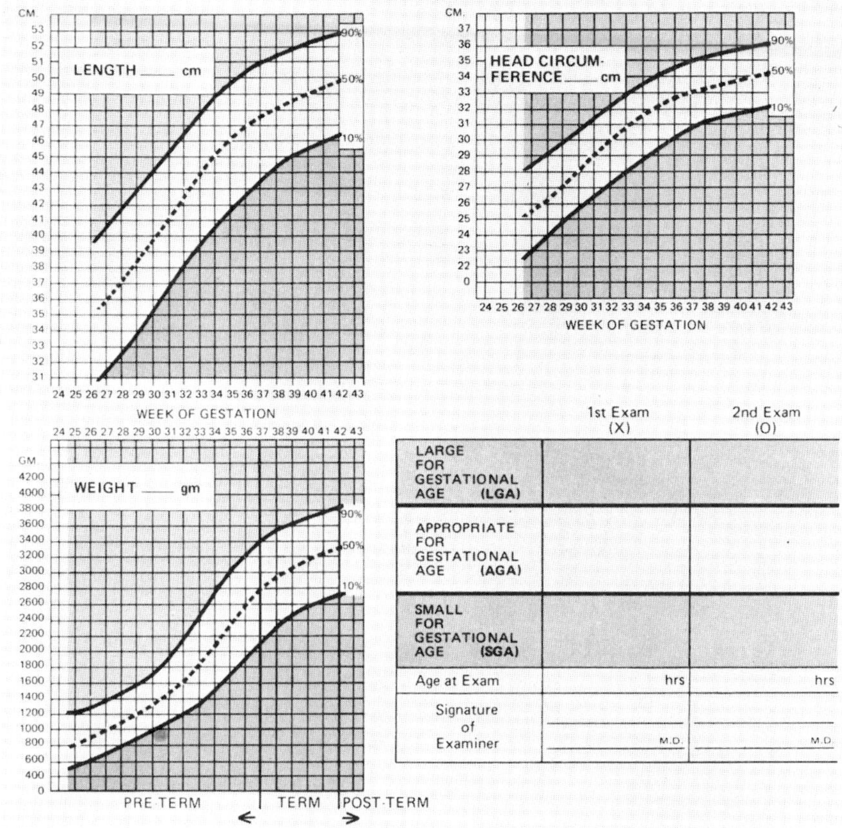

Figure 3-1. CLASSIFICATION OF NEWBORNS, BASED ON MATURITY AND INTRAUTERINE GROWTH
(Adapted from Lubchenco LC, Hansman C, Boyd E: Intrauterine growth in length and head circumference as estimated from live births at gestational ages from 26 to 42 weeks. *Pediatrics* 37:403, 1966.

assessment of progress through serial measurements in order to monitor the effect of disease or the treatment thereof.

Intrauterine Growth

Standards of normal intrauterine growth are the first and one of the more important sets of anthropometric measurements (Table 3-3). If the gestational age is known, either from a reliable history and/or from a clinical assessment based on signs of maturity (Figs. 3-1 and 3-2) (2), these weight standards make it possible to determine whether an infant was born appropriate or small for gestational age. The most widely used standards for evaluation of birth weight are by Lubchenco (3), who also

Table 3-3. Intrauterine Growth in Weight, Length, and Head Circumference as Estimated from Live Births at Gestational Ages from 24 to 42 Weeks (3, 4)

	80%							*80%*				
			50%			*Weeks of*				*50%*		
Number	P_{10}	P_{25}	P_{50}	P_{75}	P_{90}	*Pregnancy*	*Number*	P_{10}	P_{25}	P_{50}	P_{75}	P_{90}
	Males: Weight (kg)[a]						Females: Weight (kg)[a]					
13	0.610	0.730	0.830	1.020	1.230	24	11	0.490	0.645	0.760	0.980	1.250
12	0.685	0.790	0.880	1.040	1.260	25	15	0.600	0.740	0.845	1.050	1.295
43	0.760	0.875	0.965	1.110	1.330	26	25	0.700	0.830	0.935	1.125	1.350
38	0.835	0.970	1.080	1.215	1.435	27	34	0.790	0.925	1.035	1.210	1.420
64	0.915	1.075	1.205	1.350	1.570	28	54	0.870	1.020	1.140	1.320	1.530
80	0.995	1.180	1.330	1.495	1.720	29	63	0.945	1.115	1.255	1.455	1.690
61	1.085	1.290	1.465	1.650	1.875	30	48	1.025	1.215	1.380	1.600	1.880
88	1.195	1.415	1.600	1.830	2.050	31	59	1.125	1.330	1.515	1.760	2.100
66	1.320	1.550	1.760	2.045	2.280	32	58	1.250	1.465	1.675	1.970	2.330
62	1.470	1.710	1.970	2.310	2.575	33	56	1.400	1.630	1.875	2.275	2.620
74	1.645	1.920	2.220	2.620	2.920	34	71	1.550	1.825	2.155	2.555	2.920
104	1.875	2.180	2.520	2.885	3.190	35	84	1.730	2.060	2.410	2.795	3.160
118	2.105	2.410	2.745	3.090	3.385	36	84	1.960	2.320	2.630	2.980	3.335
188	2.330	2.625	2.930	3.245	3.540	37	184	2.220	2.520	2.800	3.120	3.450
354	2.505	2.795	3.080	3.380	3.665	38	282	2.405	2.680	2.940	3.235	3.545
504	2.630	2.915	3.200	3.505	3.780	39	506	2.540	2.810	3.060	3.340	3.640
576	2.700	2.995	3.290	3.610	3.880	40	588	2.630	2.905	3.160	3.440	3.720
312	2.735	3.035	3.330	3.670	3.940	41	320	2.660	2.950	3.210	3.520	3.795
164	2.730	3.005	3.310	3.660	3.995	42	172	2.630	2.940	3.210	3.550	3.840

Males and females: Length (cm)[a]							Males and females: Head circumference (cm)[a]					
30	30.8	32.9	35.5	37.5	39.9	26	24	22.4	23.6	25.2	26.6	28.5
21	31.8	34.1	36.6	38.6	41.0	27	20	23.2	24.4	25.8	27.2	28.9
46	33.0	35.5	37.8	39.8	42.2	28	40	24.3	25.4	26.7	28.0	29.4
53	34.4	36.8	39.0	40.9	43.1	29	49	25.3	26.4	27.6	28.8	30.2
47	36.1	38.3	40.3	42.2	44.5	30	49	26.2	27.4	28.6	29.7	31.1
54	37.5	39.7	41.6	43.5	45.9	31	53	26.9	28.2	29.6	30.5	31.9
62	38.8	41.1	43.2	45.0	47.2	32	58	27.6	29.0	30.4	31.4	32.7
69	39.9	42.3	44.7	46.2	48.4	33	65	28.4	29.8	31.2	32.1	33.4
111	41.0	43.4	45.8	47.3	49.4	34	103	29.2	30.6	31.9	32.9	34.0
149	42.0	44.6	46.7	48.1	50.2	35	149	30.0	31.3	32.5	33.4	34.5
189	43.1	45.6	47.4	48.8	50.9	36	186	30.6	31.8	32.9	33.8	34.9
345	44.1	46.5	48.0	49.3	51.3	37	353	31.1	32.3	33.2	34.1	35.2
595	44.9	47.1	48.4	49.8	51.7	38	611	31.4	32.5	33.4	34.3	35.4
957	45.5	47.6	48.8	50.1	52.0	39	961	31.6	32.8	33.7	34.6	35.7
1084	45.8	47.9	49.2	50.5	52.3	40	1097	31.8	33.0	34.0	34.8	35.9
589	46.0	48.1	49.5	50.8	52.6	41	587	32.0	33.2	34.2	35.0	36.0
315	46.2	48.2	49.7	51.0	52.8	42	315	32.1	33.4	34.3	35.1	36.2

[a] SOURCE: Adapted from Lubchenco et al: *Pediatrics* 32:793, 1963 and 37:403, 1966.

NEUROMUSCULAR MATURITY

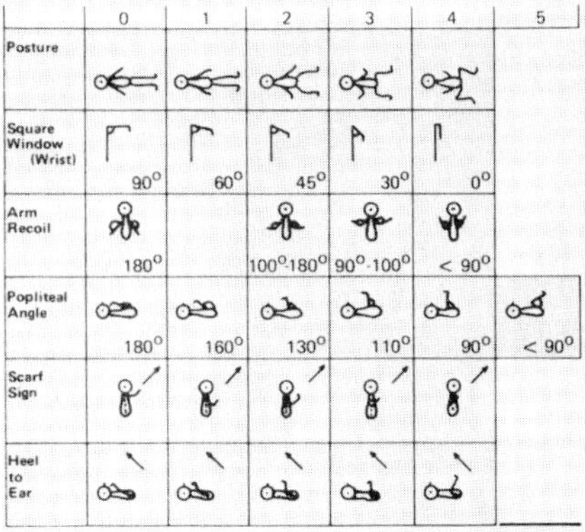

PHYSICAL MATURITY

	0	1	2	3	4	5
SKIN	gelatinous red, trans-parent	smooth pink, visible veins	superficial peeling &/or rash, few veins	cracking pale area, rare veins	parchment, deep cracking, no vessels	leathery, cracked, wrinkled
LANUGO	none	abundant	thinning	bald areas	mostly bald	
PLANTAR CREASES	no crease	faint red marks	anterior transverse crease only	creases ant. 2/3	creases cover entire sole	
BREAST	barely percept.	flat areola, no bud	stippled areola, 1–2 mm bud	raised areola, 3–4 mm bud	full areola, 5–10 mm bud	
EAR	pinna flat, stays folded	sl. curved pinna, soft with slow recoil	well-curv. pinna, soft but ready recoil	formed & firm with instant recoil	thick cartilage, ear stiff	
GENITALS Male	scrotum empty, no rugae		testes descend-ing, few rugae	testes down, good rugae	testes pendulous, deep rugae	
GENITALS Female	prominent clitoris & labia minora		majora & minora equally prominent	majora large, minora small	clitoris & minora completely covered	

Gestation by Dates ______________ wks

Birth Date __________ Hour __________ am / pm

APGAR __________ 1 min __________ 5 min

MATURITY RATING

Score	Wks
5	26
10	28
15	30
20	32
25	34
30	36
35	38
40	40
45	42
50	44

SCORING SECTION

	1st Exam=X	2nd Exam=O
Estimating Gest Age by Maturity Rating	______ Weeks	______ Weeks
Time of Exam	Date ______ Hour ______ am/pm	Date ______ Hour ______ am/pm
Age at Exam	______ Hours	______ Hours
Signature of Examiner	______ M.D.	______ M.D.

Figure 3-2. ESTIMATION OF GESTATIONAL AGE BY MATURITY RATING (Scoring system from Ballard JL: A simplified assessment of gestational age. *Pediatr Res* 11:374, 1977; based on the method of Dubowitz L, Dubowitz V, Goldberg C: Clinical assessment of gestational age in the newborn infant. *J Pediatr* 77:1, 1970. Figures from Sweet AY: Classification of the low-birth-weight infant, in Klaus MH, Fanaroff AA (eds): *Care of the High-Risk Neonate*. Philadelphia, WB Saunders Co, 1979, p 79.)

collected normative data for height, head circumference, and weight/length ratio (calculated from Röhrer's ponderal index) for infants from 24 to 42 weeks' gestation (3,4). Weight is a very practical measure of intrauterine growth, because it can be obtained easily and accurately and reflects abnormality of intrauterine growth whether height is affected or not. However, height and head size should be evaluated in conjunction with weight because of the prognostic implications (Chapter 1).

Body Weight

Infants should be weighed in the nude and older children, in their underwear. When daily measurements are required, weighing should be performed before breakfast to minimize weight fluctuation from variable gastrointestinal content. Large fluctuations are nevertheless common, especially in infants and young children recovering from malnutrition. A starved child or one recovering from an intercurrent illness may show a sudden, major weight increase right after admission to the hospital that does not represent a true increase in tissue mass. Sudden changes may reflect the weight of intestinal contents, recovery from dehydration, or retention of water, which occurs not uncommonly in marasmic children. Irregular bowel evacuation may be responsible for continued large daily fluctuations. The determination of weight gain due to anabolic processes therefore may require prolonged observation and the use of a plot of daily weights. The average gain per day is determined by approximating a straight line to the weight curve and dividing the total increment per period by the number of days.

Weight in percent of the mean for age (or weight age/chronological age) is not a useful measure since it is often misleading. An example is the 1-year-old girl with familial short stature who has a height just below the third percentile and a normal weight for height. Her weight for age is 83% of normal, a value that would place the infant in the malnourished range if her height were normal.

Weight for height is commonly used as an index of nutritional status (Fig. 3-3) but also must be interpreted with caution. Errors are avoided if

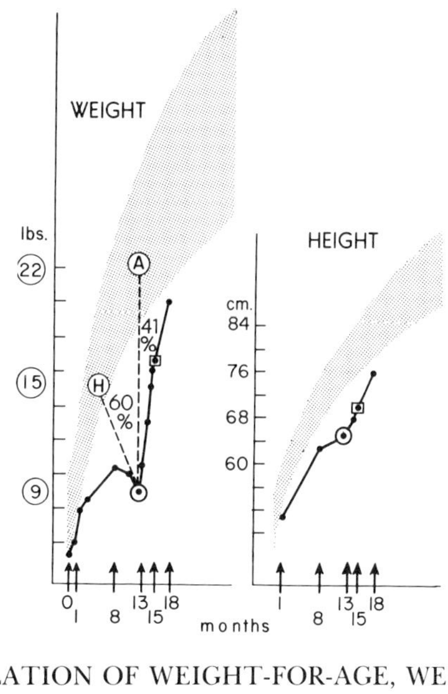

Figure 3-3. CALCULATION OF WEIGHT-FOR-AGE, WEIGHT-FOR-HEIGHT, AND HEIGHT-AGE

Example of a 13-month-old infant—weight is 41% of the normal mean for age and 60% of normal mean for height; height-age is 8 months.

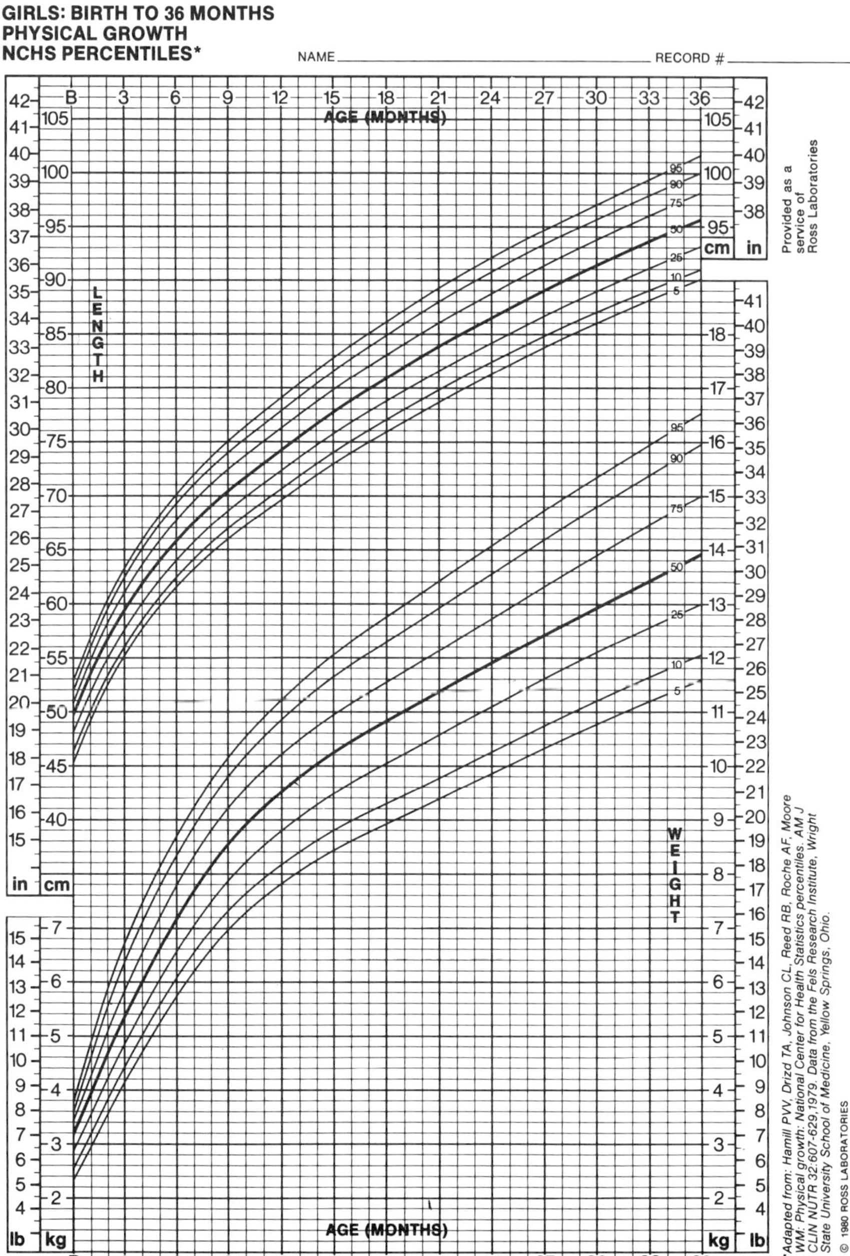

Figure 3-4 and 3-4a. PHYSICAL GROWTH PERCENTILES
Example is for girls, birth to 36 months. (Data from National Center for Health Statistics: *NCHS Growth Charts, 1976*, Monthly Vital Statistics Report, vol 25, no 3 Supp (HRA) 76-1120, Rockville, Maryland, Health Resources Administration, June 1976. Data from the Fels Research Institute, Yellow Springs, Ohio.) Graph, courtesy of Ross Laboratories.

GIRLS: BIRTH TO 36 MONTHS
PHYSICAL GROWTH
NCHS PERCENTILES*

NAME ________________ RECORD # ________

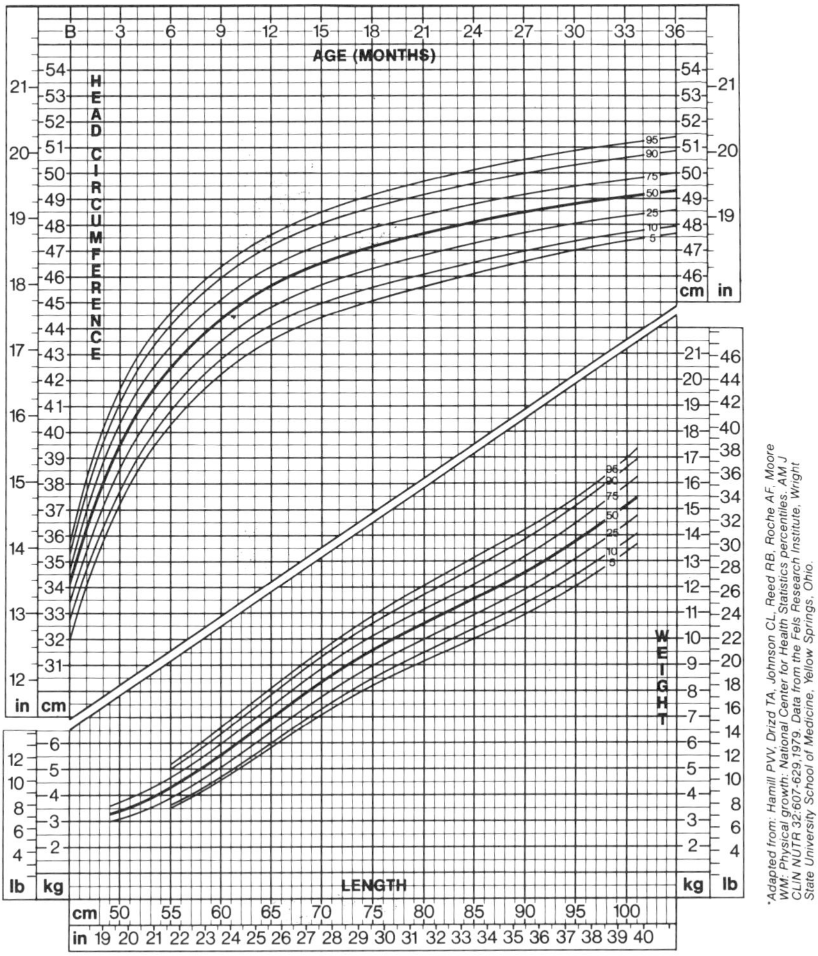

DATE	AGE	LENGTH	WEIGHT	HEAD C.
	BIRTH			

DATE	AGE	LENGTH	WEIGHT	HEAD C.

---

serial measurements of weight for height are plotted on standard growth charts (Figs. 3-4 and 3-5). This will often reveal the characteristic "channel" of the patient (Fig. 3-6). Postnatal deviations from the individual norm are then easily recognized. A weight above 85% of the mean for height can be "normal" for individuals with an "asthenic" body habitus.

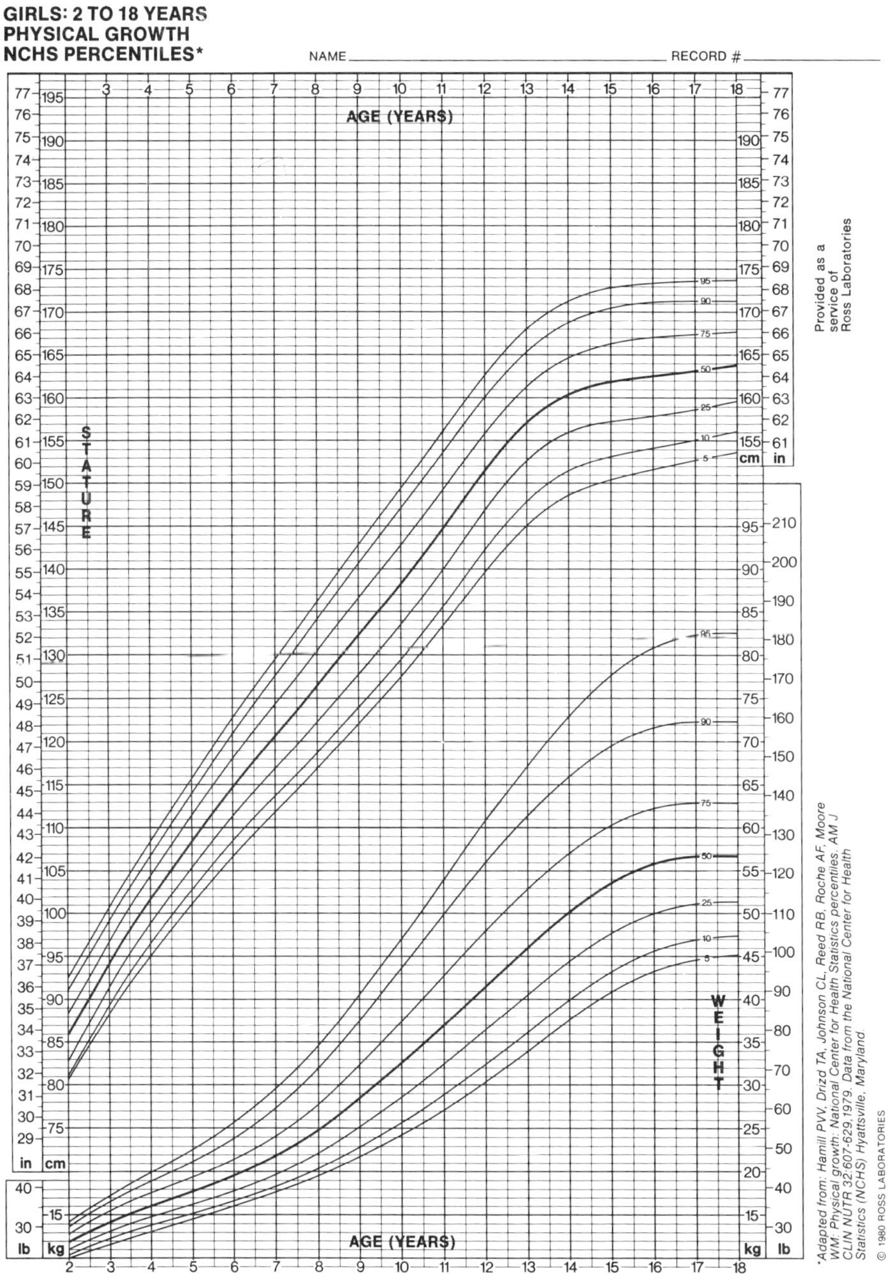

Figure 3-5. PHYSICAL GROWTH PERCENTILES: Example is for girls 2 to 18 years (same source).

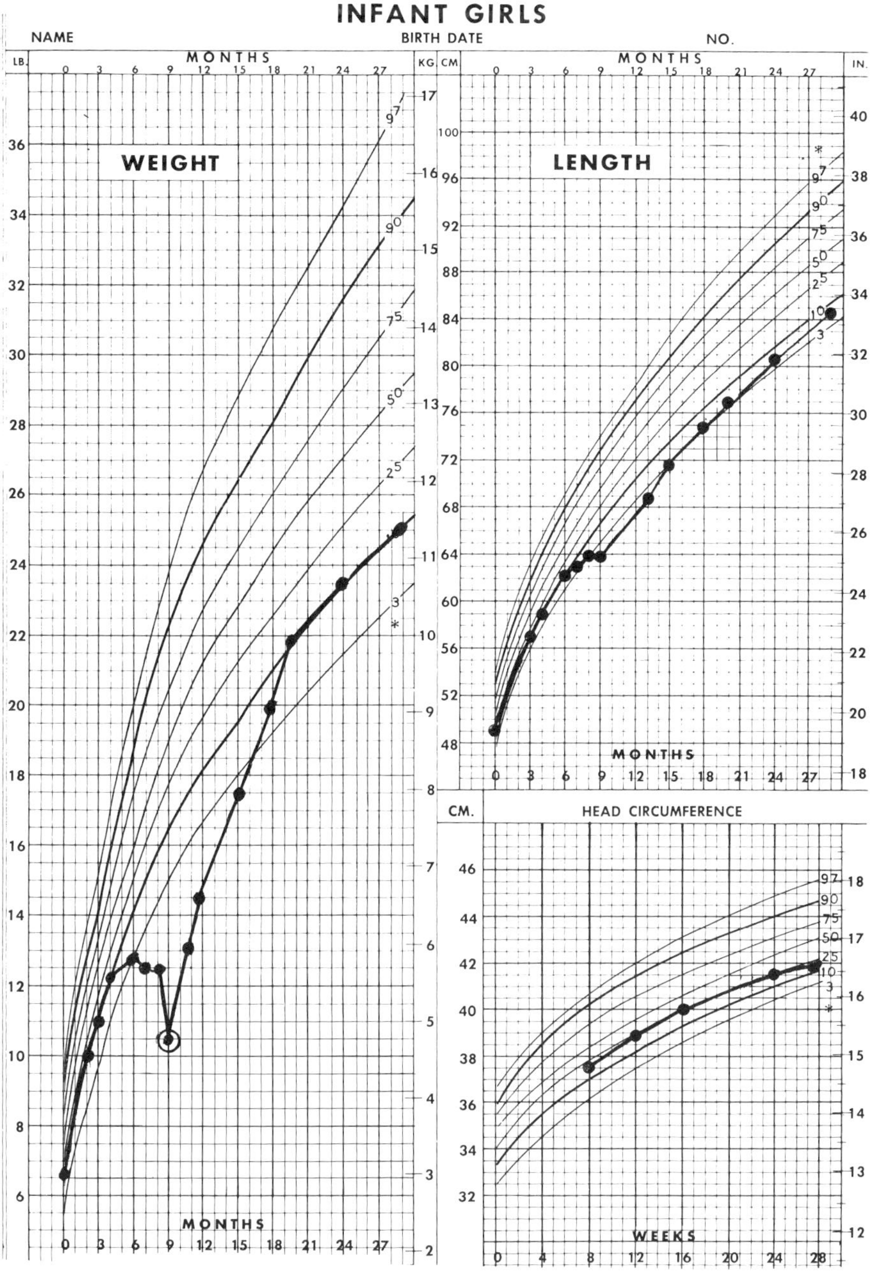

Figure 3-6. LONGITUDINAL GROWTH RECORD OF AN INFANT, SEVERELY MALNOURISHED AT 9 MONTHS
Graphed on Stuart growth chart (7). The "channeling" of weights and heights up to 4 months of age reflects her individual norm.

Recumbent Length

Recumbent length refers to measurements taken of the infant in a horizontal position and should be distinguished from height or stature, which is used in children and measured standing. Due to orthostatic compression of the vertebral column, height is less than recumbent length by approximately 1 cm. Special care must be taken to obtain reproducible measurements. Proper equipment consists of a table with a fixed vertical headboard and a footboard that moves perpendicular to the table surface, so that it can be pressed firmly against the soles of the feet. A measuring tape is attached to the table, the zero end aligned with the headboard. Two people are needed to obtain accurate measurements. One person must hold the patient's body in the midline and keep the neck slightly hyperextended, so that the infant's gaze is vertically upward. The other person extends the knees and positions the footboard for measurement.

Stature

The term *stature* is equivalent to *height*. It can be measured against any office wall that does not have a baseboard. A wooden strip, preferably with a groove to guide a right angle headboard, is attached to the wall together with a measuring tape. The patient should be barefoot and standing straight, with knees together and the buttocks, shoulders, and occiput against the wall. Head posture is correct if the patient's gaze is horizontal.

Standards for height, weight, and height and weight velocity have been developed for U.S. children 6 to 17 years old by the National Center for Health Statistics (5,6). The Stuart growth charts (7) are popular as standards for graphing infants. The method of plotting measurements serially relative to the percentiles of the normal reference population allows recognition of the individual's own particular growth characteristics. Normally, a trend becomes established soon after birth. When the indices of a child move from one channel to another, a change in growth velocity, which may be nutritional in origin, has occurred.

Interpretation of single height and weight measurements is difficult. Generally, a random anthropometric measurement is considered abnormal when the value is at or beyond ±2 SD of the population mean, or below the third or above the 97th percentile. The physician who monitors progress through serial measurements will already recognize growth failure when height or weight drops by no more than 1 SD. In the example of Fig. 3-6, the individual norm was apparently the tenth percentile until 4 months of age. By 6 months, growth failure was obvious, although weight had dropped less than 1 SD. Interpretation of changes in growth velocity is more difficult during puberty. Early-maturing children, who begin their pubertal growth spurt early, appear to have abnormally accelerated growth. The converse is true for late-maturing children.

Deficits are often expressed as a percentage of the age- and sex-specific median or mean. This is useful only in an individual case and when used in the comparison of data for children of similar ages, because a particular percentage has a different significance at different ages since the variance changes with age. It is also inappropriate to compare the difference between height age and chronological age, because a given deficit is not the same at all ages, especially if expressed as a percentage. Height-age is a practical means of describing individual deficients.

Sitting Height or Crown–Rump Length

Sitting height and crown–rump length are useful measures in patients with an abnormal upper/lower ratio and may be used when leg deformities preclude accurate measurements of linear growth. As a percentage of total height, the values for the newborn, the 3-year-old, and the adolescent are 70%, 57%, and 52% respectively. Crown–rump length is measured on a table the same as recumbent length except that the legs are lifted straight up by flexing the hips of the infant and moving the board firmly against the buttocks. Sitting height is obtained after age 2 by use of a box measuring $2\frac{1}{2}$ by $3\frac{1}{2}$ by 4 ft. The box is turned so as to make its height approximately equal to the length of the child's lower leg. The box is moved against the measuring wall, and the child sits comfortably on the box, with thighs placed horizontally and the back against the measuring strip.

Upper/Lower Ratio

The midpoint of stature in the newborn is at the level of the umbilicus, whereas in the adult it is at the symphysis pubis. This ratio, which changes from 1.7 to 1.0 during growth, can be used as a measure of proportionate growth. Excluding bowing of the legs due to rickets, abnormal ratios are never due to nutritional causes.

Head Circumference

In infants under 3 years of age, head circumference is a convenient index of brain growth providing hydrocephalus is ruled out (8). An insertion tape is available for circumferential measurements like those of the head and midarm. One end of the tape is expanded, and the other is fed through an opening in the expanded end, where a line indicates the completion of the circumference. The tape should be passed anteriorly above the eyebrow and placed over the occipital protuberances so that it measures the maximum circumference. Care must be taken that the plane of the tape is the same on both sides of the head.

Skinfold Thickness

This measurement is a popular tool in assessing fatness and grading undernutrition. Values correlate with total body fat, as measured in underwater weighing. A variety of calipers are available. Measurements are not exactly the same with each. The Lange caliper is recommended in the United States because appropriate reference data are available (9,10,11). Preferred sites are the triceps and the subscapular area. Triceps skinfold thickness is measured at the midpoint of a line drawn posteriorly between the acromion and olecranon. The arm should be hanging relaxed at the side of the trunk, with the elbow extended. Subscapular skinfold thickness is measured just inferior to the angle of the scapula. The calipers are compressed over a double fold of the skin and subcutaneous fat, which is picked up with the thumb and index finger of the examiner. Pressure should not be excessive, and the reading should not be delayed. Three readings should be taken and averaged. (Table 3-4.)

Upper Arm Circumference

The upper arm circumference is a measure of both the fat and muscle mass of the arm. It should be obtained at the level of the triceps skin-fold, and the arm should be in the same position as for that measurement. Care

Table 3-4. Percentiles for Upper Arm Circumference and Triceps Skinfolds

			Arm Circumference Percentiles, mm					*Triceps Skinfold Percentiles, mm*				
Age Group	*Age Mid-point, (years)*	*No.*	*5th*	*15th*	*50th*	*85th*	*95th*	*5th*	*15th*	*50th*	*85th*	*95th*
					Males							
0.0–0.4	0.3	41	113	120	134	147	153	4	5	8	12	15
0.5–1.4	1	140	128	137	152	168	175	5	7	9	13	15
1.5–2.4	2	177	141	147	157	170	180	5	7	10	13	14
2.5–3.4	3	210	144	150	161	175	182	6	7	9	12	14
3.5–4.4	4	208	143	150	165	180	190	5	6	9	12	14
4.5–5.4	5	262	146	155	169	185	199	5	6	8	12	16
5.5–6.4	6	264	151	159	172	188	198	5	6	8	11	15
6.5–7.4	7	309	154	162	176	194	212	4	6	8	11	14
7.5–8.4	8	301	161	168	185	205	233	5	6	8	12	17
8.5–9.4	9	287	165	174	190	217	262	5	6	9	14	19
9.5–10.4	10	315	170	180	200	228	255	5	6	10	16	22
10.5–11.4	11	294	177	186	208	240	276	6	7	10	17	25
11.5–12.4	12	294	184	194	216	253	291	5	7	11	19	26
12.5–13.4	13	266	186	198	230	270	297	5	6	10	18	25
13.5–14.4	14	207	198	211	243	279	321	5	6	10	17	22
14.5–15.4	15	179	202	220	253	302	320	4	6	9	19	26
15.5–16.4	16	166	217	232	262	300	335	4	5	9	20	27
16.5–17.4	17	142	230	238	275	306	326	4	5	8	14	20
17.5–24.4	21	545	250	264	292	330	354	4	5	10	18	25
24.5–34.4	30	679	260	280	310	344	366	4	6	11	21	28
34.5–44.4	40	616	259	280	312	345	371	4	6	12	22	28

Table 3-4. (Continued)

Age Group	*Age Mid-point, (years)*	*No.*	*Arm Circumference Percentiles, mm*					*Triceps Skinfold Percentiles, mm*				
			5th	*15th*	*50th*	*85th*	*95th*	*5th*	*15th*	*50th*	*85th*	*95th*
					Females							
0.0–0.4	0.3	46	107	118	127	145	150	4	5	8	12	13
0.5–1.4	1	172	125	134	146	162	170	6	7	9	12	15
1.5–2.4	2	172	136	143	155	171	180	6	7	10	13	15
2.5–3.4	3	163	137	145	157	169	176	6	7	10	12	14
3.5–4.4	4	215	145	150	162	176	184	5	7	10	12	14
4.5–5.4	5	233	149	155	169	185	195	6	7	10	13	16
5.5–6.4	6	259	148	158	170	187	202	6	7	10	12	15
6.5–7.4	7	273	153	162	178	199	216	6	7	10	13	17
7.5–8.4	8	270	158	166	183	207	231	6	7	10	15	19
8.5–9.4	9	284	166	175	192	222	255	6	7	11	17	24
9.5–10.4	10	276	170	181	203	236	263	6	8	12	19	24
10.5–11.4	11	268	173	186	210	251	280	7	8	12	20	29
11.5–12.4	12	267	185	196	220	256	275	6	9	13	20	25
12.5–13.4	13	229	186	204	230	270	294	7	9	14	23	30
13.5–14.4	14	184	201	214	240	284	306	8	10	15	22	28
14.5–15.4	15	197	205	216	245	281	310	8	11	16	24	30
15.5–16.4	16	187	211	224	249	286	322	8	10	15	23	27
16.5–17.4	17	142	207	224	250	291	328	9	12	16	26	31
17.5–24.4	21	836	215	233	260	297	329	9	12	17	25	31
24.5–34.4	30	1153	230	243	275	324	361	9	12	19	29	36
34.5–44.4	40	933	232	250	286	340	374	10	14	22	32	39

SOURCE: Adapted from Frisancho AR: *Am J Clin Nutr* 27:1052, 1974.

must be taken to fit the tape snugly around the arm (Table 3-4). The diameter, circumference, and area of the muscle may be calculated from upper arm circumference and triceps skinfold (12,13). The calculation is based on the assumption that the area for muscle and bone is circular (see nomogram for rapid calculation—Fig. 3-7). Muscle area is superior to skinfold thickness as a measure of nutritional status in populations with normal degrees of fatness.

Sexual Maturity

Since growth is closely related to sexual maturation, this becomes an important parameter to monitor after the onset of puberty. Stages of maturation are determined from the development of the breast in girls and the external genitalia in boys. Deviations from the norm are usually due to endocrine or genetic influences. Undernutrition delays the onset and decreases the extent of the pubertal growth spurt. (Figs. 1-1 and 1-2).

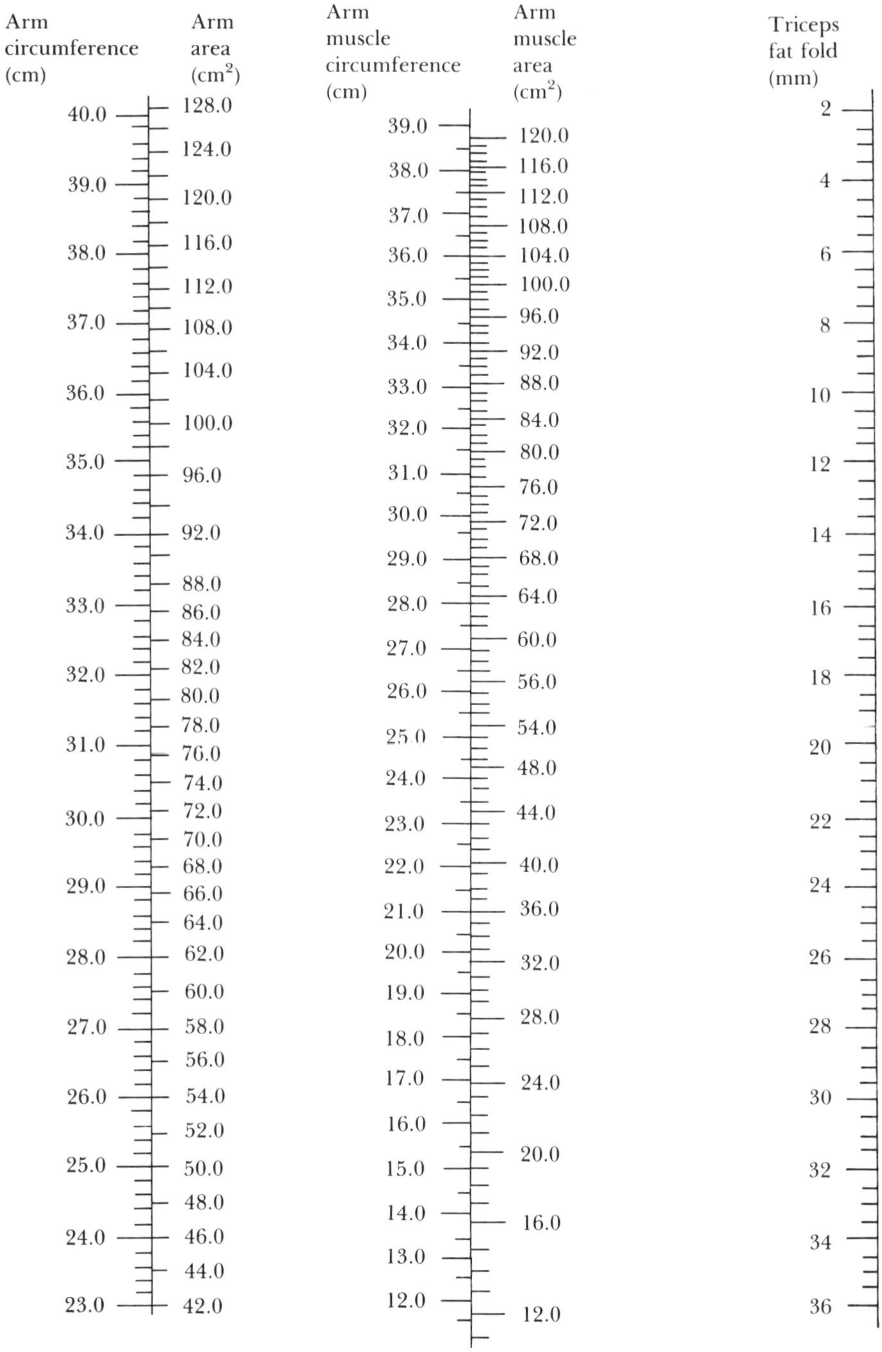

Figure 3-7. ARM ANTHROPOMETRY: NOMOGRAM FOR RAPID CALCULATION OF MUSCLE CIRCUMFERENCE AND CROSS-SECTIONAL AREA
To obtain muscle circumference, place ruler between the values for arm circumference and fat fold, and read muscle circumference and corresponding muscle

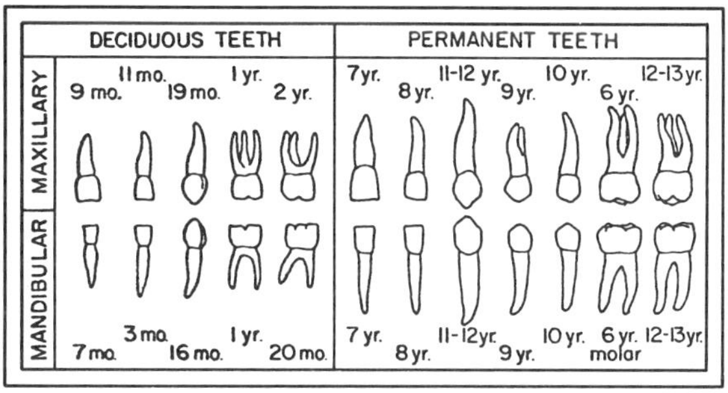

Figure 3-8. AVERAGE ERUPTION OF TEETH

Skeletal Maturity

The determination of skeletal maturity is extremely useful in the nutritional evaluation of growing individuals. In patients with linear growth failure due to malnutrition, bone age is invariably retarded. A number of methods of determination are available (14,15). Since each requires considerable training, the method to be recommended is that with which the examiner is most experienced. Accurate scoring is difficult. Interpretation must take into account the fact that the standard error and degree of variance in the reference population are large.

The appearance of epiphyseal ossification centers is used to determine bone age during infancy. Epiphyseal closure is part of the assessment during puberty. Comparison with chronological age reveals how much time is left for growth, since adult stature is reached once all the epiphyses of long bones are closed. Thus, plotting stature against bone age is a convenient method of observing growth in relation to growth potential.

It is possible to predict adult stature in normal individuals, using a calculation based on chronological age, height, weight, bone age, and parents' height (16). However, this assessment is often inaccurate in patients with growth failure due to undernutrition and chronic disease. Whenever linear growth deviates from normal, misjudgments of adult height are common, because it is difficult to predict the onset and amount of linear growth during puberty and the effect of therapeutic intervention strategies.

Dental age consists of grading the degree of development of either four or seven permanent teeth. The test is conceptually similar to the determination of skeletal maturity but less reliable (see also Fig. 3-8). In the Ten-State Nutrition Survey eruption of deciduous and permanent teeth

←

cross-sectional area at the intercept of the middle line. (From Gurney JM, Jelliffe, DB: Arm anthropometry in nutritional assessment: Nomogram for rapid calculation of muscle circumference and cross-sectional muscle and fat areas. *Am J Clin Nutr* 26:912, 1973.

was not significantly related to nutritional status. There is no association between time of tooth eruption and skeletal maturation.

ASSESSMENT OF NUTRIENT INTAKE

Long-Term History of Nutrient Intake

An accurate account and reconstruction of events that influence nutrition are extremely important, but should be interpreted within the context of the entire nutritional assessment. Since one has to rely on the memory and honesty of the reporter, it is not uncommon for histories taken on the same day by two competent interviewers to be totally different, although each judged the historian as "reliable." A history taken under stressful circumstances or when the historian is tired is bound to be unreliable. The physician may misinterpret what was actually said or meant, especially when the use of terminology is different between lay and professional people. Judgment of the historian's reliability is too often based on characteristics that reflect social class and level of education. An example is depriving parents who give misleading information. Finally, it may be unrealistic to expect a parent of several children to remember what was fed to one of them months or even years earlier.

Nevertheless, the history often provides important clues that, taken together with other observations, eventually lead to the diagnosis. An example is the child whose growth curve fell off at 4 months, which was also the time when gluten-containing cereals were added to the diet. Or the child who lost weight after 8 months of age, when the mother offered, prematurely, both table food and milk from the cup—causing decreased milk intake, spillage, and wasting of food. An attempt should always be made to piece together as many bits of information as possible, and compare the nutritional with the growth history, especially in cases where the insult is of long duration, evidenced by the fact that both height and weight are deficient.

Estimate of Current Nutrient Intake

An assessment of current intake can be made in several ways—including a 24-hour recall (Table 3-5), a 7-day diary, and observation in the hospital. The 24-hour recall is more accurate than the long-term history only to the extent that it relies on recent memory. Other pitfalls are the same, including those caused by parents who like to "look good," a characteristic that is not necessarily particular to depriving parents. For instance, an insecure or rigid parent may not be able to accept the "failure" of being unable to handle a child with organic feeding difficulties. In obtaining the 24-hour recall, a common source of error is to ask about the intake of the preceding day, not realizing that it may not reflect the average intake over time if the child had an intercurrent, brief illness that brought the parents

Table 3-5. Food Intake Questionnaire

Foods Consumed (Use reverse side if necessary)

How many meals are taken per day? __________ time of day ______________
How many snacks per day? __________________ time of day ______________
Are these schedules adhered to regularly? __________
How much milk is taken regularly per day? __________
Type of milk or formula ____
Have different milks/formulas been tried in the past? ___________________

Type	From – to (age)	Effect of change

Is the patient's food specially prepared? __________
Describe how ____
Choice ____
Enrichment ____
Consistency ____
What foods are consumed in insufficient amounts?
______________________ How much per day or week? ______________
______________________ ______________
Are foods consumed in excess and to the exclusion of others?
______________________ How much per day? ______________
______________________ ______________

Describe a typical 24-hour food intake: Use precise measures for each food item (level table(tea)spoon, 8-oz measuring cup, $\frac{1}{4}$, $\frac{1}{2}$, full baby-food jar, 8-oz glass, juice glass, portions of meat cuts, etc.)

Breakfast

Lunch

Dinner

Snacks

to the doctor in the first place. Not infrequently, much energy is wasted on food diaries, which are meaningless unless precise measures are used. The emotional climate in the home is not a healthy one if a parent must keep a record of food intake over a long period of time. Two or three 7-day periods, separated by free intervals, are sufficient for this estimate.

Finally, it may be necessary to admit the child to the hospital for observation of eating habits and measurement of intake. (See Chapter 5.) Accurate calorie counting requires recording of the amount of food offered and refused, preferably by measuring weight rather than using common household volume measures. This effort is meaningful only if the child's physical and emotional state of health during hospitalization is comparable to that at home and if the parent confirms that the appetite is similar. It is also desirable that the type of food and preparation be unchanged. Few hospitals are equipped to provide reliable intake data on any patients except for small infants who consume milk and simple baby foods.

BIOCHEMICAL AND OTHER MEASUREMENTS

There is no simple battery of screening tests that allows an estimate of nutrient stores. A number of biochemical tests are generally advised for the assessment of nutritional status (Table 3-6). They include tests of vitamin nutriture and mineral status. Unfortunately, these tests are not readily available, and their reproducibility is often poor—either because of technical difficulties or variable biological circumstances of the individual at the time the sample was taken (e.g., the effects of the preceding meal, use of drugs, circadian rhythm).

Most of these tests therefore are only indicated when the individual shows symptoms of deficiency or is at risk because of diet history or predisposing biological conditions. To circumvent the vagaries of these tests and clinical difficulties in recognizing borderline deficiency states, physicians often treat prophylactically. However, this is justified only in populations at risk of having vitamin deficiency. Prophylaxis is dangerous as a substitute for making a diagnosis in suspected mineral deficiency states (see also Chapters 8, 10, and 11).

Biochemical tests are not very helpful in the diagnosis of total body protein deficiency, as seen in chronic undernutrition that is associated with muscle wasting. In the United States, serum albumin is generally not diagnostically decreased in undernourished infants and children. Rather, a low serum albumin suggests disorders like nephrotic syndrome or protein-losing enteropathy. A number of carrier proteins have been used as an index of protein nutriture. Among these, serum transferrin is considered a good index (17) but has not been adequately tested as such in infants and children. Immunoglobulin levels and tests of cellular immunity also have been recommended for the assessment of protein nutriture. However, normal ranges for infants are uncertain, and a significant abnormality is more likely due to intestinal protein loss than insufficient protein intake.

Nitrogen balance measurements are used to monitor the therapeutic response of patients with protein-calorie malnutrition. A simplified method has been recommended for adults that uses only calculations of nitrogen intake—based on the protein content of foods—and measurements of urinary urea nitrogen, which is the major portion of the total nitrogen lost in urine (17), but omits measurement of fecal nitrogen. The feasibility of this approach has not been tested in the pediatric age group. Knowing whether nitrogen retention occurs is helpful in cases where lack of weight

Table 3-6. Laboratory Assessment of Nutritional Status

Determination	*Normal*	*Deficient*
Protein		
Serum protein (g/dl)[a]		
0–11 months	>5.0	<5.0
1–5 years	>5.5	<5.5
6–17 years	>6.0	<6.0
Serum albumin (g/dl)[a]		
0–11 months	>2.5	<2.5
1–5 years	>3.0	<3.0
6–17 years	>3.5	<3.5
Serum transferrin (μg/dl)		
(Total iron-binding capacity)	>250	<225
Iron		
Hemoglobin (g/dl)[a]		
6–23 months	>10.0	<9.0
2–5 years	>11.0	<10.0
6–12 years	>11.5	<10.0
13–16 years, male	>13.0	<12.0
13–16 years, female	>11.5	<10.0
Hematocrit (%)[a]		
6–23 months	>31	<28
2–5 years	>34	<30
6–12 years	>36	<30
13–16 years, male	>40	<37
13–16 years, female	>36	<31
Serum iron (μg/dl)[a]		
6–23 months	>30	<30
2–5 years	>40	<40
6–12 years	>50	<50
12 years, male	>60	<60
12 years, female	>40	<40
Transferrin saturation (%)[a]		
6–23 months	>15	<7
2–12 years	>20	<7
12 years, male	>20	<7
12 years, female	>15	<7
Serum ferritin (ng/ml)	>10	<10
Water-soluble vitamins		
Thiamine		
Urinary thiamine (μg/g creatinine)[a]		
1–3 years	>176	<120
4–6 years	>121	<85
7–9 years	>181	<70
10–12 years	>181	<60
13–15 years	>151	<50
RBC transketolase (19)[b]		
All Ages	<15	>25

Table 3-6. (Continued)

Determination	*Normal*	*Deficient*
Riboflavin		
Urinary riboflavin (µg/g creatinine)[a]		
1–3 years	>500	<150
4–6 years	>300	<100
7–9 years	>270	<85
10–15 years	>200	<70
Niacin		
Urinary N-methylnicotinamide (mg/g creatinine)		
Adults	>1.6	<0.5
Pyridoxine		
Urinary pyridoxine (µg/g creatinine) (19)[b]		
1–3 years	>90	<90
4–6 years	>75	<75
7–9 years	>50	<50
10–12 years	>40	<40
13–15 years	>30	<30
16 years	>20	<20
Erythrocyte glutamic pyruvic transaminase (19)[b]		
Adult (ratio)	<1.25	>1.25
Vitamin B_{12}		
Serum vitamin B_{12} (pg/ml) (19)[b]		
All ages	>150	<100
Vitamin C		
Serum Vitamin C (mg/dl) (19)[b]	>0.3	<0.2
Fat-soluble vitamins		
Vitamin A		
Plasma vitamin A (µg/dl)[a]		
All ages	>30	<20
Plasma carotene (µg/dl)[a]		
0–5 months	>10	<10
6–11 months	>30	<20
1–17 years	>40	<30
Vitamin E		
Serum vitamin E (mg/dl) (19)[b]		
All ages	>0.7	<0.5
Red cell hemolysis in H_2O_2 (19)[b]	10	20
All ages		

[a] From *Ten State Nutrition Survey*.

[b] See Reference 19. Note that normal values may vary with other methodologies.

gain after realimentation may be due to shifts in body composition or edema masks increases in tissue mass.

Knowledge of body composition, mainly fat and fat-free body mass, is desirable in the assessment of abnormal nutritional states, but it is by and large technically difficult, expensive, and usually not readily available. Measurements include whole body counting for potassium-40 (^{40}K) as an index of fat-free body mass, urinary excretion of endogenous creatinine as a measure of muscle mass, basal oxygen consumption as a measure of metabolically active tissue mass, and total body water or extracellular fluid space. Urinary excretion of hydroxyproline reflects collagen turnover and has been shown to correlate positively with linear growth.

Aside from technical difficulties, each of these measurements has its limitations for use in individuals with an abnormal body composition. For instance, bromide space and other measures of body water compartments cannot be used for the calculation of fat-free body mass in conditions where the relation between the two may be abnormal. Basal oxygen consumption is influenced by changes in the relation between tissues with high and low metabolic activity as well as thyroid function. Following exclusion of thyroid abnormality by appropriate tests, values for basal oxygen consumption (i.e., metabolic rate) may be used as a measure of changes in body composition. Providing the measurements are taken 12

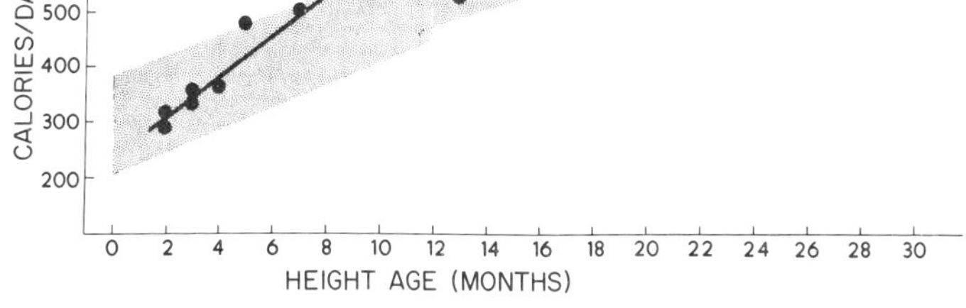

Figure 3-9. METABOLIC RATE (KCAL/DAY) OF INFANTS AND CHILDREN, AGE 3 MONTHS TO 10 YEARS, WITH GROWTH FAILURE DUE TO MALNUTRITION

Plotted on height age. Maternal deprivation, less than 3 years (circles); psychosocial deprivation, over 3 years (squares). (From Krieger I: Endocrines and nutrition in psychosocial deprivation in the U.S.A.: Comparison with growth failure due to malnutrition on an organic basis, in Gardner LI, Amacher P: *Endocrine Aspects of Malnutrition*. Santa Ynes, Calif, The Kroc Foundation, 1973.)

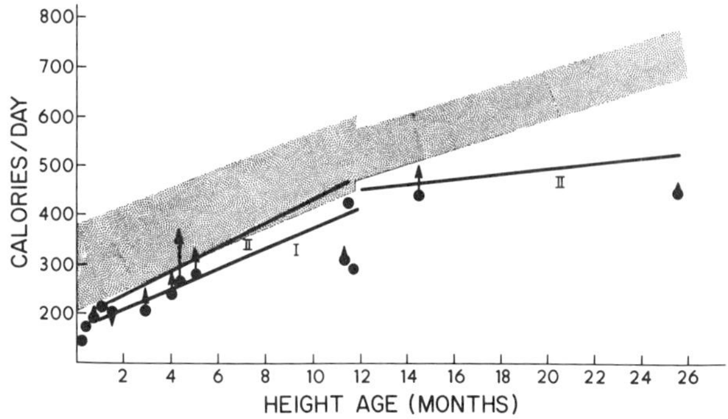

Figure 3-10. METABOLIC RATE (KCAL/DAY) OF INFANTS AND CHILDREN, AGE 4 MONTHS TO 4 YEARS, WITH GROWTH FAILURE OF PRENATAL ONSET

Plotted on height age, before (circles) and after (arrow) weight gain (n = 14). (From Krieger I, Taqi MS: Free serum thyroxine level and basal metabolic rate. *Am J Dis Child* 129:830, 1975.) Regression line I is for a separate group of patients with dwarfing syndromes, and regression line II is for infants with growth failure of prenatal onset (small-for-gestational-age Dwarfism). (From Krieger I, Woolley PV Jr: The basal metabolic rate in growth failure of prenatal onset. *Am J Dis Child* 127:340, 1974.)

hours after a meal to eliminate effects of postprandial heat production due to growth, the basal metabolic rate (BMR) reflects body cell number rather than cell mass (18), a fact that can be used to distinguish growth failure of prenatal onset from growth failure due to postnatal malnutrition (Chapter 5 and 6). A high BMR per unit of body weight is associated with loss of adipose tissue and muscle wasting. This abnormality is not evident when height age or weight for height are used as the reference standard. Patients less than 3 years with linear growth failure due to chronic postnatal malnutrition have normal values of the BMR per unit of height, height age, or weight for height. (Fig. 3-9). By contrast, patients with growth failure of prenatal onset have low values (Fig. 3-10).

REFERENCES

1. Frankenburg WK, Dodds JB, Fandal A: *Denver Developmental Screening Test*, Denver, University of Colorado Medical Center, 1970.
2. Dubowitz LMS, Dubowitz V, Goldberg C: Clinical assessment of gestational age in the newborn infant. *J Pediatr* 77:1, 1970.
3. Lubchenco LO, Hansman C, Dressler M, et al. Intrauterine growth as estimated from live born birth weight data at 24 to 42 weeks of gestation. *Pediatrics* 32:793, 1963.
4. Lubchenco LO, Hansman C, Boyd E: Intrauterine growth in length and head circum-

ference as estimated from live births at gestational ages from 26–42 weeks. *Pediatrics* 37:403, 1966.

5. Hamill PVV, Johnston FE, Lemeshow S: *Body weight, stature, and sitting height. White and negro youths 12–17 years*, DHEW Publication (HRA) 74-1608, Series 11, No 126. U.S. Dept of Health, Education and Welfare, National Center for Health Statistics, 1973, p 16.
6. Malina RM, Hamill PVV, Lemeshow S: *Selected body measurements of children 6–11 years*, DHEW Publication (HSM) 73-1605, Series 11, No 123. US Dept of Health, Education and Welfare, National Center for Health Statistics, 1973, p 19.
7. Stuart HC: Standards of physical development for reference in clinical appraisement. *J. Pediatr* 5:194, 1934.
8. Nellhaus G: Composite international and interracial graphs. *Pediatrics* 41:106, 1968.
9. Committee on Nutrition: Measurement of skinfold thickness in childhood. *Pediatrics* 42:538, 1968.
10. Johnston FE, Hamill PVV, Lemeshow S: *Skinfold thickness of children 6–11 years*, DHEW Publication (HSM) 73-1602, Series 11, No 120. US Dept of Health, Education and Welfare, National Center for Health Statistics, 1972, p 20.
11. Johnston FE, Hamill PVV, Lemeshow S: *Skinfold thickness of youths 12–17 years*, DHEW Publication (HRA) 74-1614, Series 11, No 132. US Dept of Health, Education, and Welfare, National Center for Health Statistics, 1974, p 20.
12. Frisancho AR: Triceps skinfold and upper arm muscle size norms for assessment of nutritional status. *Am J Clin Nutr* 27 (10):1052, 1974.
13. Gurney JM, Jelliffe DB: Arm anthropometry in nutritional assessment: Nomogram for rapid calculation of muscle circumference and cross-sectional muscle and fat areas. *Am J Clin Nutr* 26:912, 1973.
14. Greulich WW, Pyle SI: *Radiographic Atlas of Skeletal Development of the Hand and Wrist*, 2. Stanford, Calif, Stanford University Press, 1959, p 61.
15. Roche AF, Wainer H, Thissen D: *Skeletal Maturity. The Knee Joint as a Biological Indicator.* New York, Plenum Medical Book Co, 1975, p 91.
16. Roche AF, Wainer H, Thissen D: *Predicting Adult Stature for Individuals, Monographs in Paediatrics.* Basel, Karger, 1975, p 69.
17. Blackburn GL, Bistrian BR, Maini BS, et al: Nutritional and metabolic assessment of the hospitalized patient. *J Parent Enteral Nutr* 1:11, 1977.
18. Krieger I: Relation of specific dynamic action of food (SDA) to growth in rats. *Am J Clin Nutr* 31:764, 1978.
19. Sauberlich HE, Dowdy RP, Skala JH: *Laboratory Tests for Assessment of Nutritional Status*, Cleveland, Ohio, CRC Press, 1973.

4
Infant Feeding Disorders

WORKUP

In the United States feeding disorders are a more common cause of undernutrition during the first year of life than deprivation or poverty. Common causes are the inability to eat due to anatomic or neuromuscular disorders, vomiting on either a psychogenic or organic basis, and food refusal or disinterest in food for psychological reasons. If an organic cause is not recognized, feeding problems are easily misinterpreted as psychogenic. On the other hand, certain psychogenic problems, such as gagging or refusal of solid food resemble manifestations of organic diseases. Recognition of the causal relationships becomes very complicated when organic feeding difficulties are improperly managed and result in secondary psychogenic complications. Proper management requires knowledge of the primary cause.

History

A thorough investigation of past events is necessary, as it determines the extent of necessary physical and laboratory investigations. Thus, a good history may show conclusively that an extensive search for anatomical lesions is not required or, in cases where the problem started at birth, that psychogenic causes need not be considered.

The history should attempt to answer the following questions*:

Did the problem start right after birth, and were the manifestations already evident to nursery personnel?

Are there now or were there at any time signs suggestive of psychological problems (rocking, head banging, nightmares, tempers, nail biting, or the like)?

In postnatally acquired disorders, were associated events evident (febrile illness; an accident or significant environmental change like moving, divorce, death in the family)?

Did the acquisition of feeding skills follow a normal sequence and time schedule?

What corrective measures were taken and with what degree of success (formula changes, punishment)?

Describe mealtimes (eating alone? multiple dislikes expressed at the table? coaxing?).

Describe the parents' attitudes toward the child and the feeding problem (frustration? rigidity? concern? nervousness?).

In case of vomiting, describe the relation to meals and the type of food ingested, whether solid or liquid. Describe the type of vomiting, whether effortless flowing out or projectile. Describe the color, bilious or not, and

* Questionnaires may be filled out by the parent in advance—Tables 4-1 and 4-2.

Table 4-1. Questionnaire

Eating Skills

Is your child able to:
suck? _________ swallow? _________ eat pureed foods well? _________
Is it necessary to push the food back in repeatedly? _________
Is this upsetting to the child? _________
use tongue to lick? _________ or to take food into the mouth? _________
chew _________ Or does child munch on foods, leaving most uneaten? _______
handle liquids as well as solids? _________
solids better? _________ liquids better? _________
eat finger foods? _________ drink well from a cup? _________
make attempts but spills a lot? _________
sit alone? _________ sit propped up? _________
spit out pureed food? _________ playfully? _________ or in temper? _______
Describe the motor problem (if any) ______________________________
____

At what age were the following foods introduced?
Cereal or pureed foods _________ finger foods _________ fluid from a cup _________

List times of day when milk and/or other foods are fed ____________________
____

List age when able to go 8 hours without food or drink ____________________

estimate the quantity. Would the infant eat after vomiting, or does the infant appear sick afterward?

Rule out rumination. Does the infant seem to strain before regurgitation, either by making motions of the abdominal muscles or noises in the throat? Does the infant rechew or reswallow the regurgitated food?

In case of polyphagia, are there bizarre cravings? Eating binges interrupted by periods of normal or decreased intake? Does the child overeat single food items, like a loaf of bread or a jar of jam at a time; or does the child overeat regularly? All types of food or favorite foods only? (See Chapters 5 and 11.)

In case of polydipsia, is it constant or intermittent? Is the patient able to tolerate a 12-hour period without liquids? Is there associated polyuria? Measure both fluid intake and output at home.

In case of crying and regurgitation ("colic"), is this a "bottle baby"—that is, one who has the milk bottle all day as a pacifier? What type of pacifier is used? At what time of day does crying occur mostly? Does the infant feed itself? Does the infant burp well? Is crying relieved by picking the infant up? Or by passage of flatus or stool? Is the infant getting enough sleep? Is the meal schedule adhered to regularly? What is the largest interval between meals? Does it take more or less than 20 to 30 minutes to feed an 8-oz bottle of milk?

The Physical Exam

A routine physical is sufficient, but special emphasis should be placed on the neurological exam, and feeding should be observed. A thorough neurological exam and developmental assessment are done to rule out mental retardation and neurological deficit, which are commonly associated with feeding problems.

The examiner should observe the parent feeding the infant and, if this observation indicates it, should feed the infant to analyze the tone of lip closure, the strength of suck over the inserted finger, and the ability to swallow and chew (see Chapter 1). The presence of drooling may be significant. A hypersensitive gag reflex should be looked for during the routine oral exam. The examiner may wish to check the infant's ability to handle a small piece of solid food placed on the tip of the tongue. The lateral mobility of the tongue can be examined by asking the child to move the outstretched tongue to each corner of the mouth or to follow the examiner's finger.

Table 4-2. Questionnaire

Eating Behavior

Is or does your child:
act hungry at feeding time? ________ how? cry loud? ________ act fussy? __
demand food during the night? ________ what time? ________
use pacifier now? ________ in the past? ________ how many hours per day?
________ at bedtime only ? ________
overeat? ________ favorite foods only? ________ which? ____________
____
eat an excess of all types of foods? ________
eat poorly? ________ picky? ________ demand other foods but not eat them?
________ gag on food? ________
act tired at mealtime? ________ get distracted during meals? ________
eat at the family table? ________
act disruptive at mealtime? ________ play with food? ________ dawdle? ___
When did it start? ________
Was the child demanding for food as a small infant? ________
How do you handle the problem? ____________________
ignore it? ________ keep child at table longer? ________ how long? ____
send child away from table? ________ where to? ____________
withhold dessert or favorite foods? ________ hide food from child? ______
offer different foods? ________ plead? ________ bribe? ________
Are you consistent in your handling of this problem? ________
Do both parents agree on handling of problem? ________
Do other family members get involved? ________ who? ____________
Describe effect on siblings, if any? ____________________

Laboratory and Other Tests

The tests needed for the investigation of dysphagia, food refusal, and vomiting unaccompanied by nausea vary, depending on the nature of the problem. A history and physical exam should show whether any of the following tests are indicated:

Chest x-ray
Soft tissue study of the neck
Fluoroscopic study of the esophagus with contrast medium
Upper GI series
Cinematographic studies of breathing and swallowing
Angiography, if vascular anomalies are suspected
Esophagoscopy, if these studies are inconclusive

If allergy is suspected, no skin tests are needed. Instead, diagnosis should be made through the use of elimination diets, starting with a casein hydrolysate formula and eliminating all other foods and juices for about 2 weeks. If the child improves, rechallenge with the suspected allergen is necessary. To confirm the diagnosis of milk protein intolerance a lactose tolerance test should be performed, because casein hydrolysate formulas are currently free of both lactose and milk protein (see Chapter 9).

MANIFESTATIONS AND CAUSES

Psychogenic Disorders

Mismanagement of general infant care and of feeding and nutrition can lead to a variety of feeding problems and, ultimately, to undernutrition. These difficulties are common in an emotionally unstable environment. They also occur as a result of inadequate instruction of an inexperienced parent or one who raised other children with apparent success, only because they were more resistant to mismanagement. The parent who allows serious undernutrition to occur before seeking help is depriving the infant. Very often, however, parents of infants with psychogenic feeding problems have consulted many physicians and do seem to be concerned. This type of parent should be distinguished from the one who does not care and is unable to relate and love the infant. Children of such parents fail to develop physically as well as intellectually and emotionally (see Chapter 5). In this so-called maternal deprivation syndrome, feeding problems are not common. By contrast, the tense anxious parent, who cares but is insecure and therefore overconcerned, tends to create an environment where feeding problems develop. However, since she or he handles and stimulates the infant, development is usually not retarded. Mismanagement should also be suspected if feeding problems develop in the infant of a psychotic parent or one who is preoccupied with psychoneurotic conflict. These parents tend to handle their infants nervously and inconsistently, and if they are not able to relate and care, feeding problems may be allowed to get out of hand. Thus growth failure is often severe and associated with developmental retardation, because the infants of these parents are left alone a good part of the day and lack stimulation.

The causal relationships between a particular type of mismanagement and the resulting symptom are often not clear. It is therefore important for the physician not to fix the blame but rather to handle the problem globally and to assure that all aspects of feeding are handled properly and according to current concepts of care. This includes (*1*) adherence to a flexible demand feeding schedule, which develops in the infant the security of knowing that a cry for food is answered; (*2*) adherence to a physiological sequence in the development of feeding skills; and (*3*) use of proper feeding techniques.

Colic

In infants, failure to adhere to these management principles can lead to a variety of problems, commonly referred to as "colic." Infants with colic look unhappy, are fussy, and may cry for prolonged periods. They are not relieved by being fed, cuddled, having their diapers changed, or being made comfortable in other ways, such as being rocked or walked. Paroxysms of crying may last for hours. The term *colic* derives from the impression that there is indeed pain due to spasms of the colon, since relief sometimes follows the passage of feces or flatus. The abdomen may be tense, and the legs are intermittently drawn up. Often these attacks do not end until the infant is completely exhausted. The fact that they commonly occur toward the end of the day suggests that events in the household play a role. Allergy is the cause in occasional cases. Excess intestinal air may be the result of carbohydrate fermentation, possibly lactose intolerance. However, changing the diet rarely helps. Recovery occurs spontaneously, at about 3 to 4 months of age. Attacks may be so severe as to require sedation in order to relieve both the parent and the infant.

It may be difficult to judge whether an attack is due to abdominal pain. Hospital admission to rule out an acute surgical condition of the abdomen is sometimes necessary. On the other hand, the infant who is generally fussy and keeps the parents up night after night without crying violently is also often called "colicky." In these cases, unhappiness may be the result of irregular feedings or too early weaning, since each deprives the infant of the oral satisfaction and security that are attached to sucking regularly from the breast or bottle. Allowing the child to suck all through the day, either from the bottle or a pacifier, also can cause problems. Air swallowing results when the infant continues to suck when the bottle is empty or when an unplugged nipple is used as a pacifier. Whether the regular use of a pacifier is harmful by itself is questionable. Rather, allowing a pacifier may indicate that the parent does not want to be bothered; she or he "plugs up, rather than picks up" the baby. This type of parent also tends to keep the infant too long exclusively on milk and thus misses the best time for introduction of solids. Aside from air swallowing and colic, the excessive reliance on sucking can establish a pattern of overeating and the use of oral satisfaction as a substitute for mature gratifications. Allowing the infant to feed itself from the bottle too early in life on a regular basis is also suggestive of the type of parental behavior that is likely to cause feeding problems. Improper techniques that can lead to colic because of intestinal air distension are (*1*) failure to burp, (*2*) frequent interruption of sucking by withdrawing the nipple, which is a common habit of the tense and nervous parent; and (*3*) use of a nipple with a hole that is either too small or too large. An infant swallows air when frustrated by interruptions or by laborious sucking through a small hole. The infant who has to gulp down an excessive flow of milk also tends to swallow air. The consequences are either eructation of the air, which may be accompanied by forceful regurgitation of stomach content, or passage into the intestines where distension can cause spasms. Finally, an overtired infant will also cry. With the forceful inspiration after a prolonged cry, air may be swallowed. A vicious cycle ensues, where the infant is carried around, bounced, cuddled, and kept awake, only to get more tired. The result is a syndrome consisting of an agitated infant who cries a lot, regurgitates, vomits with a burp, sometimes projectile, and occasionally manages to reswallow the regurgitate in a manner reminiscent of rumination.

Regurgitation

The term *regurgitation* refers to the return of a small amount of food during or soon after eating. It is never associated with nausea and should never be considered a cause of undernutrition. Within limits, regurgitation of small quantities with a burp is normal in small infants. Asymptomatic reflux through the cardia seems common in infants (1–3), and this phenomenon explains the physiologic occurrence of regurgitation. Due to functional immaturity of the cardia, larger amounts may be regurgitated, providing certain other predisposing factors coexist. Anatomical defects must be ruled out in such cases. Improper burping by holding the baby on the lap and face down may be a simple explanation. In the absence of such factors, regurgitation of larger quantities with every feeding is suggestive of chalasia, which refers to relaxation of the lower end of the esophagus and cardia.

Chalasia is considered a neurogenic disorder by most observers, especially since it occurs more often in infants with CNS disorders (see later). However, air swallowing is often a contributing factor. Reflux of contrast medium under fluoroscopy cannot be considered diagnostic of chalasia, since it occurs in asymptomatic infants (2). Weight loss and the amount of regurgitated material distinguish significant chalasia more reliably from transient physiologic regurgitation than an x-ray does. Parents who are repulsed by the continuous sour smell of their infant tend to exaggerate the severity of regurgitation. Therefore, in the absence of weight loss, the physician need not be overly concerned if such a parent complains of "large" regurgitation. Treatment of chalasia and regurgitation is aimed at reducing the amount of swallowed air and at preventing regurgitation by keeping the infant erect for about 1 hour after feeding. Since bouncing should be avoided, use of a special, semireclined infant chair is preferred to holding. If a large quantity is regurgitated in spite of these efforts, parents are encouraged to refeed the infant. If these strategies fail, thickened formula may be tried—that is, formula mixed with cereal and other strained foods. The relative benign nature of this self-limited disorder should be pointed out to the parent in order to avoid added anxiety, which may already be a factor contributing to air swallowing.

Overflow Vomiting

Overflow vomiting is extremely rare and reflects a pathologic emotional environment where the infant overeats, usually after being starved. Although overeating is sometimes blamed for regurgitation and colic, it is an unlikely cause. Vomiting due to overeating should not be diagnosed unless the signs of maternal or psychosocial deprivation coexist (Chapter 5). These children are or have been undernourished in the past and frequently have bizarre cravings and severe behavior problems.

Rumination

The term *rumination* is, unfortunately, used rather loosely for chronic vomiting not accompanied by nausea and sickness. It should be reserved for a very specific type of regurgitation that occurs repeatedly after a meal and is followed by attempts to rechew or retaste and reswallow the regurgitate. When these attempts are regularly unsuccessful, undernutrition results. Cases have been reported where loss of weight and dehydration were so severe and conservative treatment so unsuccessful that death was or would have been unavoidable without parenteral alimentation. Many infants seem to induce the regurgitation by straining the stomach muscles or pharynx. In others, food comes up effortlessly. It is this author's impression that effortless rumination is more common in infants under 6 months of age. The physiologic dysfunction and immaturity of gastric closure (1,2) may be the explanation.

The behavior of ruminators suggests that there are two types (4). Infants in one group are younger, bright-eyed, hyperactive, and responsive to the environment. They come from homes where careful investigation does not uncover signs of deprivation. To the contrary, overstimulation may play a role. These infants are the focus of the entire family; they are passed around, bounced, and played with—often late into the night by a parent who wants to get a share of the infant after a day's work. Infants of the other group are obviously more preoccupied with the habit. They enjoy retasting the regurgitate and behave much like infants who get oral gratification out of thumb sucking or other types of self-stimulating behavior. This type of rumination may be the only sign of psychopathology, or it may coexist with other signs in the maternal deprivation syndrome.

These observations caution against the common attitude of suspecting psychopathology in all ruminators regardless of age. The gastric pH of small infants is less acid than of adults. Hypochlorhydria, which seems common in ruminators (5), may make the regurgitate "almost" palatable. Rumination seems to occur with increased frequency in anatomic lesions, like sliding hiatal hernias, which predispose to gastric reflux. Thus, reswallowing the regurgitate may be a "healthy" mechanism to conserve food. Brockbank (5) noted in 1907 that the cardia and lower esophagus were dilated on postmortem exam of some of his patients. If dilation had been the result of rumination, one would have expected esophageal strictures due to gastric acidity distal to it. Rumination thus may have been the result of chalasia on an organic basis. Hereditary rumination (6) and occurrence in successive generations (5) have been described.

Treatment for the hyperactive, alert ruminator is similar to that for chalasia—that is, maintaining the child in an upright position for 1 hour postprandially in a semireclined infant chair. The deprived ruminator needs, in contrast, stimulation and distraction from the habit through being held. If undernutrition is severe, feeding through an indwelling duodenal tube may be lifesaving. It should be carried out for a minimum of 2 weeks and must be combined with intensive stimulation. Pacifiers should be avoided. Often infants no longer ruminate after the tube is withdrawn. Such excellent results may be attributable to an effect comparable to that of behavior modification, especially in cases where prior treatment attempts with only sensory stimulation were unsuccessful. Although some infants continue to attempt rumination of gastric secretions, most will stop while they are unable to ruminate food during duodenal feeding and thus seem to "forget" the habit.

Food Refusal

Food refusal is often associated with other expressions of negativism like tempers, spitting, and throwing food. Recognition of negativism is more difficult in the child who dawdles, gags, and chews unnecessarily long. Anatomic lesions must be ruled out in such cases. One should also consider that dawdling may be normal for the infant who is exploring self-feeding. If it is, however, a sign of negativism, where the child means to harass and manipulate the caretaker or to attract attention, other manifesations of psychopathology may provide a diagnostic clue. It is commonly seen in psychosocial deprivation, where coprophagy, garbage eating, and self-mutilation may be other signs of rage (Chapter 5).

Bribing and pleading, which takes the all-too-familiar form of coaxing the infant with "one bite for Daddy, one bite for Granny," may also lead to a negativistic reaction. Thus, what may start out as a legitimate refusal to eat may become a negativistic attitude. This occurs frequently toward the end of the second year, when caloric requirements for size decline, and some degree of negativism is a normal phenomenon and an expression of developing independence. Whatever the reason for coaxing—be it inadequate knowledge of the infant's needs or insecurity and eagerness to please—it is bound to cause problems, including manipulative responses in other areas of social interaction. The positive reinforcement of behavior modification techniques is a justified form of "bribing" only in children who have an anatomic or neuromuscular problem that requires extra effort and justifies a reward for success.

Therapy varies depending on the cause of food refusal. For instance, a rigid parent should ease restrictions and allow eating from a variety of foods placed before the infant like a smorgasbord. The opposite strategy is needed for the child who needs attention or supervision and discipline.

Anorexia

Disinterest in food may develop in any age group. Only in teenagers is it a well-defined entity—*anorexia nervosa.* It may also be a classical manifestation of depression. Although rare in children, depression with anorexia occurs in chronically ill or handicapped children. In psychosocial deprivation, anorexia may occur intermittently, together with other signs of depression like withdrawal, sadness, and inactivity.

These are unlikely reasons for anorexia in otherwise healthy infants and young children. Most often, when parents claim, "My child does not eat," it is because their expectations of a normal intake are unrealistic. This commonly occurs toward the end of the second year, when requirements decrease because growth begins to decelerate. Among other causes, by far the most common one is decreased intake due to a decreased growth potential, as in primordial growth failure (Chapter 6). Here, too, requirements are less than expected. Thus, these infants are able to suck and eat normally, but quickly get disinterested. If all these causes of anorexia can be ruled out, mismanagement of feeding, which results in passive negativism, must be considered.

Pica

Pica denotes the eating of items that are, in our culture, not meant for eating. Three major causes are recognized. It can be a manifestation of normal oral exploratory behavior. Thus, it need not be an ominous sign in children less than 1½ years old. In large families from lower socioeconomic groups, where siblings often have to take over supervision of the younger child, pica in a toddler may be an expression of lack of training and supervision. Toward the end of the second year of life, the normal child should have been taught restrictions on improper infantile exploratory behavior. If pica persists, it may be caused either by the infant's inability to learn because of mental deficit or by failure to respond positively to socializing pressures for psychological reasons.

Nutrient deficiency has been blamed for pica involving dirt and materials that contain specific nutrients, such as zinc, copper, or calcium. This explanation of pica is highly questionable. Indeed, eating clay, contrary to original reports, may cause zinc deficiency rather than being a sign of it. An increased incidence of iron deficiency has been reported in pica (7). This, too, need not reflect a direct causal relationship, because pica and iron deficiency both may result from an abnormal parent–child interaction, with prolonged reliance on milk from the bottle as the sole food. This practice caused iron deficiency in the past because formulas were not iron-fortified.

Anatomic Lesions

Feeding Difficulties

Tumors or other obstructive lesions of the mouth, nose, or pharynx cause feeding difficulties. Nasal obstruction interferes with breathing, more during sucking from the bottle than with chewing and swallowing. Tumors of the tongue may be caused by cysts, hemangiomas, or ectopic thyroid tissue. Diffuse enlargement (macroglossia) occurs in myxedema or may be due to lymphangiomas and rhabdomyomas. A large tongue, as seen in acromegaly, gargoylism, and Beckwith syndrome, is rarely the cause of poor feeding. The same holds true for Down's syndrome, where the tongue is large relative to the size of the oral cavity. Pharyngeal obstructions to swallowing may be due to acquired lesions, such as abscesses and neoplasms, or to congenital lesions, such as teratomas, cystic malformations, and lymphangiomas. Congenital cysts, including branchial cysts, may cause problems any time after birth when they fill with secretions and enlarge.

Respiratory distress of any sort may cause feeding difficulties, because too much time and effort must be spent on breathing; the time needed for a swallow and effective suck—especially in tachypnea—is too long to leave enough time for the required breaths per minute. Breathing has priority, and food intake diminishes.

Micrognathia may cause problems because the small mandible causes the base of the tongue to obstruct the pharynx. It is always a major factor in the feeding difficulties of Pierre Robin syndrome because of the associated cleft palate. Since the tongue obstructs easy flow of liquid, food is pushed through the cleft. Feeding devices that are helpful in cleft palate are therefore of less benefit in Pierre Robin syndrome.

Clefts of palatal fusion may be unilateral or bilateral. They vary in extent, involving only the soft palate or, in addition, one or more of the following structures—hard palate, premaxilla, and lip. Palatal clefting causes difficulty sucking because a negative pressure cannot be achieved. The infant with intact lips can learn to compensate in time by creating negative pressure with the lips alone (Chapter 1). Feeding tends to be prolonged, even with the help of feeding devices. Fatigue, hunger, air swallowing, coughing, choking, and vomiting are common. Since corrective surgery of a cleft palate should not be attempted until the patient is 2 years of age, management of such infants represents a challenge.

Chronic Vomiting

The vomiting of nonbilious material, unaccompanied by nausea, fever, or diarrhea, may be due to such anatomic lesions as diaphragmatic hernias, esophageal stenosis (achalasia), or strictures and tracheoesophageal fistulas. Pyloric stenosis causes projectile vomiting because the full force of the distended gastric muscles is behind it. Occasionally, normal infants may have projectile vomiting. It is usually associated with a burp and may occur as often as several times a week, especially in infants who swallow air. In these cases, refeeding is generally successful. By contrast, in pyloric stenosis, projectile vomiting becomes regular, and refeeding causes repeat vomiting. Weight loss and dehydration ensue. Metabolic alkalosis and hypokalemia are typical consequences.

Tracheoesophageal fistula is a common congenital anomaly and occurs in five varieties. The two most common, which make up 95% of all types, cause severe problems when the first swallow is taken by the newborn, because they are associated with atresia. Fluid returns, and the child struggles, coughs, and turns cyanotic. The two least common types, which together constitute 1%, also are associated with atresia. In one type, the esophagus opens into the trachea, and the infant practically "drowns" with the first feeding. The H-type fistula, which has a frequency of 4 in 100 fistulas, causes chronic problems with feeding, including vomiting that may start any time after birth. The anomaly consists of a small connection between esophagus and trachea. The intake of fluids, as opposed to solids, causes respiratory embarrassment, coughing, choking, and vomiting. There are repeated episodes of pneumonia. Gastric distension is another characteristic sign. Treatment is surgical in all these anatomic lesions. Treatment of strictures may require dilatation by use of bougies.

Palatopharyngeal incompetence causes loss of liquid through the nose, choking, and occasionally vomiting. The manifestations are not unlike those in H-type fistulas. However, this disorder is characteristically associated with nasal speech of pressure consonants (*b, p, d, t, f, v,* etc.) and an inability to produce the pressure necessary to blow out a candle. On physical examination, the soft palate may be short or asymmetrical and show minimal movement during gagging. If there is a total absence of the musculature, the soft palate will look translucent. A bifid uvula or a notch in the posterior border of the hard palate is often other evidence of an anatomical defect in this area. This problem is due to a bony or muscular defect, which prevents the formation of an effective seal between the nose and the oropharynx. The disorder may be caused or precipitated by an adenoidectomy.

Neuromuscular Dysfunction

Neurogenic feeding difficulties are common in diseases of the central and peripheral nervous system. Immature neonates and infants with diffuse CNS damage frequently have nonspecific feeding problems due to poor coordination of oropharyngeal muscles. Oropharyngeal dysfunction is also a manifestation of neuromuscular diseases, which can be divided into movement disorders and disorders associated with hypotonia. Feeding difficulties are characteristic in each type.

Neonatal Oropharyngeal Dysfunction

Feeding difficulties in newborn infants, which are evident at birth, may be due to poor coordination of sucking, swallowing, and breathing. This occurs in small infants, who may show no evidence of CNS disease or may have only "soft" neurological signs. Diagnosis and management are difficult because the feeding problems mimic the psychogenic disorders already listed. Prognosis is uncertain. Some affected infants develop normally with time, providing severe undernutrition in early infancy can be prevented. The transient dysfunction of these infants is probably a sign of immaturity. In others, mental retardation becomes obvious within the first 3 to 6 months. Etiologies include congenital infection, defects of brain development, and metabolic diseases.

Chalasia is a relaxation of the cardia due to neuromuscular dysfunction that causes gastroesophageal reflux (GER) and a variety of complications if untreated. The disorder usually becomes evident within a few days after birth and is transient, lasting up to 4 months. Since GER can be demonstrated by x-ray (2) or pH-meter (1) in asymptomatic infants, diagnosis of chalasia requires demonstration of consistent reflux or consistent decrease in lower esophageal pressure below 20 mm Hg. Testing for reflux under fluoroscopy is done by applying manual pressure to the stomach or lowering the thorax below the level of the stomach. Crying and struggling also cause reflux fairly consistently in affected infants.

The disorder is common in institutionalized retarded infants (8). Typically, onset is at a later age in this group, suggesting that it may be an acquired disorder. It is also prevalent in infants and children with hiatus hernia (9) and sliding hiatus hernia and in young infants with bronchopulmonary dysplasia. The causal relationship with pulmonary disease is not clear. Chalasia may cause aspiration and repeated pneumonia. On the other hand, it is possible that bronchopulmonary dysplasia predisposes to chalasia because of large intrathoracic pressure swings with labored respirations. A small percentage of cases has associated esophagitis, which may cause blood vomiting and aggravate the functional disorder by further decreasing lower esophageal pressures (8). According to Herbst et al., apnea is a potential complication of chalasia, which can be reproduced by instilling dilute acid into the esophagus (1).

Most cases respond to medical management. This must be initiated before failure to thrive and esophageal irritation develop. Infants should be placed in a semireclined infant chair for 1 hour after feeding. Thickened feeding may also be used. Anatomic causes should be corrected, but surgery for GER is not advised unless conservative measures have been tried for a minimum of 6 weeks and failure to thrive is severe.

The term *achalasia* refers to a disorder of the cardia or lower esophagus, which is narrowed. There is aperistalsis, increased resting sphincter pressure and incomplete relaxation after swallowing. Fibrosis and disorganization of the lower esophageal musculature have been described in long-standing cases. Such changes may be caused by esophagitis or preceding chalasia with reflux of acid gastric content. A sudden, temporary obstruction to swallowing with reverse peristalsis may occur which is usually initiated by emotional stress. Patients have chronic difficulty swallowing and regurgitate undigested food; frequent coughing spells occur that are caused by an overflow of fluids into the larynx. Ultimately, growth failure results. Pulmonary infections are common. Diagnosis is made radiologically with a contrast medium that outlines the dilated esophagus, terminating in a fine point at the obstruction. Treatment consists of dilation with a pneumatic bag or bougie. Belladonna derivatives may be tried. Severe and resistant cases may require esophagocardial myotomy.

Movement Disorders

Disease of the upper motor neuron or extrapyramidal tract may cause feeding problems at any age. If there is hyperreflexia and spasticity, primitive oral reflexes may persist past the time when inhibition should occur. In such cases, persistence of a strong bite reflex may interfere with spoon feeding. An exaggerated gag reflex interferes with the introduction of solid food and may cause problems when a long nipple is used. Persistence of the protrusion reflex past the age of inhibition, at about 4 months, results in a tendency to push out food that is placed on the tongue. In spastic children, tongue thrust is common and may seriously interfere with swallowing and especially with chewing. These children slam the tongue against the teeth during a swallow. Tongue thrust also interferes with lateral movement of the tongue during chewing. Movement disorders manifested by chorea, athetosis, and dystonia usually have their onset in the second year of life or later. The tongue and the muscles of the face, neck, and shoulder are involved in chorea. A high incidence of undernutrition has been reported (see Chapter 7), which is probably related to food spillage and higher energy needs due to involuntary muscular activity. Patients with chronic diseases causing chorea (Wilson's hepatolenticular degeneration and hereditary dystonia musculorum deformans) require close supervision and help during feeding to prevent spillage. Ataxia is a manifestation of chronic diseases, such as Friedreich's ataxia and ataxia telangiectasia. Food spillage is also a major cause of negative energy balance in this group of disorders. However, if these patients move less to avoid falling due to ataxia, they have generally decreased calorie requirements. Undernutrition is consequently less common.

Hypotonia

Generalized hypotonia that involves the facial muscles causes feeding problems in infancy because the muscle strength needed for sucking is decreased. Disorders that cause hypotonia in this group include Werdnig–Hoffmann disease, carnitine deficiency, nonketotic hyperglycinemia, and so on. In severe cases, cheeks sag to produce a jowl and a tented triangular shape to the upper lip. Facial expression is bland, and there is no nasolabial fold. The suck reflex, which is present at birth and disappears between 3 and 4 months, is rarely suppressed, but the strength of the reflex is decreased. There is little resistance to pressure on the mandible, and the bite reflex is weak. Milk may drool out at the side of the mouth, because the lips do not create an effective seal around the nipple. Spontaneous drooling may be a sign of hypotonia, but it also occurs in healthy children and in cases of macroglossia.

TREATMENT

In general, the approach to treatment is either psychologically oriented or mechanical. The psychological approach is an important aspect of treatment even if the problem is anatomical or neurogenic in origin. Mechanical devices, on the other hand, should not be used in psychogenic disorders unless they are lifesaving or otherwise indicated, as in severe rumination. The choice of treatment is determined by the prognosis, which differs in transient, chronic, or progressive diseases. For instance, the training of oral feeding skills would be futile in progressive degenerative CNS diseases, which have a poor prognosis for the retention of learned skills. Individualization is necessary in all cases, taking in account the child's home environment.

Psychological Approach

In normal as well as defective infants, minor psychological feeding problems are not uncommon. They must be recognized and treated before behavior patterns result that are difficult to correct. Proper management of feeding and care should be stressed before unusual corrective measures are tried. The commonly used change of formula only convinces the parents that the child is ill, heightens their anxiety, and diverts parental attention from the real cause, which may be their own handling of the child. Diet changes must have a rational basis and should consist of more than a change in proprietary names of formulas. To reduce anxiety and avoid guilt feelings in cases where the diagnosis is uncertain, it is wise to suggest "immaturity" as the explanation until the correct etiology has been determined or until the problem has disappeared.

Overall management should stress the sequence of food introduction, proper meal schedules, and feeding techniques. These matters should be discussed even with parents who have raised other children with apparent success, since the environment does not remain the same, stress increases with family size, and siblings may have been more resistant to mismanagement. Parents with multiple children may be more harassed and may not take time to burp the infant, reserve enough time for feeding, or sit comfortably. They may use a nipple that is too fast or allow self-feeding too early.

In older infants and toddlers, behavior therapy is frequently recommended for psychological feeding problems. Within limits, this form of training is as old as mankind. Parents have always used the behavioral approach, called *positive reinforcement,* when they praise and reward the child for new accomplishments. This should not take the form of a bribe wherein the infant feels the parent can be controlled. Positive reinforcements used inappropriately can be harmful. For example, if a negativistic child who refuses a vegetable is "reinforced" with a favorite food for every bite of vegetable eaten (10), it may well aggravate the problem. Negative reinforcement has to be appropriate for the intelligence level of the child. A stern, nonpunitive slap on the hands is the only thing that a 1-year-old will understand, preferably coupled with a threatening *no* that the infant will learn in time. The punishment must follow the deed immediately. Withholding dessert and other measures often cannot be linked with the offense by the small child, who has a short memory and poor comprehension of cause and effect. Lectures on nutrition are not appreciated, even by schoolchildren who understand the content of the lecture. The problem becomes more difficult when dealing with mentally defective children. They require tangible rewards or restrictions that they can understand.

Since it is often difficult to be certain of the specific etiologic mechanism, it may be necessary to try more than one psychological approach. For instance, in cases of psychogenic passive food refusal, a casual "take it or leave it" attitude may be advisable, providing the parent can be reassured that a period of suboptimal intake will do no harm. If unsuccessful, extra attention coupled with firm insistence, but no begging or pleading, may be tried. The extra attention should always be carried over into other activities. However, these two basically different approaches should never be tried alternately; each should be given a trial of sufficient length, and all family members should act alike. Demonstrative, active food refusal should be punished in a matter-of-fact fashion without hostility—preferably by sending the child away from the table into a room alone. The parents must be consistent and not feed the child until the next meal. To compensate for this seemingly punitive response, positive reinforcement should be used liberally for other deserving behaviors. Prolonged problems of this kind indicate significant psychopathology of the parent(s) that requires psychiatric attention. If the negativistic eating behavior is associated with growth failure, psychosocial deprivation should be suspected.

Food refusal may not be as pathologic a sign as perceived by a rigid parent. The physician therefore must find a balanced attitude. Minor complaints should be viewed as such, and isolated food preferences of the child should be respected, especially if the nutrient content of the few refused items can be compensated for by other foods. In general, nutritional dogmatism should be avoided.

Mechanical Approach

The mechanical approach takes various forms, including surgery, dietary manipulations, and use of special feeding devices or techniques. The choice is determined by the objectives, which vary depending on the type and severity of the disorder, the prognosis, and the degree of associated malnutrition. Enteral or parenteral alimentation is indicated as an acute measure in severe malnutrition and as a means of gaining time for more conservative treatment. Maintenance of adequate growth takes priority in young infants over adherence to otherwise sound management principles. Thus, increasing caloric density through the addition of sugars or fat may be advisable on a temporary basis in malnourished infants with limited volume capacity.

Variations in feeding technique are required in cases of neuromuscular disorders. For instance, in hypotonia, sucking is aided by supporting the jaw with the free hand and pushing it up and backward over the nipple, thus creating a milking effect. In infants who hold the jaws tightly together due to spasticity, gently pulling and pushing the nipple partially back and forth also has a milking effect. To aid swallowing, the head should be anteflexed and the trunk semireclined, so that fluid can flow down by gravity. Swallowing is induced reflexly when the liquid touches the posterior oropharyngeal walls. It is a common mistake to retroflex the neck, not realizing that this position makes it difficult to use the tongue for swallowing. To induce swallowing of pureed foods, one may use a backward stroke under the chin with slight pressure to provide a stimulus for the tongue. For infants with a hyperactive gag reflex, a special small spoon may be used in order to avoid touching the palatopharyngeal and palatoglossal arch. The tongue must be pushed down with the spoon to accomplish this. By lifting the end of the handle, the tongue is pushed down; and upon withdrawing the spoon, food is placed anteriorly into the mouth, avoiding a reflex gag and thus leaving it to the infant to manage the rest. Soft food textures are required.

Feeding devices include special spoons, cups, bowls, bottles, and nipples. Bowls are designed to allow food to be scooped up against the sides of the bowl, which should be higher than those of standard utensils. The use of suction cups, Velcro, or carpet tape underneath the bowl anchors it. Special spoons are available for children who cannot close the fist or coordinate the grasp and movement to the mouth. A homemade device is a foam rubber curler that is slipped over the handle to prevent slipping and facilitate the grasp. Cups are available with two handles or with a spout and cover. For children with a poor grip, a pliable, plastic-coated handle, which is attached to an adjustable ring, can be used. The ring can be fitted over any size glass.

Special-purpose nipples are a great help in improving sucking efficiency. The so-called primi nipple may be tried for any infant with a poor suck. However, primary attention should be paid to proper function of the nipple hole. Cross-cut holes may stick, especially when the nipple is soft. Correct function of the nipple hole can be tested in two different ways. The feeding of 4 to 8 oz per meal, depending on age, should take between 20 and 30 minutes. Holding the bottle upside down at shoulder level should result in a drop of milk leaving the nipple hole when the preceding drop hits the floor.

For infants with a cleft palate, several special-purpose nipples are available. The lamb's nipple should be tried first. When not enough hard palate is intact, a nipple with a built-in obstructor is advisable. A "ducky" nipple is used for patients with a cleft lip. If none of these devices can be used successfully by the infant in producing sufficient negative pressure, it may be helpful to try a Playtex feeder with disposable plastic bags, against which pressure can be applied throughout the feeding process (11). For patients with Pierre Robin syndrome, a J-shaped glass feeder has been suggested (12). It is used to feed the infant in a prone position, because this allows the jaw to drop forward. With the same intent, these infants may be fed upright, but bent slightly forward.

Infants who do not suck at all and who require relatively small amounts of food can be fed successfully for some time with an eyedropper or a syringe. The syringe is attached to a short feeding tube that is placed in the side of the mouth.

Exercises are occasionally indicated, but realistic goals must be set or else they will do more harm than good. An example is the older infant who drools and may benefit from improving the orbicularis oris muscle tone by sucking on a straw. The aid of a speech therapist may be sought for the development of appropriate exercises.

REFERENCES

1. Herbst JJ, Minton SD, Book LS: Gastroesophageal reflux causing respiration distress and apnea in newborn infants. *J Pediatr* 95:763, 1979.
2. Blank L, Pew WL: Cardioesophageal relaxation (chalasia) studies on the normal infant. *Am J Roentgenol* 76:540, 1956.
3. Strawczynski H, Beck IT, McKenna RD, et al: The behavior of the lower esophageal sphincter in infants and its relationship to gastroesophageal-regurgitation. *J Pediatr* 64:17, 1964.
4. Krieger I: Personal observations.
5. Brockbank EM: Meryeism or rumination in man. *Br Med J* 1:421, 1907.
6. Runge EC: Three cases of hereditary rumination. *Boston Med J* 132:515, 1895.
7. Gutelins MF, Millican FK, Layman EM, et al: Nutritional studies of children with pica. *Pediatrics* 29:1012, 1962.
8. Sondheimer JM, Morris BA: Gastroesophageal reflex among severely retarded children. *J Pediatr* 94:710, 1979.
9. Abrahams P, Burkitt BFE: Hiatus hernia and gastroesophageal reflux in children and adolescents with cerebral palsy. *Aust Pediatr J* 6:41, 1970.
10. Palmer S: Feeding problems in children, in Palmer S, Ekvall S (eds): *Pediatric Nutrition in Developmental Disorders.* Springfield, Ill, Charles C Thomas, 1978, p 111.
11. Paradise JL, McWilliam BJ: Simplified feeder for infants with cleft palate. *Lancet* 53:566, 1974.
12. Takagi, Y, McCalla JL, Bosma, JF: Prone feeding of infants with the Pierre Robin Syndrome. *Cleft Palate J* 3:232, 1966.

5
Growth Failure Without Organic Disease

UNDERNUTRITION IN INFANTS

Definitions

A variety of terms are used interchangeably in the literature to describe nutritional deficiencies.

Malnutrition is the most general of terms, because it includes undernutrition and overnutrition, as well as abnormalities caused by an excess or deficit of specific nutrients. Unfortunately, it is common practice to use the term *malnutrition* synonymously with *undernutrition.*

Undernutrition signifies both insufficient delivery of body-building and energy-providing nutrients to the tissues, and the condition resulting from it. Undernutrition should not be confused with underfeeding or undereating. Deficient nutrient delivery may be the result of inadequate intake, absorption, or delivery to the tissues or of failure of utilization by the tissues.

Marasmus is a severe form of undernutrition with physical evidence of acute deprivation (i.e., a weight for height less than 80% of the mean). The term is used predominantly in underdeveloped countries. It comes from the Greek word for "waste" and refers to the severe muscle wasting that is one of its manifestations. Marasmus usually includes elements of both chronic and acute malnutrition with evidence of weight loss, often precipitated by intercurrent illnesses, such as gastroenteritis.

Kwashiorkor is a disorder that is common in underdeveloped countries and may be associated with marasmus, in which case one refers to the disorder as *marasmic kwashiorkor.* Kwashiorkor is a nutritional deficiency disease with specific manifestations, some of which are an expression of hypoalbuminemia.

Protein-calorie malnutrition (*PCM*) is a term that reflects the deficiency of protein and calories without defining exactly whether one or the other nutrient was more deficient during the development of malnutrition, since this is rarely known with certainty. The term is apparently being used to describe both, cases of kwashiorkor and marasmus. In as much as the imbalance between protein and calorie intake may not be the major cause of kwashiorkor and since the clinical picture of marsmus may change into kwashiorkor within a few days, making a distinction between the two disorders is difficult, and the term *PCM* is convenient.

Failure to thrive (*FTT*) is aptly descriptive, but its use in the medical literature has caused confusion. *FTT* describes merely the general effects of undernutrition on body mass, statural growth, and development in young infants. Since the term was intended to reflect a delay in both growth and development, it is rarely used to refer to older children and never to individuals who have passed the age for growth and development. The term was not intended to define a type of insult, or to imply deficient care by the parent or caretaker. It is unfortunate that the name is often used interchangeably with *maternal deprivation syndrome*. FTT can result from organic disease, because illness or malnutrition by itself restrict the social stimulation necessary for normal development and thus can cause delay in both growth and development. FTT should be a preliminary diagnosis. It is often used on admission to the hospital and indicates the need for further etiologic classification.

Growth failure refers to a deficient rate of gain in weight and/or height. The term does not describe the cause as being nutrient related, as it may be due to any one of a number of disorders, including endocrine, metabolic, or genetic diseases.

Diagnosis of "Failure to Thrive Without Apparent Cause"

In a majority of cases with failure to thrive (FTT), neither history nor physical examination reveals a definite cause. If a child like this comes from an unstable economic and emotional environment, deprivation syndrome is frequently diagnosed, although psychosocial disruption per se is not proof of a causal relationship with FTT. Misdiagnosis has tragic consequences when it leads to removal of the child from the home in cases where this is not indicated. Careful investigation and evaluation by qualified health care personnel are therefore necessary to rule out other causes of FTT, including hidden organic disease, cerebral dwarfism, small-for-gestational-age (SGA) dwarfism, and metabolic disease.

Starting with the admission interview, attempts should be made to determine whether the deficiency in growth and development is indeed the result of environmental deprivation, why the patient was deprived, and what steps can be taken to prevent further deprivation. This requires a thorough history and environmental evaluation.

History

The attitude toward the parents while taking the history is extremely important. The physician must convey a desire to understand and help and must avoid being judgmental or else the parents will not cooperate.

Of the historical data that are routinely obtained as part of any clinical workup, some are especially pertinent in FTT. They are (*1*) evidence of prenatal insults; (*2*) birth weight, height, and head circumference for length of gestation; (*3*) injury or disease that could have damaged the CNS and caused the developmental delay; (*4*) past heights, weights, and developmental milestones, preferably documented with records from other physician contacts; (*5*) evidence for other causes of growth failure; and (*6*) a family history of short stature, siblings born small for length of gestation, and so forth.

A description of eating behavior is an important part of the nutritional history. It is helpful to ask whether the child demands food or sleeps through mealtimes, since deprived infants tend to become undemanding with time. The reason for the physician contact may be revealing, because the parents tend to be unconcerned and may bring the child for minor complaints or upon urging of the social worker rather than for malnutrition. Equally informative may be the parents' explanation of the cause of growth failure, which is often bizarre in cases of maternal deprivation. Their account of the child's daily routine, if checked against other data, like the 24-hour diet recall, may reveal major discrepancies. Parental recall and knowledge of the child's past record of immunizations, illnesses, and so on will reflect their concern for the child. Environmental factors like housing, income, marital discord, alcoholism, and so on are important in the evaluation, but adverse findings are by themselves not diagnostic of deprivation. Finally, the history taking provides an opportunity to observe the parents' behavior and interactions with the child.

Physical Examination

A thorough neurological exam should be conducted in each case and should include an evaluation for the presence of "infantile posture" or catatonialike posturing. Baseline anthropometric measurements must be taken with extreme care, because important judgments will be based on the observation of changes in weight and height during the therapeutic trial. Behavior should be described, and the degree of mental retardation should be evaluated objectively, using the Denver Developmental Screening Test for infants and preschool children and the Stanford–Binet Intelligence Test for older children.

Laboratory Workup

The initial workup need not be extensive and can be done on an outpatient basis. Tests that require fasting must be avoided as much as possible. A major objective of these tests is the exclusion of hidden organic disease of the renal, cardiopulmonary, endocrine, and metabolic systems. The initial workup should be restricted to a few basic tests: blood count, urinalysis (including pH, specific gravity, ketones, reducing substances, and spot tests for metabolic diseases), colony count, serum CO_2, Na, K, Cl, P, Ca, alkaline phosphatase, BUN, FBS, SGOT, serum albumin and globulin, serum thyroxine, urine and serum amino acid screen by paper electrophoresis, a chest x-ray, bone-age determination, and a bone survey to rule out physical abuse. If the stools are normal by history and gross inspection, no further workup for malabsorption is needed. It is also not necessary to conduct an intravenous pyelogram or renal function tests when BUN, pH, and electrolytes are normal, because in the absence of waste retention and disturbances in acid–base balance, renal anomalies that may be found cannot be considered a cause of the growth failure.

The Therapeutic Trial

If the outpatient investigation of the growth failure does not reveal a cause that can be corrected in the home, or if there is abundant circumstantial evidence suggestive of deprivation, hospital admission is necessary to conduct a therapeutic trial in order to rule out maternal deprivation. The hospital provides the setting where nurses, social workers, psychiatrists, dietitians, and physical therapists can all contribute to the diagnostic process and the development and institution of therapeutic measures.

The therapeutic trial has three major objectives: (*1*) documentation of the patient's ability to gain weight at an accelerated rate, without special therapeutic efforts; (*2*) evaluation of dietary manipulations necessary to accomplish weight gain in cases where it does not occur spontaneously; and (*3*) observation of general behavior and eating habits, as well as changes in behavior that occur during hospitalization.

Ideally, a management conference should be held on admission, or all members of the health care team should be apprised of the patient's needs and objectives to be accomplished during hospitalization, which may include specific observations necessary to diagnose feeding problems or behavior abnormalities.

The patient should be offered a minimum of 150 kcal/kg/day or the recommended amount for age calculated from the predicted weight for height (i.e., 90 to 120 kcal/day/kg predicted weight). On the other hand, it is simpler to order an excess (a double tray) of a suitable diet for the patient's maturational age. Deprived infants generally eat well and gain readily. Consequently, counting calories for diagnostic purposes is not necessary in patients with a good appetite. Diet orders should specify (*1*) number of meals and snacks per day, (*2*) interval between meals, (*3*) food consistency (based on maturational age!), (*4*) caloric density (high-calorie foods are advised in patients with limited volume capacity for food), and (*5*) assistance at mealtimes (infants should be held for bottle feedings).

Diagnosis of Emotional Deprivation

A firm diagnosis of an emotional deprivation syndrome can be made only by observing the following responses to the therapeutic trial:

1. Weight gain occurs without unusual dietary manipulations in patients who had a weight deficit for height.
2. Weight gain is followed by a linear growth spurt in patients who had a height deficit for age, providing they remain in a growth-promoting environment.
3. A rapid advance in psychomotor development occurs, and behavior abnormalities disappear (infants show definite changes within a few weeks).

A number of pitfalls are common: (*1*) The prescription of a "diet for age" is frequently not appropriate for the maturational age of the developmentally retarded infant with maternal deprivation syndrome. These infants may not be able to handle the volume or consistency of the diet for age and continue to do poorly in the hospital. (*2*) Since these infants have increased calorie needs for their size, they are often not given as much food as they would eat. (*3*) The significance of weight gain is misinterpreted when it occurs in a child who lost some weight prior to the therapeutic trial due to intercurrent illness. Consequently, maternal deprivation may be diagnosed incorrectly. To make a firm diagnosis of a deprivation syndrome, weight gain must be sustained, preferably until a normal weight for height is achieved. (*3*) The weight curve is often misinterpreted when the child shows large weight fluctuations from day to day. It is advisable in these cases to graph the daily weights and to draw a line to the weight curve from which the average gain for a period of about 2 weeks should be calculated.

Manifestations of Undernutrition

Marasmus and Kwashiorkor

The terms *marasmus* and *kwashiorkor* are used for two types of severe undernutrition that differ with respect to etiology and clinical manifestations. According to the traditional viewpoint, calorie deficiency is the major cause of marasmus because all foodstuffs are taken in insufficient amounts. By contrast, the characteristic feature of kwashiorkor is protein deficiency of sufficient severity to cause hypoalbuminemia (below 2.5 g/dl). However, the etiology seems to be more complex, since total body protein is equally or even more severely depleted in marasmus than in kwashiorkor. Other factors, such as the age of onset, precipitating illness, mineral imbalance or specific nutrient deficiencies, and the ability to adapt, may play a role.

Marasmus is a term used mostly in tropical and subtropical countries for severe malnutrition without edema (Fig. 5-1). According to the classifica-

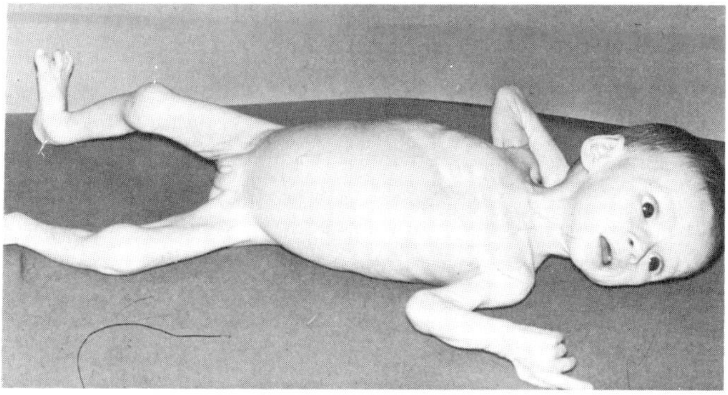

Figure 5-1. SEVERELY MALNOURISHED INFANT (MARASMUS) Caused by underfeeding in the maternal deprivation syndrome.

tion of Gomez, severe or third-degree malnutrition means that body weight is less than 60% of the mean for age (1). This classification was challenged by Waterlow (2), who recommended that height for age be used to gauge the duration of undernutrition and that weight for height is a means to assess wasting. Primordial dwarfs are an example of cases where weight for age is inappropriate. They may have a weight for age in the "marasmic" range without being wasted because they are short. Undernourished infants in the United States not infrequently have weight reductions to 80% of the normal mean for height. The diagnosis of marasmus would be appropriate in these cases, but the term is infrequently used. Endocrine adaptations, which are considered typical of marasmus, are seen in the type of undernutrition common in the United States, (i.e., undernutrition due to organic disease or maternal deprivation).

Edema is the single clinical feature that is universally present in *kwashiorkor*. Other features, such as hepatomegaly and skin and hair changes, are not uniformly present. Endocrine abnormalities do not seem to distinguish kwashiorkor from marasmus, possibly because elements of both often coexist. The term *marasmic kwashiorkor* has been recommended for patients who are edematous and who have a weight that, as in marasmus, is less than 60% of the normal mean for age. Hepatomegaly and edema sometimes develop during recovery from severe undernutrition; yet when this occurs in the United States, a diagnosis of kwashiorkor is usually not made.

Causes

In essence, the unavailability of nutrients is the cause of marasmus. This, in turn, may be due to inadequate intake, absorption, or delivery to the tissues or to failure of utilization by the tissues. Marasmus is therefore not unique to the developing countries, although it is more common there than in the United States. Infants are usually weaned too early, and breast milk is replaced with dilute formulas or other low-calorie liquids, such as rice water. Frequently, the condition is suddenly aggravated by an infection of the gastrointestinal or urinary tract, by pneumonia, otitis media, or septicemia. Multiple factors that feed into the poverty cycle contribute to the problem, including lack of education and cultural child-rearing practices. Diarrhea is another important contributory factor. The incidence of malnutrition is thus relatively low in primitive societies where diarrhea is not endemic. Since malnutrition measurably alters the immune response (Chapter 8), a decreased host defense system in conjunction with poor hygienic conditions probably starts a vicious cycle of infection, diarrhea, malabsorption, further malnutrition, and so on. Infection is not a major contributing cause to malnutrition in American cities. There is evidence that resistance is related to better zinc nutriture (Chapter 11).

Marasmus develops relatively slowly. Onset in infants can usually be traced to weaning soon after birth. By contrast, kwashiorkor starts more suddenly and at a later age, when the infant is weaned to a very low protein diet with relatively high calorie content. It has been suggested that there is an inefficient regeneration of plasma albumin and that muscle proteins cannot be used for "proteinogenesis" by the liver because of endocrine maladaptions (3).

General Manifestations

Muscle wasting and loss of adipose tissue in marasmus are blatantly obvious on inspection. There are, in addition, abnormalities of structure and function in almost every system, including the CNS. Most important among these functional changes are endocrine and gastrointestinal abnormalities. In kwashiorkor there is, in addition, edema; the liver may be enlarged; hair is sparse with reddish discoloration, and the skin shows dermatitis and pigment changes. Liver enlargement is attributable to fatty infiltration. The dermatitis may be due to deficiency of any one of a number of specific nutrients, including zinc and the B vitamins.

Protein-calorie malnutrition also affects bone growth and maturation. There is a delay in the appearance of carpal and epiphyseal ossification centers (4), and the sequence of ossification is disrupted (5). Head circumference is decreased, reflecting a corresponding decrease in brain size and DNA content (6). Following improved dietary intake, marasmic infants may show a rapid increase in head circumference, causing suture separation that simulates a space-occupying lesion (7). In one study, patients with kwashiorkor who were examined 4 weeks after realimentation by means of echoencephalography had enlarged cerebral ventricles, whereas marasmic infants showed no deviation from the norm (8).

Many of the laboratory abnormalities that occur in protein-calorie malnutrition, including signs of vitamin deficiency, reflect the patient's current diet. This also pertains to the plasma amino acid profile. Essential amino acids decline, including valine, leucine, and isoleucine, while nonessential amino acids, like glycine and alanine, increase (9). Because of the close relation to food ingested during the days preceding the blood sampling (10), these changes cannot be used as a measure of malnutrition.

Endocrine Abnormalities

Studies of endocrine function in marasmus and kwashiorkor were reviewed by investigators from several countries, including the United States, at a symposium (11) that showed consensus in many respects. Some discrepancies were noted, but they appeared to be due to changes that occur during recovery, since not all studies were conducted on admission or before realimentation.

Growth hormone levels were uniformly elevated in all studies of patients with kwashiorkor, whereas variable results were reported for patients with marasmus, ranging from low baseline values in Chile to high normal values in South Africa, Mexico, Jamaica, and the United States. With the exception of the group from Chile, these patients were able to respond to arginine, insulin-induced hypoglycemia, and stress. Growth hormone was poorly suppressed by glucose, but a mixed meal caused a fall of growth hormone levels. The introduction of protein feedings appears to be responsible for this fall (12). These and other endocrine changes may occur as early as 3 days after realimentation. Studies of patients with low values, including those from Chile, were apparently conducted after introduction of protein feedings (13). Plasma somatomedin activity is low in kwashiorkor (14,15), possibly because of the presence of somatomedin inhibitors (14). The phenomenon of "no growth despite growth hormone" can thus be explained, especially since there is now convincing evidence that somatomedin contributes directly to mammalian growth (16).

Insulin secretion is low in both marasmus and kwashiorkor (13,11). Fasting blood sugar is normal or slightly decreased, and clearance after a glucose tolerance test is slow. The insulin response following an oral glucose load is delayed, and the ratio between insulin and glucose is low, suggesting impaired insulin secretion or release. Improvement in insulin levels may take several months, especially in marasmus. These findings, in conjunction with the data on growth hormone, suggest that hormonal changes occur in malnutrition as an adaptive mechanism to provide fuel, where low levels of insulin promote lipolysis and mobilize protein from muscle for gluconeogenesis.

Whereas earlier studies—including histopathologic observations of people dying of cachexia—were indicative of pituitary hypofunction, this was not borne out by recent work showing not only elevated growth hormone levels but also increased activity of other tropic hormones, including adrenocorticotropic and thyroid stimulating hormone. A so-called pseudo hypophysectomy may develop, however, in extreme cases of marasmus, especially in adults.

Plasma cortisol levels were elevated in most studies of kwashiorkor and marasmus, both from abroad (11) and in the United States (17). However, total plasma cortisol levels may be decreased in kwashiorkor, although the free and presumably active portion is elevated. Data on adrenocortical function in response to ACTH stimulation are conflicting. The duration of stimulation is a factor, because responsiveness may decrease in severe malnutrition if the adrenals are stimulated for more than 3 days. Dexamethasone does not suppress the pituitary. The metapyrone test was normal in cases of malnutrition from the United States, providing enough of the drug was given to block all cortisol production and thus to stimulate the pituitary effectively through negative feedback (18). These studies do not support the hypothesis, suggested by rat experiments (3), that hypoalbuminemia in kwashiorkor is related to cortisol deficiency.

Comparison of thyroid function studies from different countries show disagreement. In a careful study of marasmic infants from Peru, thyroxine was low, thyroxine-binding globulin was normal, and free thyroxine values showed a wide scatter from low to normal values (19). Several investigators reported low thyroxine values in kwashiorkor, but since thyroxine-binding globulin was low, free thyroxine values tended to be normal. Marasmic infants from the United States (20), including infants with undernutrition due to organic disease, also had low serum thyroxine values. Normal or supranormal secretion of thyroid stimulating hormone and findings suggestive of mild primary hypothyroidism were reported from South Africa (11).

In contrast to some earlier studies (21), most investigators now agree that the basal metabolic rate (BMR) is not elevated in either of the two forms of protein-calorie malnutrition. The values are high when weight is used as a reference standard in marasmus or falsely low in kwashiorkor because of the edema. A high BMR per body weight is due to the preponderance of tissues with a high metabolic rate and the loss of muscle and fat, which have a relatively low metabolic rate. Moreover, metabolic rate measurements, which in infants are commonly conducted 4 hours after a meal, are high when malnourished infants are beginning to gain weight and retain nitrogen (22). This is due to the effect of the so-called specific dynamic action, which is a function of growth (22,23). The degree and the acuteness of malnutrition also influence the basal metabolic rate, as suggested by a study from the United States, where only infants with redundant skinfolds had a low BMR (20). The decrease of the metabolic rate is an obvious lifesaving adaptation to the lack of fuel, although the mechanism is not clear. The low BMR does not appear to be directly related to the decrease in thyroid function, because the BMR rises during recovery before there is a rise of serum thyroxine (20). The low BMR during the acute phase of malnutrition is not a reflection of energy needs; it is an adaptive phenomenon and rises with realimentation.

Gastrointestinal Abnormalities

There is a large body of literature on gastrointestinal changes in portein-calorie malnutrition showing that mucosal abnormalities and corresponding deficiencies of mucosal enzymes occur, as well as a decrease in pancreatic secretions and abnormalities of the intestinal flora. Atrophy of the gastric mucosa may cause hypochlorhydria, which decreases the bactericidal barrier. Together with the deficient immunodefense system, this abnormality causes bacterial overgrowth and may lead to bacterial invasion.

There is still controversy over the cause of malabsorption, whether it is a direct consequence of malnutrition or is related to diarrhea and infection. Morphological changes reported from the developing countries include cellular infiltrates, villous atrophy with shortening of the brush border, and replacement of villi by abnormal ridges (24). However, these abnormalities are not specific and may persist after recovery from malnutrition for as long as a year and possibly longer (25).

Similar changes of a nonspecific nature that occur in well-nourished infants and adults without a history of malnutrition are called *tropical enteropathy* or *tropical jejunitis*. They persisted in Peace Corps volunteers for as long as a year or more after they left a contaminated environment (26). This similarity and the prolonged persistence of histopathologic changes after recovery from malnutrition suggest that the nutritional insult is not necessarily the cause of intestinal changes in malnutrition. This seemingly theoretical issue has practical implications with regard to the need for antibiotic prophylaxis of malnourished children in unhygienic tropical environments.

Bacterial overgrowth appears to be responsible for a decrease in conjugated bile acids and an increase in free bile acids that may cause intestinal cell injury, fecal loss of bile acids, and a reduction in fat micelle formation (27). Fat malabsorption, which is occasionally observed in protein-calorie malnutrition, is probably due to these changes in bile acids as well as a decrease in pancreatic secretions (28).

According to most reports, protein digestion and absorption are not abnormal, although in severe cases of marasmus in the tropics, almost all absorptive functions may be affected (29). Nitrogen balance studies of marasmic infants from the United States showed that they were able to absorb nitrogen normally and had excellent nitrogen retentions, ranging from 120 to 300 mg/kg/day, starting with the first day of admission to the hospital. Since the infants did not have diarrhea, they were given and accepted a calorie-sufficient diet of 150 kcal/kg/day and protein intakes of 2.7 to 5.6 g/kg/day. Nitrogen absorption ranged from 80 to 92% of intake, which reflects excellent digestive capacity in view of the large protein load. Malnourished infants with diarrhea have increased fecal nitrogen excretion. In one study of malnourished infants, 24-hour fecal weight was positively correlated with fecal nitrogen (24). Lactose intolerance and poor glucose absorption (30) are the most common gastrointestinal dysfunctions in protein-calorie malnutrition. Normalization follows dietary treatment. However, return of lactase activity to normal is slow, and a proportion of infants do not recover from lactose intolerance (31).

Treatment

Early treatment is dependent on the presence of such associated conditions as dehydration, diarrhea, and infections, which require appropriate attention. The state of hydration is difficult to evaluate in a patient who has lost subcutaneous fat. Unnecessary intravenous fluid therapy that delays institution of a calorie-sufficient diet should be avoided. Consequently, if there is no history of diarrhea, if electrolytes are normal, and if the BUN is not indicative of hemoconcentration, intravenous therapy is not necessary. Infants with moderate malnutrition, that is not caused by organic illness, should be offered a regular diet for their maturational age immediately and should be allowed to eat as much as they wish. By contrast, in infants with severe malnutrition, buildup should be slower, and it may be wise to treat initially with a formula that decreases the load on the intestinal capacity to digest and absorb fat and carbohydrates. Therefore, a formula like Similac 24 LBW, which is used with low birth weight infants, may be used in less dilute form to make 30 kcal/dl. A diet that provides 100 kcal/kg is usually tolerated by the end of the first week; within the next week, intake should be stepped up to 150 kcal/kg and then more if the patient is willing to take more. When a steady rate of weight gain has been achieved and stools remain normal, the patient may be switched to regular formula or, in children over 1 year of age, to homogenized milk and pureed foods. Vitamin supplements must be given if the patients are not on proprietary formulas. Iron is also advised, because iron stores are quickly used up when the rate of weight gain is high.

EMOTIONAL DEPRIVATION

Hospitalism

References to sad-looking, malnourished infants who were dying of illness and starvation in foundling homes are plentiful in the American literature. Physicians called it *atrophy* or *cachexia* and attributed the condition to a lack of overall care, nutrition, and a wretched environment where infection was rampant because of poor hygiene. As early as 1908, Chapin linked the handling of infants with their well-being (32). Later, Bakwin (33) suggested a more direct relationship between psychological factors and failure to thrive. He claimed that institutionalized infants "ingested diets. . . . which in the home are entirely adequate for growth"; yet he described an "indifferent appetite" and the fact that food was "accepted without enthusiasm." Although Bakwin recognized anorexia, he apparently made the assumption that food intake had been "adequate."

In 1945, Spitz (34) described a syndrome characterized by anaclitic depression, anorexia, and failure to thrive, which he called *hospitalism*, a term used earlier by Chapin. He compared a group of infants raised in foundling homes without mothers or mother substitutes with another group that was cared for in prison by their own mothers. The foundling home infants were sad-faced and undergrown and had a developmental quotient of 79, compared to one of 105 for the control group. Spitz recognized that they deteriorated because they lacked the handling and cuddling of a warm human relationship. On follow-up, 37% had died, whereas all infants in the control group were still alive. In a second report, Spitz (35) described severe emotional disturbances and intellectual deficit in the surviving foundling home infants. His classical analysis of their personality has been confirmed in many subsequent reports. Prominent features were selfishness, attention seeking, aggressive or self-destructive behavior, and an inability to give or receive affection and to form meaningful relationships. Reference to the availability of good food is made, but Spitz did not provide an account of food intake. It is therefore unlikely that he meant to imply that growth failure can develop in the face of an adequate nutrient intake. However, many reports have appeared in the literature since then that imply just that, although no report documents actual food intake to substantiate the claim.

For example, differences in the growth of children in two postwar German orphanges were attributed by Widdowson (36) to the quality of care rather than to the quantity of food intake. Children in the home that was supervised by a kindly matron gained more weight than those in the orphanage whose matron was a stern disciplinarian. The observer assumed that basic food rations were evenly distributed among the children, although the same report states that the stern matron had a group of favorites who grew better than others. This observations should, in fact, suggest that these favorites received more and better food than the remaining infants.

Provence and Lipton (37) studied infants who were raised in an institution where special care was taken to assure regular feeding. Although the infants remained for almost 2 years in a sterile hospital environment, isolated from each other and cared for in a perfunctory manner by the usual rotation of attendants, they grew normally, but they demonstrated all the behavior abnormalities considered characteristic of hospitalism. This observation strongly suggests that emotional deprivation affects development and behavior, while growth is a function of food intake. Provence also drew attention to the fact that infants living in families may develop a syndrome similar to hospitalism.

Solkoff et al. (38) looked for evidence of hospitalism in neonates confined to isolettes. They provided tactile stimulation for five newborn infants, 5 minutes every hour of the day for 10 days, and compared them with five control subjects. The stimulated infants were more active and physically healthier; they cried less and regained their birth weight faster than the control subjects, who were cared for in the usual manner. The authors do not mention whether the stimulated infants also sucked more vigorously and ate more.

Parent–Infant Bonding: Relation to Emotional Deprivation

The effects of tactile stimulation on newborns observed by Solkoff (38,39) seemed to be independent of the person providing the stimulation, since infants under 2 months do not discriminate among people (40). After that time, infants begin to respond differently to one caregiver than to another and show well-defined attachment by 6 months of age. It is therefore not surprising that Schaffer (41) noted behavior disturbances only if the separation from the primary caregiver occurred after 6 months.

In the early 1960s evidence began to accumulate that prolonged separation right after birth also carried a risk, mainly because it led to parenting difficulties. Deficient parent–infant bonding, in turn, seemed to be responsible for a higher incidence of battering and failure to thrive (42). Later studies pursued the effect of early separation on the mother and the attachment process (43). Blau (44) had reported already in 1963 that mothers of premature infants were different from mothers of full term infants. They felt distant from the baby and insecure in their role as mother. Subsequent studies documented profound differences between the behavior of mothers who were allowed direct contact right after birth and those who were not admitted into the nursery until several weeks later (45). Early contact mothers soothed and fondled their infants more and exhibited different language behavior. Long-range effects of deficient parent–infant bonding were suggested by studies that indicated an effect on the IQ and language scores of children as late as 5 years of age.

While these data do not suggest that the early days after birth are the only time for optimal bonding, they do indicate that the process is facilitated in the newborn period. Studies on the importance of early attachment and on the adverse effects of a barren environment have led to profound changes in attitudes toward infant care during hospitalization, especially in the newborn period. Whereas neonates used to be kept in enclosed incubators without sensory input, many institutions now permit parents to feed newborns, including prematures, and make rooming-in available to parents of older infants and children.

Various behaviors have been associated with successful parent–infant bonding, including the attitude toward feeding. Thus, breast feeding seems to be eased, and early contact mothers have reported increased satisfaction with feeding (46). This may explain the high incidence of failure to thrive in premature infants who were separated from their mothers for a prolonged period after birth. Failure to develop a meaningful attachment facilitates the development of maternal deprivation syndrome.

Maternal Deprivation Syndrome and Psychosocial Dwarfism: Clinical Comparison

The *maternal deprivation syndrome* (*MDS*) is characterized by growth failure, developmental retardation, and affective abnormalities that develop in an adverse environment and improve after removal from that environment. The patients are, as the term indicates, infants who are dependent on their mother or caretaker for nurture. This syndrome has also been called emotional deprivation, sensory deprivation, and environmental retardation. By contrast, the term *psychosocial dwarfism* (*PSD*) has been used to single out patients who not only exhibit the symptoms of MDS but also demonstrate unusual and bizzare behavior patterns such as garbage eating, polydipsia, night wandering, tempers, and self-abusiveness (47,48). All patients described in the literature have been at least 2 but generally more than 3 years old.

Undernutrition is responsible for the growth failure; sensory and emotional deprivation caused behavior abnormalities and psychomotor retardation. Neglect plays a major role in MDS, whereas punitive interaction is more predominant in PSD, evidenced by a high incidence of physical abuse (49).

Growth

Deficient gains in weight and height are the most obvious features and the ones that usually lead to the detection of these cases. Weight is generally more severely affected than height in MDS. By contrast, school-age children and adolescents with PSD may be proportionate or even obese. Children with PSD in the 2- to 5-year-old age group tend to be underweight, like infants with MDS (Figs. 5-2 and 5-3). Even the patients who are proportionate at the time of first contact often have been malnourished in infancy. Bone maturation is delayed and corresponds roughly to height age. Skeletal proportions, facial features, and head size usually are also appropriate for height age, giving the appearance of "infantilism" (Fig. 5-4). Onset of growth failure in MDS appears to be at or very soon after birth. Weight records of patients with PSD show that onset is frequently in the latter part of infancy.

Development

Motor and language development are slow in both MDS and PSD. Deprived infants and children do mature eventually and in time acquire motor skills. This allows them to venture beyond the sphere of the abusing parent, where they are subjected to modifying influences. Consequently, some disease manifestations may improve spontaneously.

Speech and language are affected in PSD. Articulation is poor, and some children refuse to talk altogether. Flirtatious nonverbal communication of some older patients suggests an ability for more advanced

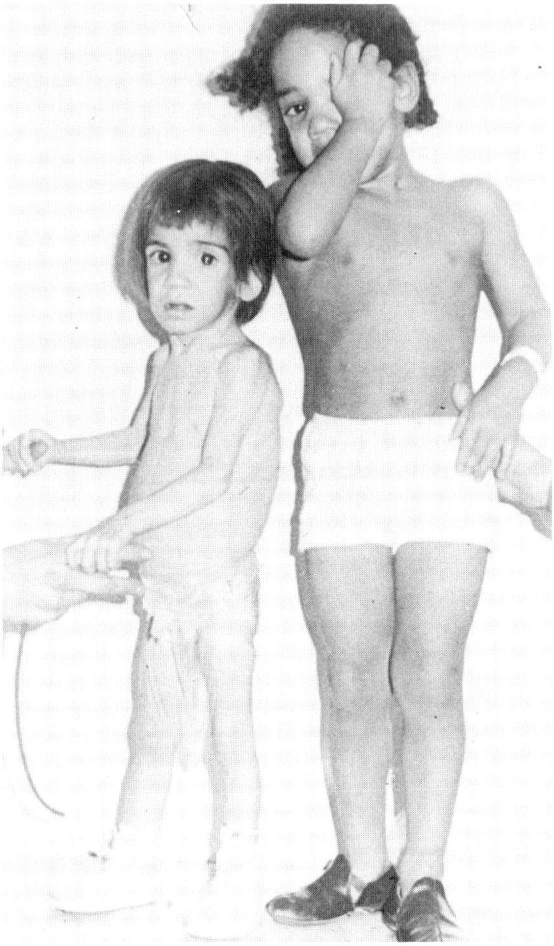

Figure 5-2. MARASMUS IN PSYCHOSOCIAL DEPRIVATION DWARFISM
37-month-old girl, weight 5.59 kg, height 75 cm, standing next to a normal girl of the same age.

function than that reflected by their language performance. Infants often have a watchful look, termed *radar gaze,* which also belies the degree of retardation measured by standard intelligence tests. An alert facial expression helps to distinguish deprived from mentally defective individuals.

Behavior

Affect and behavior are abnormal in both MDS and PSD. Infants are generally withdrawn and apathetic. They do not reach out with their hands to explore and actively seek attention, nor do they assert themselves by crying and fighting. Thus, they may give the impression that they are autistic. However, they respond when held, and they seem to enjoy body contact, a finding that is not compatible with autism. Since they are undemanding, they are considered "good babies." This lack of assertiveness is also reflected in their eating behavior. They can be passed around to anyone willing to hold them, seemingly fearless of strangers. Although these infants withdraw, they find ways to amuse themselves through repetitive motions, such as rocking and rhythmic head nodding or shaking. Autoerotic behavior takes more vehement forms in older patients with PSD, who may have scars on the forehead from repetitive head banging.

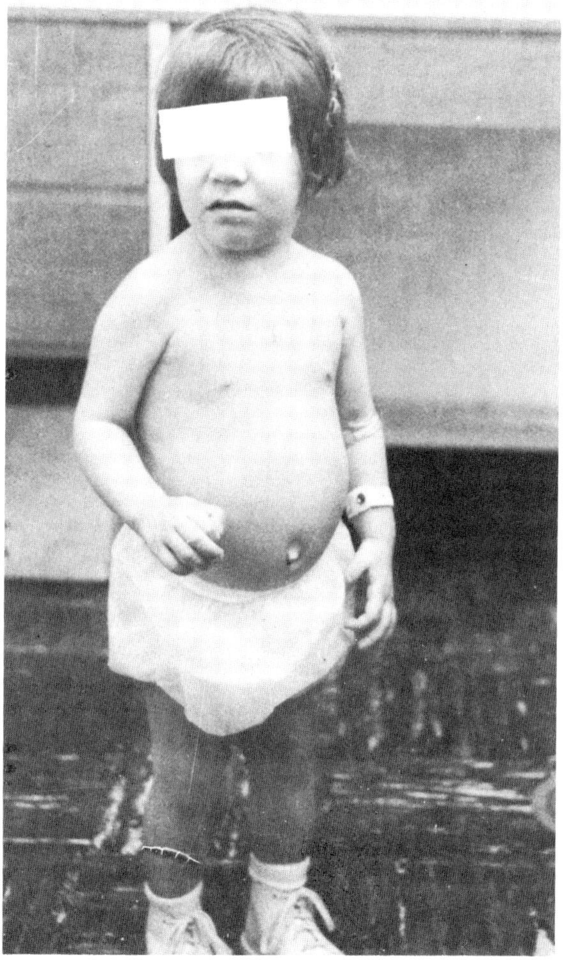

Figure 5-3. 38-MONTH-OLD GIRL WITH PSYCHOSOCIAL DEPRIVATION DWARFISM
Same as Figure 5-2, after 4 weeks of hospitalization.

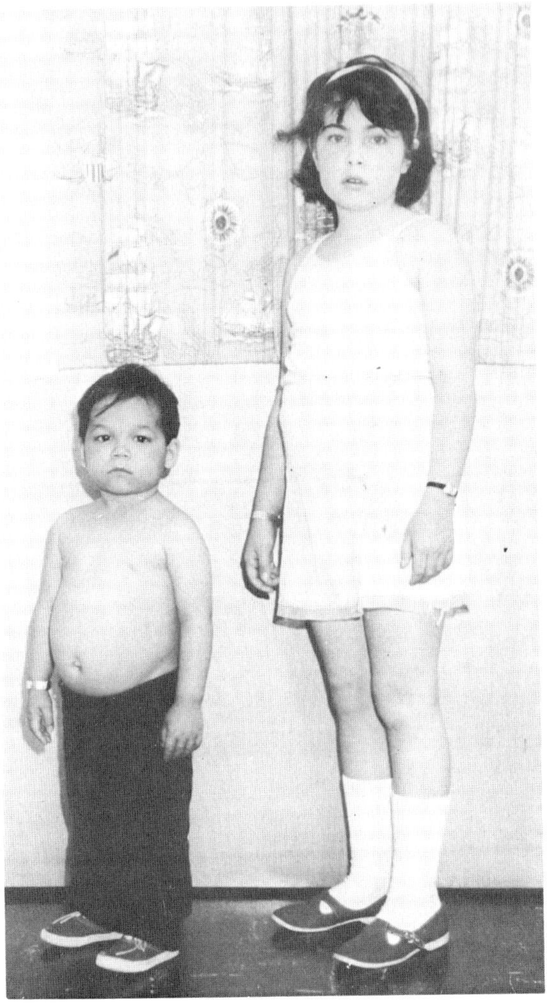

Figure 5-4. 10-YEAR-BOY WITH PSYCHOSOCIAL DEPRIVATION DWARFISM
Standing next to a normal girl of the same age.

Patients with PSD may be intermittently withdrawn and depressed. Although they may appear affectionate and well behaved, closer analysis invariably reveals that this behavior is not consistent. Some are abnormally compliant most of the time and allow themselves to be manipulated, only to throw a violent temper tantrum at another time. Frequently, aggression is turned toward the self. Whereas some investigators attribute self-inflicted injuries to pain "agnosia" (50), an inability to perceive appropriate warning through pain, others feel that it reflects a need for extremes of stimulation and masochistic gratification. Self-abusive behavior has been observed in monkeys reared in isolation. What seems to be a close parent–child relationship on casual observation is thus, in reality, infantile dependency or an abnormal need to win approval. The impression given by parent or child during the first office visit is often misleading, especially since information of negativistic behavior, such as tempers, fecal soiling, oppositional food refusal, and garbage eating, are usually withheld, especially if the parent is not directly questioned about these signs.

Neurological Signs

When lying supine, neonates adopt a posture in which arms are abducted, externally rotated, and supinated (Fig. 5-5). Infants with MDS adopt this infantile posture and maintain it for extended periods of time, even while sitting upright or standing (51). A sign of similar significance can also be provoked in older children with PSD. When placing an extremity in any position, these patients will maintain it for several minutes in catatonialike fashion without being asked to do so. The infantile posture appears to be

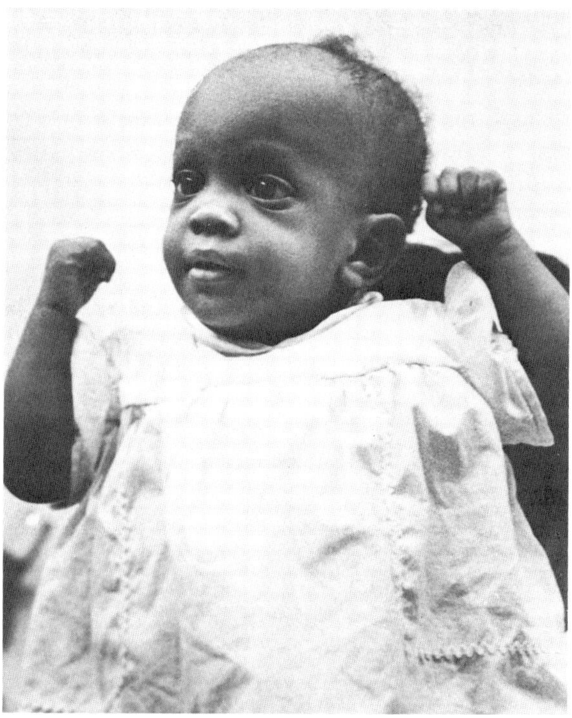

Figure 5-5. INFANTILE POSTURE IN A 14-MONTH-OLD INFANT WITH MATERNAL DEPRIVATION SYNDROME AFTER WEIGHT RECOVERY
This pathologic posture disappeared one week later, 6 weeks after hospital admission.

a manifestation of cerebral function at a subcortical level. The sign is nonspecific, since it has been described in severe organic brain disorders as well as in maternal deprivation syndrome.

Eating Behavior

Infants with MDS are undemanding and do not cry for food (52). When fed, they eat ravenously to the extent that there may be overflow vomiting. In describing the child's appetite, parents frequently say that the infant "eats like a wolf," "eats until the stomach looks like bursting," "eats more than an adult," and the like. While this may be a sign of hunger, the phenomenon has been attributed to an inability to recognize satiety because of an impairment of body image and sense of self (53). Anorexia is not common in infants (52). This is probably attributable to the fact that these infants are, at this early phase, not reactive and negativistic.

Eating behavior in PSD is more bizarre than in MDS. These children scavenge through garbage cans, eat scraps of rotten food, and drink from toilet bowls or rain puddles. These cravings have been variously interpreted as a sign of hunger or as a need for excessive stimulation and punishment. Although the majority eat repulsive matter with caloric value, some will eat nonnutritive things like crayons and foam rubber. Like infants with MDS, patients with PSD require large volumes of food and drink. Polydipsia is common but appears to be psychogenic in most cases. The combination of ravenous appetite and growth failure in a child who does not have a malabsorption syndrome is characteristic of one of the two deprivation syndromes—MDS or PSD.

Pathogenesis

Developmental, affective, and behavioral abnormalities in MDS are a direct result of the infants' lack of stimulation and social interaction. By contrast, "abnormal" social interaction—rather than the lack of it—seems to be the cause of behavior abnormalities in many cases of PSD, although incarceration has been documented in some instances. Mental retardation results mainly from the emotional deprivation. Malnutrition in early infancy may be a contributing factor. Lack of significant retardation in some cases of PSD can be attributed to persistent interaction—distorted as it may be—and to later onset of undernutrition. There is considerable controversy over the cause and pathogenesis of growth failure. A direct effect of psychic influences on growth has been proposed. Endocrine functions are abnormal, but the observed changes also result from undernutrition. There are multiple factors operative that can explain malnutrition, including anorexia or food refusal, intentional starvation by the parent, gastrointestinal losses, and relative hypermetabolism.

Endocrine Function

It was originally proposed that growth failure in MDS and PSD is the result of a direct effect of psychologically induced nervous stimuli on metabolism and endocrine function, and that these patients indeed consistently receive the excessive amount of food that the parents claim they eat. This concept came about as a result of psychiatric studies of infants in institutions who were assumed to have taken adequate amounts of food simply because it was available. Unfortunately, food intake was not measured in any of these studies. The hypothesis, which links psychological problems and growth, later appeared to gain support from endocrine findings of irregular growth hormone release (54). It is still not known whether the observed growth hormone abnormalities are sufficiently severe and consistent to cause growth failure of the degree seen in PSD, whether they are the result of chronic and/or intermittent malnutrition, or whether a specific and purely emotional insult is indeed operative via a direct effect on growth-regulating centers in the hypothalamus.

Unresponsiveness of the pituitary gland to stimuli for growth hormone release has been a consistent finding in all reported studies of psychosocial dwarfs, but only slightly more than half of the cases were affected. The high incidence of decreased growth hormone response led some observers to coin the name *reversible hyposomatotropism* (50). Random tests of plasma growth hormone on the day of hospital admission revealed elevated values in one study (55). Unresponsiveness to Metapirone, which is also a sign of hypopituitarism, was reported by Powell (54) in his study of patients with growth hormone deficiency, but this finding has since been attributed to insufficient dosage rather than to actual failure to respond to the negative feedback stimulus (18). Growth hormone therapy has been tried in a few cases and does not cause a growth spurt.

Infants with MDS generally have elevated plasma growth hormone levels that rise further after provocative stimulation with hypoglycemia (55), arginine, or exercise (11). Other abnormalities have been found in both patients with MDS and those with PSD, including low somatomedin (14), decreased total and free throxine, and high basal metabolic rates per unit of body weight (20). These alterations are not the cause of the growth failure; they are also found in primary malnutrition and malnutrition due to organic disease. Elevated cortisol secretion rates, on the other hand, were observed in infants with MDS and in patients with PSD, but not in those with malnutrition due to organic disease (17).

Nutrition

Growth failure in MDS is, according to most observers, the result of caloric undernutrition. This was demonstrated in an experiment where understimulation was continued for a brief period, either in a hospital isolation room or in the infant's home. Food was provided in a perfunctory manner, and any kind of stimulation was avoided. A majority ate well and gained accordingly at an accelerated rate; only a few infants took an insufficient amount of calories and did not gain (52). This suggests that notwithstanding histories to the contrary, most infants were not given enough food by their caretakers. Histories of ravenous eating thus seem to reflect the good appetite of these infants but not the actual intake. A good appetite is readily confirmed in the hospital and facilitates rehabilitation. The eating behavior is incongruous in view of the malnourished physical condition of these infants.

The reasons that infants with good appetites are not nurtured and fed while cared for in the home are usually related to the parents' psychological status. The majority have a personality disorder and are unable to perceive and relate to the needs of others, including the infant (56). The behavior of these infants facilitates underfeeding, as they are frequently undemanding or become so with time. The conclusion that can be drawn from these observations on the pathogenesis of growth failure is supported by a primate study showing that monkeys reared in isolation eat well and grow normally even though the emotional insult is severe enough to cause fear, absence of social play, and autistic posturing (57).

Observers have found it difficult to explain how growth failure can persist once these infants mature sufficiently, since they are then no longer completely dependent on the parents and are usually able to compete for food. The persistence of growth failure under these circumstances requires unusual conditions. These conditions are apparently not common, since the incidence of PSD is low compared to that of MDS. Food deprivation in older children with PSD occurs through several mechanisms: (*1*) food restriction as a form of abuse, (*2*) oppositional food refusal by the child, (*3*) anorexia during periods of depression, and (*4*) iatrogenic food restriction imposed during treatment of diarrhea, which is common in PSD because the large, mushy stools of the children are frequently misdiagnosed as being due to malabsorption. Published accounts all mention similar means and rationalizations for food restrictions, such as making the child wear a sign when out of doors telling neighbors, "Don't feed me!"; placing food where it is out of reach of the patient; or reasoning that eating excessively is bad for the child because of diarrhea, a bloated stomach, or for other health reasons. Admissions of intentional starvation from parents who had originally reported large food intakes have been reported (49). Home feeding experiments conducted in three patients with PSD gave results similar to those obtained in the isolation experiments for MDS and showed that patients with PSD can gain if they are given enough calories (18).

Environmental Factors, Including Maternal Characteristics

Parents who are unable to nurture their infants sufficiently to promote growth and development usually have psychological disorders that explain this deficit. Psychotics fail because they are frequently out of touch with reality, while neurotics are consumed by intrapsychic conflict. The parent with a personality disorder is unable to perceive and relate to the needs of others, including the child. Due to the nature of these three disorders, these parents may not be aware that they are failing in their parental responsibility because they are either not motivated or not able to care enough or do not perceive the infant's condition realistically.

Situational stress may be equally incapacitating. Parent's who find themselves in an undesirable situation economically, emotionally, or otherwise may be overcome by a feeling of hopelessness and futility. This, in turn, often leads to apathy and withdrawal or to feelings of anger and resentment, thus further impairing parental capacity and positive interaction with the child.

Parental behavior that leads to deprivation of the child is frequently rooted in experiences of the past. Thus, parents who were inadequately nurtured by their own parents may simply not be aware of the full complement of roles they must play. Parents who were not given the opportunity to mature and develop realistic goals have remained "infants" themselves, with dependency needs that prevent them from being effective in caring for their child.

There appears to be a high incidence of personality disorders among parents of infants with MDS (56). They tend to neglect the child and do not interact enough. On the other hand, parents of children with PSD do interact with the child but in a manner deterimental to the child's emotional development. They share certain characteristics with parents who batter their children, evidenced by the high incidence of fractures and proven battering in PSD (49). The parents' attitude toward the child is restrictive, manipulative, and punitive. They have rigid child-rearing ideas and make unreasonable demands that the child cannot meet, thus providing for themselves a reason for venting their hostilities. The child is viewed as the antagonist, and any deviant behavior is, therefore, often misconstrued as a cunning device to test the parents' patience or to challenge their authority.

In contrast to parents of infants with MDS, parents of psychosocial dwarfs often exhibit an affective relationship with the child that makes a good impression during the initial interview. These parents are usually able to give an informed history and show that they have provided adequate health care, such as immunizations and health checkups, and seem to lead stable lives. Hidden under the veneer of the "good parent" however, are insecurity, identity problems, or repression of conflict. Careful observation may show that the children are handled inconsistently, with demonstrative cuddling at one time and severe punishment the next. It is not surprising that the product of this upbringing is a child with equally inconsistent behavior: violently oppositional on one hand and overly compliant on the other. During the office visit, these children frequently make a good impression, acting well behaved and friendly. This behavior is deceptive and delays recognition of the syndrome.

Energy Balance

The role of energy expenditures is an important consideration in patients who have a ravenous appetite and are supposed to have a good food intake in the face of growth failure. The basal metabolic rate (BMR) in MDS is low for age and, by and large, normal for height, height age, or weight predicted from height, but is elevated in relation to actual body weight. A high BMR per actual body weight is caused by a preponderance of metabolically active tissues, such as the brain and parenchymal organs, over fat and muscle tissues with lower metabolic rate. The BMR per body weight decreases during recovery, as fat and muscle weight increases. By contrast, the BMR per weight predicted from height remains close to normal and is stable during weight recovery (58). The exception is in patients with clinical signs of severe malnutrition, evidenced by redundant skin folds, who have a low BMR for height age (20). After realimentation this value usually rises within 1 or more weeks to a normal range, where it then holds steady throughout the period of weight recovery.

Since caloric intake and BMR are customarily judged by norms using body weight as a reference standard, it is understandable why observers gain the impression that calorie requirements are abnormally high in MDS. Requirements seem higher still in PSD because many patients have elevated BMRs both for weight predicted from height (Fig. 3-8) and for actual body weight. Inefficiency of cellular metabolism is not the reason for the high BMR, because absolute values do not decrease during recovery.

The relation between intake and weight gain has been studied in infants with MDS, and it was found that the energy cost for weight gain is not different from that in control subjects with malnutrition due to organic causes, including congenital heart disease (59). These data cannot be extrapolated to PSD because insomnia, restlessness, and intermittent diarrhea increase caloric expenditures.

Gastrointestinal Function

A negative energy balance may develop in those patients with PSD who have a history of loose stools, However, tests of absorptive and digestive function have not shown abnormality (47). It is possible, therefore, that the loose stools merely reflect an irritable colon. Malnutrition or gastrointestinal infections caused by garbage eating probably influence gastrointestinal function in isolated cases. It is also possible that a mixed meal with natural roughage is handled differently than single foodstuffs that are used in routine absorption tests. This possibility was suggested by findings of decreased nitrogen absorption in two of three cases tested (18).

Malnutrition seems to precede the appearance of loose stools. Recovery occurs in the hospital despite persistence of loose stools for several weeks, providing the patients are given as much food as they want. Unfortunately, patients are frequently placed on restrictive diets because of the loose stools; consequently, malnutrition is aggravated. These observations suggest that malabsorption is not the primary cause of growth failure, although intestinal losses contribute in some cases to the caloric deficit.

Diagnosis

There is no symptom complex that establishes the diagnosis of MDS or PSD conclusively, because all described findings may be the result of other diseases that cause mental retardation and are associated with feeding problems that lead to malnutrition. It is also not possible to establish the diagnosis by identification of psychological factors that are conducive to, or consistent with, environmental deprivation. This is evidenced by the finding that siblings of affected children often do not show the signs of grossly inadequate parenting. Moreover, reliance on weight for age as a sign of FTT is misleading, because it is low in other conditions, including primordial and small-for-gestational-age dwarfism. Since the incidence of these disorders is highest among underprivileged inner-city populations, where MDS is also prevalent, misdiagnosis is common, especially if too much emphasis is placed on environmental factors conducive to deprivation. Consequently, diagnosis of MDS or PSD rests mainly on the therapeutic trial, demonstration of a growth spurt and improvement of developmental and affective status upon removal from the growth-retarding environment.

Improvement is readily detected in underweight infants and children because they usually start to gain weight immediately when they are offered enough calories. Moreover, since there is normally a clustering of developmental milestones in infancy, improvement is easily recognized. For example, a 2-year-old who is unable to sit alone may learn, during a short hospitalization, developmental tasks that normally take much longer to achieve (i.e., to sit, stand, pull up, walk, etc.). Diagnosis through observation of improvement is more difficult in PSD when these children are no longer underweight, because rapid weight gain cannot be expected if the child's weight is already proportionate for height. Consequently, a significant increase in linear growth rate and developmental improvement remain as the only means for a positive diagnosis. These changes may not be recognizable for several months. It is, therefore, not feasible in these cases to use a hospital stay to establish the diagnosis through the therapeutic trial.

Treatment

Intervention strategies should be based on the assessment of a number of interrelated factors: (*1*) the cause of the parents' dysfunction, (*2*) the severity of the dysfunction, (*3*) the prognosis for correcting the existing problem, and (*4*) the time necessary to achieve meaningful change. In addition, one must evaluate whether parental dysfunction is confined to the child in question, whether parents are willing to participate in the intervention plan, and whether the child is at risk of sustaining physical abuse by remaining in the home.

The two major intervention options are (*1*) working to help the parents overcome the psychological problems that cause their ineffectiveness and (*2*) finding a temporary or permanent parental substitute, either among relatives or through foster home placement. If meaningful change cannot be accomplished within a reasonable time, it is advisable to place the child temporarily in foster care, especially when the child is at risk of starvation or physical abuse. When the infant does stay at home, it is mandatory that progress be monitored through assessment of development, affective status, and physical growth. Theoretically, at least, parents can be induced to feed their children without significantly changing their overall functioning. It is therefore important that one does not rely solely on growth recovery as an indicator of environmental change.

Physicians and social workers must be aware that negative attitudes and biases toward the parents are detrimental to an effective intervention process. Although it is necessary to confront the parents with evidence that they have underfed and understimulated the child, it is counterproductive to communicate criticism and condemnation, either overt or implied, since this only serves to alienate them and create a barrier to establishing the type of relationship that is necessary for successful treatment.

Depending on the underlying problem, one can try to eliminate environmental stresses or to eliminate the impact of adverse psychological factors through psychotherapy and supportive casework. It is helpful to reduce the demands on the parents to a level within their capacity, perhaps through day-care placement of the infant or provision of a housekeeper and babysitter. Parents with character disorders need help in all phases of life, since they are often not able to assess the requirements of the child or the family. An effective program should extend over a long period of time in order to assist such parents in learning to conceptualize and deal with their roles as parents to their children and as people in a complex society.

In cases with PSD, prospects of trying to rehabilitate the family are, unfortunately, very poor. These parents hold on to the child because they have a need to act out their own problems through the child, who becomes the scapegoat. They consequently tend to resist psychotherapy, fight foster home placement, do not keep appointments, and frequently move away. A careful, tactical approach is needed, aimed at gaining cooperation while maintaining surveillance to safeguard the child until a solution can be worked out. It is often counterproductive to focus all attention on the child, because this may be resented by the parents, who need help themselves. Development of a treatment plan and cooperation are facilitated if one can start by fulfilling some self-recognized needs of the parents.

ANOREXIA NERVOSA

Clinical Description

Etiology

The term *anorexia nervosa* was first used in 1874 by Sir William Gull (60), who also suggested an alternate name, *anorexia hysterica*. He attributed the disorder to "willful starvation." Investigators have since sought to prove that this disorder is due to primary hypothalamic dysfunction, which they thought was responsible for the patient's refusal to eat as well as for other manifestations known to be of central origin (i.e., amenorrhea, hypothermia, and hyperactivity). However, all investigations so far indicate that these manifestations are secondary, since they are recognized sequelae of malnutrition and disappear in anorexia nervosa upon weight recovery. Thus, concepts concerning the etiology of anorexia nervosa have come around full swing since the first description; most observers now feel that this is a psychiatric disorder that leads to starvation as only one sign of psychological conflict.

Psychodynamics

Major dieting is endemic and epidemic among young women in the United States. This cultural trend is utilized by troubled adolescents who carry dieting to an extreme. There may well be a continuum ranging from normal weight control and preoocupation with currently popular vegetarian diets to willful starvation. It has been estimated that 1% to 2% of young women develop anorexia nervosa (61). Incidence figures vary depending on the criteria used.

The disorder is precipitated by the adolescent's struggle for independence and identity. Characteristic predisposing factors can be identified both in the patient's premorbid personality and the milieu that created it. Thus, the age of onset is puberty. Very few young men are affected after that time, whereas women may develop the disease up to their thirties. Girls with anorexia nervosa outnumber boys 20 to 1. In Bruch's series, 50% of the children were firstborn (62). In the United States they come typically from white, middle-class families and a fairly stable environment. Either because of the parents' demands or the example they set, these children are achievement oriented and disciplined and tend to be overcritical of themselves. Self-expression has not been encouraged, and the children are introverted. Most descriptions mention that they are of above-average intelligence, which probably reflects their willingness to study more than their native intelligence. While they appear to be well-behaved, model children, they seem too compliant and too neat. Sibling rivalry usually has been very intense.

As they reach the teens, they find outside influences and the challenges of growing up disturbing, because they are afraid of what they are not able to control. As a consequence they tend not to expose themselves to the world around them, avoid strangers, and withdraw more into study and books. They are uninterested in sex and are uncomfortable with interpersonal relationships in general. It has been suggested that self-starvation is used subconsciously as a means to avoid breast development. As they struggle to keep their environment in order and impulses under control, they increase the restrictions they impose on themselves and make up new and unnecessary rules of behavior. Thus perfectionism may turn into obsessive-compulsiveness, and they may wish others around them to conform to their rules. Relations with family members consequently become strained; they are irritable, impatient with others, and often depressed. The disturbed struggle for control carries over into their eating. It is this observer's impression that many of these girls have features in common with parents who restrict food intake in their children and cause psychosocial dwarfism (see above), which may be regarded as a form of "anorexia nervosa by proxy."

Eating Behavior

Patients with anorexia nervosa frequently have been chubby prior to the onset of their disease. They may have been ridiculed and may have begun dieting for sound reasons. In the process they become knowledgeable about cooking and the nutrient content of foods. They often enjoy preparing meals for themselves and others, possibly motivated by the need to control the calorie content. In time they become pathologically preoccupied with food. They may plan the daily meals well in advance, hoard their special food items, and develop elaborate eating rituals. If they are forced to eat more than they allow for themselves, they invent routines that conceal the fact that they did not eat. Thus, they may crumble food on the plate to distribute it or hide food and lie about the amount eaten. Self-induced vomiting is not uncommon. Nevertheless, these patients intermittently go on eating binges, only to diet even more rigorously afterward or to use laxatives. As they lose weight, they deny the seriousness of their weight deficit. A disturbed body image, which is a commonly used description in the literature, refers to the fact that these malnourished youngsters may sincerely believe themselves to be too fat. To further promote weight loss, they tend to be active and exercise to a degree that is astonishing in view of their frailty. They are driven to be always on the move. Some observers have considered this to be another manifestation of a primary central nervous system disorder, comparable to the diencephalic syndrome. However, slow respirations, bradycardia, and other signs of a lowered metabolism are not compatible with this concept.

The diet of these patients differs from the common starvation-level diet in that it is usually protein rich and high in vegetables and raw fruits. The common finding of hypercarotenemia (63) is probably due to a high intake of carrots and other carotene-rich vegetables, because metabolic abnormalities that could explain it have not been found. Many patients take vitamin supplements that they believe will maintain health despite the energy deficiency.

Diagnosis and Differential Diagnosis

Although the diagnostic criteria used by different investigators vary somewhat, they all include those listed in Table 5-1. Thus, they agree that age is typical; weight deficit must be severe and due to an active refusal to eat. To rule out any justified organic reason for food refusal, unusual behavior aimed at weight reduction must be evident. Many investigators place emphasis on the presence of amenorrhea. However, this should be viewed as only one of several endocrine changes in response to severe malnutrition (see below).

Patients with anorexia nervosa are emaciated yet not lethargic. They tend to be unusually active unless they are in extremis. Manifestations of malnutrition may include bradycardia, slow respirations, hypothermia, and hypotension, which are all signs of a decreased metabolic rate. The skin is dry, and downy hair may cover the neck, cheeks, forearms, and legs. Yellow pigmentation, which tends to be more pronounced over the palms and soles but spares the conjunctiva, is evidence of carotenemia. Constipation is due to diminished food intake.

The differential diagnosis includes disorders that are capable of producing severe malnutrition, but are not associated with obvious signs of the primary disorder. Hypothalamic or suprasellar tumors should be considered, as well as occult malignancy. X-rays and scans of multiple systems may be necessary, although the clinical signs of a decreased metabolic rate speak against malignancy. Acquired lesions of the adrenal glands (Addison's disease) may be confused with anorexia nervosa. How-

Table 5-1. Anorexia Nervosa: Diagnostic Criteria

Onset between age 10 and 30 years
Weight loss, with body weights <15% of normal weight for height, with secondary manifestations of severe malnutrition, including hypothermia, bradycardia, endocrine changes (amenorrhea, etc.)
Exclusion of primary organic disease
Evidence of active refusal to eat
Unusual behavior aimed at weight reduction, including overactivity, denial of serious weight deficit, unusual preoccupations with food, and self-induced vomiting

ever, these patients are lethargic and have muscle weakness, episodes of hypoglycemia, and typical electrolytes (i.e., low sodium and chloride and elevated potassium). Signs of decreased pituitary function exist in both anorexia nervosa and primary pituitary disease. Acquired pituitary lesions therefore should be ruled out. Bartter's syndrome must be considered in cases with hypokalemic alkalosis. The age group affected by anorexia nervosa is the same that predisposes to ulcerative colitis and Crohn's disease. Since girls are frequently embarrassed by diarrhea and may hide its occurrence, it is necessary to inquire or test specifically for bowel manifestations.

Laboratory Workup

The recommended tests (Table 5-2) are designed (*1*) to rule out those disorders that enter the differential diagnosis and (*2*) to exclude common complications of anorexia nervosa, including vitamin and trace metal deficiency and, especially, electrolyte disturbances due to laxative abuse or self-induced vomiting. A not uncommon and potentially serious complication is hypokalemia (64), which may lead to muscle weakness and cardiac arrhythmias. It is probably also responsible for the gastric dilatation that may follow refeeding. The usual cause of hypokalemia and hypochloremic alkalosis is self-induced vomiting, although it has been speculated that hyperaldosteronism, induced by hypovolemia, is a factor. Physicians often

Table 5-2. Diagnostic Laboratory Workup

Test	*Reason/Finding*
1. Hemoglobin, blood smear	R/O anemia (Fe or Cu deficiency)
2. Serum albumin and globulin	R/O hypoalbuminemia (uncommon)
3. Serum chloride and potassium	R/O Addison's disease (high K) R/O self-induced vomiting (low K and Cl)
4. Blood pH	R/O self-induced vomiting (alkalosis)
5. Electrolytes, including calcium and phosphorus; BUN; urinalysis, including specific gravity after fluid restriction for 12 hours	R/O secondary renal dysfunction
6. Stool inspection	R/O bowel disease
7. Serum carotene	R/O malabsorption (low in malabsorption, elevated in anorexia nervosa)
8. X-rays: skull and CT scan, Abdominal flat plate, GI series Bone survey	R/O suture separation; erosion of sella turcica due to pituitary lesion R/O malignancy R/O malignancy; determine bone age

hesitate to confront these patients about their self-induced vomiting because they give no indication of it and are able to conceal the fact even during hospitalization. It should be realized, however, that chronic malnutrition rarely causes abnormal acid–base balance and that acute starvation causes metabolic ketoacidosis rather than alkalosis. Serum proteins, which are commonly determined to assess protein nutriture, are usually normal in these patients (65).

Tests of vitamin nutriture and trace mineral status should be performed only if indicated by clinical findings. Because the dietary preferences of these patients vary, abnormalities tend to be inconsistent. Serum iron and copper should be tested in cases with anemia. Low plasma zinc and copper values have been reported (66). Low plasma zinc values were poorly correlated with taste acuity and cannot be considered a cause of the patients' eating behavior. Plasma zinc may be low as a result of stress, although it is possible that zinc nutriture is marginal and may become critical after refeeding, when the metabolic rate rises and growth resumes. Thus, zinc deficiency may be responsible for the loss of hair that is sometimes observed during recovery. Carotenemia has been reported with unusual frequency. Since serum carotene is also a good screening test for fat absorption, it appears to be a useful test in the diagnostic workup. High values are apparently not due to deficiency of retinol-binding proteins (66) but reflect dietary habits.

Endocrine Changes

Because of the amenorrhea, which is a typical manifestation of the syndrome, endocrine functions have been the subject of intensive investigation. These studies have uniformly shown abnormalities in gonadotropin function (67,68), with a reduction in follicle stimulating hormone (FSH) and luteinizing hormone (LH) but in many cases a normal response to intravenous LH-releasing hormone (LHRH) (69). Similar abnormalities occur in nonpsychiatric patients who lose weight (70). According to Wakeling (68), amenorrhea is not associated with changes in prolactin.

The parallel between anorexia nervosa and chronic malnutrition applies also to growth hormone function. With few exceptions, growth hormone levels have been elevated. However, despite the increased secretion of growth hormone, plasma somatomedin was low in 8 of 17 cases studied by Rappaport (71). Prolonged administration of growth hormone in one case did not stimulate the generation of somatomedin activity. Observations on somatomedin activity are similar in chronic malnutrition unassociated with psychopathology as well as the psychosocial deprivation, where growth hormone administration had no effect either.

Plasma T_4 and T_3 are decreased, according to most studies (72), and the response to releasing hormone (TRH) is delayed (73). Surprisingly, in one study, T_3 was even lower than in patients with primary myxedema (74). These endocrine abnormalities account for the clinical manifestations that reflect hypometabolism: dry skin, bradycardia, and slow respirations. T_3 rises first after refeeding.

The plasma cortisol level is elevated in anorexia nervosa (75), and the diurnal rhythm may be lost. Disagreement exists over the cause of the hypercortisolism, which may be due to increased cortisol secretion or a slow turnover as a result of depressed metabolism. The response of the adrenal glands to ACTH is increased (67), and the pituitary responds poorly to suppression with dexamethasone (67).

There are other abnormalities that seem to be caused by hypothalamic dysfunction. Thus, patients with anorexia nervosa often show a partial loss of renal concentrating ability, which responds to pitressin (69). This abnormality reverses to normal upon weight recovery. In addition, catecholamine metabolism has been studied, and several reports suggest that plasma norepinephrine and urinary excretion of homovanillic acid are decreased (76).

Treatment

Most physicians agree that treatment should be primarily psychiatric, but they differ on the tactic and the degree to which adequate food intake should be enforced. Hospital admission is usually necessary once weight deficit is severe. Ideally, intervention through ambulatory psychotherapy should begin earlier, but this is rarely possible since these patients hide the fact that they do not eat, while they willingly subject themselves to medical investigations that are ordered because of the "unexplained" weight loss. Thus, the diagnosis is not made until it is finally realized that there is no organic disease and that dietary management does not work. By this time these patients are usually severely emaciated.

Upon hospital admission, correction of electrolyte imbalances is often necessary, and parenteral alimentation may be indicated unless the patient is able and willing to eat. Nasogastric tube feeding is not desirable because it represents to the patient an expression of force and domination. Oral refeeding should proceed parallel with intravenous alimentation. A regular diet may be ordered, but food preferences should be honored, providing the daily requirements can be met. However, the high-volume, low-calorie foods that are usually chosen by the patients make this difficult. Initially, meals must be small and frequent to avoid gastric dilatation. Diet orders should be specific about the number of meals per day and the management, including the "consequences" that result when the patient does not eat the entire meal within the allotted time. Personnel should be warned that these patients bargain themselves out of eating and manipulate the caretakers to make it possible for them to hide both food and regurgitated material. To give but one example, this observer once solved the "mystery" of hypokalemic alkalosis by eventually locating the vomitus inside towels that were hid regularly on the bottom of a large laundry hamper. Thus, such patients should wear only a hospital gown during meals, and an attendant should be present during the meal and for an hour thereafter. If this is not possible, a rest period may be prescribed after a meal, during which the bathroom must be locked. The patients should know that only a specified time is allowed for eating and that any deficit will be made up by increasing the intravenous alimentation.

There is considerable disagreement over the psychological approach to therapy. Some physicians advise a permissive approach that intentionally avoids all emphasis on eating. However, this is not practical when the patient is severely emaciated and when alimentation becomes a lifesaving measure. The opposite approach is one of using "consequences" for not eating that take the form of punishment, at least from the viewpoint of the patient, who is struggling for control of her life and is therefore very sensitive to any form of force or dominance.

Intravenous alimentation may be regarded as a form of negative reinforcement which is prescribed, like medication, in a perfunctory, nonpunitive manner by medical personnel not involved with psychotherapy. Drugs, such as chlorpromazine, that reduce anxiety may also be used. Thus, the patient is handled like any other case with an organic disease. It is important that insight-oriented therapy proceeds simultaneously with this type of medical management and that the patient is seen daily by the psychotherapist. Since the therapist is not involved with the medical side of management, the patient will not hold him or her responsible for supplementary alimentation or other measures. Parents should not become involved, either. The extent to which behavior therapy is used has been a subject of controversy. Bruch (77) considers it a simplistic and potentially dangerous approach that neglects the inner turmoil of the patient. On the other hand, Stunkard (78) has reported excellent results with his type of behavior therapy, at least if judged by the amount of weight gain that was accomplished. He used physical activity and permission to go outside the hospital as a reward every day the morning weight was 0.5 lb above that of the preceding day. However, long-term results of behavior therapy have not been better than those of other methods. Indeed, cooperation by the patient during hospitalization may be only a means of gaining back control by getting out of the hospital. Consequently, it is not surprising that reported recurrence rates after any form of therapy have been as high as 50%. A combination of medical, dietary, and insight-oriented therapy appears to be the most promising approach. Long-term psychotherapy is necessary after discharge from the hospital.

REFERENCES

1. Gomez F, Galvan RR, Frink S, Munoz JC, et al: Mortality in second and third degree malnutrition. *J Trop Pediatr* 2:77, 1956.

2. Waterlow JC: Classification and definition of protein-calorie malnutrition. *Br Med J* 3:566, 1972.
3. Arroyane G, Wilson D, DeFunes C, et al: The free amino acids in blood plasma of children with kwashiorkore and marasmus. *Am J Clin Nutr* 11:517, 1962.
4. Abbott OD, Townsend RO, French RB, et al: Carpal and epiphyseal development: Another index of nutritional status of rural school children. *Am J Dis Child* 79:69, 1950.
5. Dreizen S, Spirakis CN, Stone RE: Chronic undernutrition and postnatal ossification: Effect on time and sequence of appearance of the postnatal ossification centers in the human hand skeleton. *Am J Dis Child* 108:44, 1964.
6. Winick M, Rosso P: Head circumference and cellular growth of the brain in normal and marasmic children. *J Pediatr* 74:774, 1969.
7. Capitanio MA, Kirkpatrick JA: Widening of the cranial sutures. *Radiology* 92:53, 1969.
8. Vahlquist B, Engsner G, Sjögren I: Malnutrition and size of the cerebral ventricles: Echoencephalographic studies in infants and young children, preliminary communication. *Acta Paediatr Scand* 60:533, 1971.
9. Holt LE, Snyderman SE, Norton PM, et al: The plasma aminogram in Kwashiorkor. *Lancet* 2:1343, 1963.
10. Ghisolfi J, Charlet P, Ser N, et al: Plasma free amino acids in normal children and in patients with protein-caloric malnutrition fasting and infection. *Pediatr Res* 12:912, 1978.
11. Gardner LI, Amacher P (eds): *Endocrine Aspects of Malnutrition, Kwashiorkor and Psychosocial Deprivation.* Santa Yvez, Calif, Kroc Foundation, 1973.
12. Pimstone BL, Barbezat G, Hansen JD, et al: Studies on growth hormone secretion in protein-calorie malnutrition. *Am J Clin Nutr* 21:482, 1968.
13. Robinson H, Picou D: A comparison of fasting plasma insulin and growth hormone concentrations in marasmus, kwashiorkor, marasmic kwashiorkor and underweight children. *Pediatr Res* 11:637, 1977.
14. VandenBrande JL, Ducin MVL: Plasma somatomedin activity in children with growth disturbances, in Raiti S (ed): *Advances in Human Growth Hormone Research,* DHEW Publication (NIH) 74-612, Bethesda, Md, 1974, p 98.
15. Hintz RL, Suskind R, Amatayakul K, et al: Plasma somatomedin and growth hormone values in children with protein-calorie malnutrition. *J Pediatr* 92:153, 1978.
16. Van Buul SC, Dumoleijn L, Korteland AM, et al: The snell-dwarf mouse: Interrelationship of growth in length and weight, serum somatomedin activity, and sulfate incorporation in costal cartilage during growth hormone and thyroxine treatment. *Proceedings of the International Symposium on Somatomedins and Growth,* Santa Margherita, Italy, 1978. New York, Academic Press, 1978.
17. Krieger I, Good MH: Adrenocortical and thyroid function in the deprivation syndrome: Comparison with growth failure due to undernutrition, congenital heart disease or prenatal influences. *Am J Dis Child* 120:95, 1975.
18. Krieger I: Endocrines and nutrition in psychosocial deprivation in the USA: Comparison with growth failure due to malnutrition on an organic bases, in Gardner LJ, Amacher P (eds): *Endocrine Aspects of Malnutrition, Marasmus, Kwashiorkor and Psychosocial Deprivation.* Santa Ynez, Calif, Kroc-Foundation, 1973, pp 129, 154.
19. Graham GG, Baerte JM, Claeyssen G, et al: Thyroid hormonal studies in severely malnourished Peruvian infants and small children. *J Pediatr* 83:321, 1973.
20. Krieger I, Taqi Q: Free serum thyroxine level and basal metabolic rate: Aids to diagnosis in malnutrition and small-for-gestational age dwarfism. *Am J Dis Child* 129:830, 1975.
21. Montgomery RD: Changes in basal metabolic rate of the malnourished infant and their relation to body composition. *J Clin Invest* 41:1653, 1962.
22. Krieger I, Whitten C: Energy metabolism in infants with growth failure due to maternal

deprivation, undernutrition or causes unknown: II. Relation between nitrogen balance, weight gain, and postprandial excess heat production. *J Pediatr* 75:374, 1969.

23. Ashworth A: Metabolic rates during recovery from protein-calorie malnutrition: The need for a new concept of specific dynamic action. *Nature* 223:407, 1969.
24. Viteri FE, Schneider RE: Gastrointestinal alterations of protein calorie malnutrition. *Med Clin North Am* 58: 1487, 1974.
25. Stanfield JP, Hutt MSR, Tunnicliffe R: Intestinal biopsy in Kwashiorkore. *Lancet* 2:519, 1965.
26. Lindenbaum J, Gerson CD, Kent TH: Recovery of small intestinal structure and function after residence in the tropics: I. Studies in Peace Corps volunteers. *Ann Intern Med* 74:218, 1971.
27. Schneider RE, Viteri FE: Luminal events of lipids absorption in protein calorie malnourished children: Relationship with nutritional recovery and diarrhea: I. Capacity of the duodenal content to achieve micellar solubilization in lipids. *Am J Clin Nutr* 27:777, 1974.
28. Barbezat GO, Hansen JDL: The exocrine pancreas in protein-calorie malnutrition. *Pediatrics* 42:77, 1968.
29. Viteri FE, Flores JM, Alvarado J, et al: Intestinal malabsorption in malnourished children before and during recovery: Relation between severity of protein deficiency and the malabsorption process. *Am J Dig Dis* 18:201, 1973.
30. Bilir S: Acquired disaccharide intolerance in children with malnutrition. *Am J Clin Nutr* 25:644, 1972.
31. Leslie J, MacLean WC Jr, Graham GG: Effect of an episode of severe malnutrition and age on lactose absorption by recovered infants and children. *Am J Clin Nutr* 32:971, 1979.
32. Chapin HDA: A plan of dealing with atrophic infants and children. *Arch Pediatr* 25:491, 1908.
33. Bakwin H: Loneliness in infants. *Am J Dis Child* 63:30, 1942.
34. Spitz RA: Hospitalism: An inquiry into the genesis of psychiatric conditions in early childhood. *Psychoanal Study Child* 1:53, 1945.
35. Spitz RA: Hospitalism: A follow-up report. *Psychoanal Study Child* 2:113, 1946.
36. Widdowson EM: Mental contentment and physical growth. *Lancet* 1:1316, 1951.
37. Provence SA, Lipton RC: *Infants in Institutions*. New York, International University Press, Inc, 1962.
38. Sokoff N, Yaffe S, Weintraub D, et al: Effects of handling on the subsequent developments of premature infants. *Devl Psychol* 1:765, 1969.
39. Solkoff N, Matuszak D: Tactile stimulation and behavioral development among low-birth weight infants. *Child Psychiatry Hum Dev* 6:33, 1975.
40. Bowlby J: *Attachment*, Attachment and Loss Series, vol 1. New York, Basic Books Inc, 1969.
41. Schaffer HR, Callender WM: Psychological effects of hospitalization in infancy. *Pediatrics* 24:520, 1959.
42. Kennell JH, Rolnick A: Discussing problems in newborn babies with their parents. *Pediatrics* 26:832, 1960.
43. Kennell JH, Jerauld R, Wolfe H, et al: Maternal behavior one year after early and extended postpartum contact. *Dev Med Child Neurol* 16:172, 1974.
44. Blau A, Slaff B, Easton R, et al: The psychogenic etiology of premature births—a preliminary report. *Psychosom Med* 25:201, 1963.

45. Klaus MH, Jerauld R, Kreger N, et al: Maternal attachment: Importance of the first postpartum days. *N Engl J Med* 286:460, 1972.
46. Hales D, Lozoff B, Sosa R, et al: Defining limits of the sensitive period. *Dev Med Child Neurol* 19:454, 1977.
47. Silver JK, Finkelstein M: Deprivation dwarfism. *J Pediatr* 70:317, 1967.
48. Powell GF, Brasel JA, Blizzard RF: Emotional deprivation and growth retardation simulating true idiopathic hypopituitarism: I. Clinical evaluation of the syndrome. *N Engl J Med* 276:1271, 1967.
49. Krieger I: Food restriction as a form of child abuse in ten cases of psychosocial deprivation dwarfism. *Clin Pediatr* 13:127, 1974.
50. Money J: The syndrome of abuse dwarfism (psychosocial dwarfism or reversible hyposomatotropism). *Am J Dis Child* 131:508, 1977.
51. Krieger I, Sargent DA: Apostural sign in the sensory deprivation syndrome in infants. *J Pediatr* 70:332, 1967.
52. Whitten CF, Pettit MG, Fischhoff J: Evidence that growth failure from maternal deprivation is secondary to undereating. *JAMA* 209:1675, 1969.
53. Provence SA, Lipton RC: *Infants in Institutions*. New York, International University Press, Inc. 1962.
54. Powell GF, Brasel JA, Raiti S, et al: Emotional deprivation and growth retardation simulating idopathic hypopituitarism: II. Endocrinologic evaluation of the syndrome. *N Engl J Med* 276:1279, 1967.
55. Krieger I, Mellinger RC: Pituitary function in the deprivation syndrome. *J Pediatr* 79:216, 1971.
56. Fischhoff J, Whitten CF, Pettit MG: A psychiatric study of mothers of infants with growth failure secondary to maternal deprivation. *J Pediatr* 79:209, 1971.
57. Harlow HF, Rowland GL, Griffin GA: The effect of total social deprivation on the development of monkey behavior. *Psychiat Res Rep* 19:116, 1964.
58. Krieger I: The energy metabolism in infants with growth failure due to maternal deprivation, undernutrition or causes unknown: I. Metabolic rate calculated from the insensible loss of weight. *Pediatrics* 38:63, 1966.
59. Krieger I, Chen YC: Calorie requirements for weight gain in infants with growth failure due to maternal deprivation, undernutrition, and congenital heart disase: A correlation analysis. *Pediatrics* 44:647, 1969.
60. Gull WW: Anorexia nervosa. *Trans Clin Soc Lond* 7:22, 1874.
61. Crisp AH, Palmer RL, Kalucy RS: How common is anorexia nervosa? A prevalence study. *Br J Psychiatry* 128:549, 1976.
62. Bruch H: *Eating Disorders: Obesity, Anorexia Nervosa and the Person Within*. New York, Basic Books Inc, 1973.
63. Dally PJ: Carotenaemia occurring in a case of anorexia nervosa. *Br Med J* 2:1333, 1959.
64. Warren SE, Steinberg SM: Acid-base and electrolyte disturbances in anorexia nervosa. *Am J Psychiatry* 136:415, 1979.
65. Russell GFM: Metabolic endocrine and psychiatric aspects of anorexia nervosa. *Sci Basis Med Ann Rev* 14:236, 1969.
66. Casper RC, Kirschner B, Sandstead HH, et al: An evaluation of trace metals, vitamins and taste function in anorexia nervosa. *Am J Clin Nutr* 33:1801, 1980.
67. Danowski TS, Livstone E, Gonzales AR, et al: Fractional and partial hypopituitarism in anorexia nervosa. *Hormones* 3:105, 1972.
68. Wakeling A, DeSouza VFA, Gore MBR, et al: Amenorrhoea, body weight and serum

hormone concentrations, with particular reference to prolactin and thyroid hormones in anorexia nervosa. *Psychol Med* 9:265, 1979.

69. Mecklenburg RS, Loriaux DL, Thompson RH, et al: Hypothalamic dysfunction in patients with anorexia nervosa. *Medicine* 53:147, 1974.
70. Vigersky RA, Loriaux DI, Anderson AE, et al: Delayed pituitary hormone response to LRF and TRF in patients with anorexia nervosa and with secondary amenorrhea associated with simple weight loss. *J Clin Endocrinol Metab* 43:893, 1976.
71. Rappaport R, Prevot C, Czernichow P: Somatomedin activity and growth hormone secretion: I. Changes related to body weight in anorexia nervosa. *Acta Paediatr Scand* 69:37, 1980.
72. Moshang T Jr, Parks JS, Baker L, et al: Low serum triiodothyronine in patients with anorexia nervosa. *J Clin Endocrinol Metab* 40:470, 1975.
73. Miyai K, Yamamoto T, Azukizawa M, et al: Serum thyroid hormones and thyrotrophin in anorexia nervosa. *J Clin Endocrinol Metab* 40:334, 1975.
74. Moore R, Mills IH: Serum T_3 and T_4 levels in patients with anorexia nervosa showing transient hyperthyroidism during weight gain. *Clin Endocrinol* 10:443, 1979.
75. Casper RC, Chatterton RT Jr, Davis JM: Alterations in serum cortisol and its binding characteristics in anorexia nervosa. *J Clin Endocrinol Metab* 49:406, 1979.
76. Gross HA, Lake CR, Ebert MH, et al: Catecholamine metabolism in primary anorexia nervosa. *J Clin Endocrinol Metab* 49:805, 1979.
77. Bruch H: Series of behavior modification in treatment of anorexia nervosa. JAMA 230:1419, 1974.
78. Stunkard A: New therapies for the eating disorders: Behavior modification of obesity and anorexia nervosa. *Arch Gen Psychiatry* 26:391, 1972.

6
Growth Abnormalities in Organic Disease

Failure in the past to consider the role of nutrition was in part due to the belief that metabolic abnormalities were the major cause of malnutrition in chronic illness and that nutritional therapy would be of little benefit. This attitude began to change in response to experience with parenteral nutrition and to the finding that positive nitrogen balance and weight recovery were achieved in nutritionally depleted adults with chronic illness, even cancer. Similar observations were made in infants with growth failure due to congenital heart disease who were tube fed an adequate amount of calories and who gained weight (1). There is now strong evidence that recovery can be accelerated in many chronic disorders, that resistance to infection can be strengthened, and that duration of hospitalization can be decreased if attention is paid to the nutritional status of the patient throughout the entire course of illness.

Balanced nutrition is especially vital during periods of rapid growth. The first 6 months of life are most crucial because of the impact of nutrition on CNS development. This is the period when children born with congenital abnormalities often require multiple operations. Especially oropharyngeal, thoracic, and gastrointestinal malformations often interfere with nutrition. Whereas corrective surgery may have been successful, it is still not uncommon for such infants to fail to thrive and not to exceed their birth weight as late as 4 to 6 months of age because of ineffective postoperative management and failure to receive more than maintenance nutritional requirements. These children will almost certainly be left with some degree of mental retardation, be it minimal brain dysfunction or a more profound deficit. Moreover, some case observations suggest that linear growth recovery is limited when a severe nutritional insult occurs in early infancy. These considerations emphasize the need to consider nutrition in the therapy of chronic illness and the prophylaxis of secondary complications.

GENERAL CAUSES OF GROWTH DISTURBANCE

Chronic illness may be associated with either growth failure due to undernutrition or with obesity due to overeating. The growth failure is clinically similar to that caused by undernutrition without organic disease. Weight gain is usually affected first, and linear growth retardaton follows if the insult is prolonged, especially if it occurs during the periods of rapid growth. Moreover, development may be slowed because infants and young children are vulnerable to the physical limitations, decreased vitality, and psychosocial deprivaton imposed by confinement. The term *organic failure to thrive*, which describes delayed growth *and* development, is therefore appropriate for this syndrome.

The mechanism of undernutrition is frequently not readily apparent, although insufficient food intake appears to be the most common cause. Illness, especially one with uncertain course and duration, may cause depression in children. Anaclitic depression, which is accompanied by anorexia and failure to thrive, is a well-recognized disease entity of infants and occurs after prolonged hospitalization and separation from the mother. This syndrome is also called *hospitalism*.

Food intake may be insufficient in the absence of disease-specific causes, even though the caretaker is attentive and loving, because the demands imposed by the care of a chronically ill infant may surpass the capacity of the average person, causing the caretaker to become less effective in administering therapeutically to the child. An insecure or overanxious parent may misinterpret instructions and unwittingly restrict food intake by adhering too rigidly to dietary guidelines, ignoring the infant's demands. Iatrogenic undernutrition occurs in chronic diseases that require diet restrictions, such as allergies and gastrointestinal disorders.

Nutritional deficiencies result when normal intake no longer covers metabolic needs. Caloric requirements may be increased due to fever, or the disease may be associated with restlessness, discomfort, pain, and insomnia, all of which constitute stress that increases catabolism and results in negative energy and nitrogen balance. Surgery, tissue repair, and the synthesis of cells and proteins for host defense mechanisms also raise nutritional requirements because of increased metabolic activity. The imbalance between requirements and intake widens when the illness is associated with organic problems that make eating or retaining food difficult, as in functional immaturity of the oropharyngeal muscles, CNS diseases, or respiratory distress. Finally, a vicious cycle may result, where malnutrition and its attendant effect on the immunodefense system predispose to infections, which in turn aggravate the malnutrition by increasing energy needs.

Whereas undernutrition is the most common form of malnutrition in the chronically ill patient, obesity occurs in disorders that restrict activity but do not impose stress on major organ systems. Excluding endocrine and neurologic disorders, the mechanism responsible for obesity is frequently a disproportionately high calorie intake for the level of expenditure. The psychological impact of illness usually causes anorexia, but it may also lead to overeating, especially if this is a characteristic response of the patient to stress of any kind. Moreover, the so-called enough-is-enough message that normally regulates food intake often does not adjust effectively to sudden changes in activity level. Boredom may be a factor in some situations. However, persistent overeating, by and large, should be considered a sign of more serious psychological problems. Preexisting difficulties, such as a poor self-image, are often aggravated by chronic illness.

SPECIFIC CAUSES OF UNDERNUTRITION

Growth Failure in Congenital Heart Disease (CHD)

Incidence

Statistical studies of the incidence, type, and degree of growth failure in CHD show differences between the various heart conditions that provide some clues concerning the pathogenesis of the growth failure. Thus, patients with cyanotic heart disease, including tetralogy of Fallot (TF), pulmonary atresia (PA), and transposition of the great arteries (TGA), are more severely growth retarded than patients with acyanotic disease. In this group, TGA is the lesion that tends to cause the most severe growth failure. The degree of cyanosis does not correlate with the severity of the growth failure.

The incidence of growth failure in acyanotic lesions, such as patent ductus arteriosus (PDA), aortic stenosis (AS), coarctation of the aorta (CA), and ventricular septal defect (VSD), is only about half that in cyanotic lesions (2). Patients with large left-to-right shunts, pulmonary hypertension, or a history of heart failure most consistently have growth retardation (3). Only a few studies have shown a correlation between the degree of growth failure and the severity of the lesion (4).

Description

Surveys of patients with VSD, PDA, arterial septal defect (ASD), and AS show weight to be affected more often and more severely than height. This suggests that malnutrition at the tissue level is a major factor. Children with CA seem to be different, in that weight is less often affected than height. This type of proportionate growth is seen in genetic short stature and in certain cases of growth failure due to prenatal insults. By far the most common type of growth failure in infants with CHD is the one in which loss of adipose tissue and muscle wasting are very apparent.

Mechanism

Prenatal insults may be the cause of both growth failure and CHD. This is not only suggested by the early onset of proportionate growth retardation but also by the common association of growth failure and other congenital anomalies, including a small head circumference for height. An increased incidence of low birth weights for gestational age in patients with CHD (5) also suggests the operation of prenatal insults. These infants remain small despite nutritional manipulations or surgical correction (6).

In several studies from which patients with signs of prenatal insults to growth and organogenesis were excluded, no correlation was found between the hemodynamic burden and the growth failure. This suggests the operation of yet another important factor, insufficient food intake. Estimates of cell number and cell size in parenchymal organs of infants with CHD who died during the perinatal period revealed a decrease in both cell number and size, a similar pattern to that seen in congenital rubella syndrome. By contrast, older infants had organ and cellular abnormalities that are generally seen in undernutrition (7).

There is no paucity of explanations for undernutrition. A decreased calorie intake by infants with CHD has been documented, but the significance of this observation is difficult to interpret because of the tendency of patients with CHD to be physically less active. On the other hand, energy requirements may be increased because of excessive myocardial and respiratory work or pulmonary infections. Another complication that contributes to undernutrition in heart failure is malabsorption or protein-losing enteropathy incident to venous congestion in the gut.

The most conclusive evidence that undernutrition plays an important role came from a study (1) showing that weight gain and nitrogen retention of infants with growth failure and CHD were negligible during a control period on voluntary food intake. After the introduction of a higher caloric intake through the use of dietary manipulations or intragastric tube feeding, nitrogen retention became positive and accelerated weight gain occurred. Calorie intake was divided into (Fig. 6-1): (*1*) an allotment for the metabolic rate, which was actually measured in that study; and (*2*) an allotment to cover other estimated requirements such as muscular activity and fecal losses. When the remaining calories were related to weight gain, a positive linear correlation could be demonstrated. The ratio between residual calories and weight gain in patients with CHD was similar to that

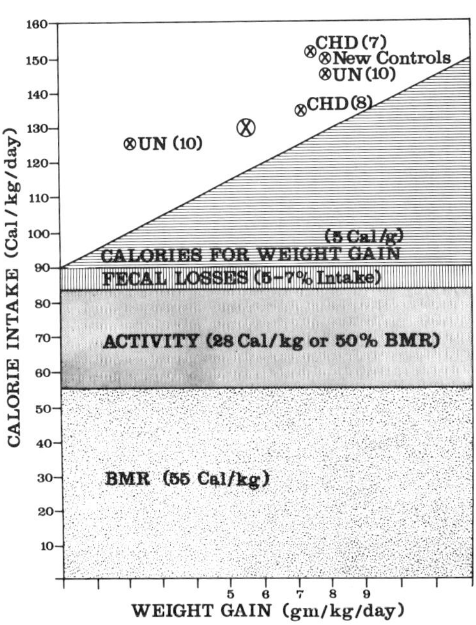

Figure 6-1. CALORIE INTAKE DURING WEIGHT RECOVERY, WITH DIVISION OF CALORIC ENERGY INTAKE INTO EXPENDITURES FOR BMR, ACTIVITY, ESTIMATED FECAL LOSSES, AND WEIGHT GAIN The higher values for malnourished infants with growth failure were attributable to a higher BMR per kilogram body weight. The BMR was calculated from oxygen consumption in seven infants with congenital heart disease, CHD(7), and in the "New Control" group. In the remaining three groups, BMR was calculated from the insensible loss of weight. (Data from studies by Krieger I, et al: *Pediatrics* 44:647, 1969; *Am J Dis Child* 120:497, 1970; *Pediatrics* 38:63, 1966.).

seen in infants with growth failure unassociated with organic disease. The basal metabolic rate per kilogram body weight was also similar in the two groups, but it was significantly higher than in normal control subjects. The relative hypermetabolism of children with growth failure due to undernutrition can be attributed to the preponderance of metabolically active tissues (8).

Growth Failure in Chronic Renal Disease

Incidence

Growth failure may develop in either congenital or acquired disease and in glomerular or tubular involvement. Recurrent urinary tract infections with or without obstructive uropathy are also a common cause of growth failure. Dialysis or renal transplantation, frequently do not correct or prevent its progression (9). The incidence of growth failure in children with renal disease ranges from 35% to 65%. It is highest in the congenital forms (10,11).

Description

Linear growth is retarded in chronic renal disease when there is osteodystrophy caused by hyperparathyroidism in response to phosphorus retention, and failure of active vitamin D formation by renal 1-hydroxylase. A low weight for height, loss of adipose tissue mass, and muscle wasting, which are seen during the active stage of growth failure due to undernutrition, are not uncommon in patients with chronic renal diseases (10). Undernutrition is masked in patients receiving stroid therapy.

Mechanism

In the absence of either uremia or a disturbed acid-base and electrolyte balance, growth failure cannot be attributed to the renal disease. However, if there are radiological changes of renal rickets or osteodystrophy, a direct causal relationship may be assumed. A low weight for height due to loss of adipose tissue and muscle wasting indicate that undernutrition at the tissue level is a factor. Bone age is decreased in both growth failure due to "exogenous" undernutrition and renal disease and consequently does not distinguish between the two causes of growth failure. Renal patients with open epiphyses, who show catch-up growth after institution of therapy, have been described (12). However, children with open epiphyses and renal osteodystrophy generally show less than the expected linear growth with skeletal maturation and loose adult stature, a finding which reflects the complex nature of the growth failure mechanism.

Undernutrition in renal disease can be attributed to the metabolic derangements accompanying renal insufficiency, mainly uremia and acidosis. This effect of acidosis was demonstrated in an experiment where rats made acidotic with ammonium chloride grew more slowly than pairfed control rats (13). Children with short stature due to a tubular acidification defect can be induced to grow at an accelerated rate, but attainment of normal stature for age requires sustained alkali therapy with larger doses than are genrally given (14).

A glomerular filtration rate of 25 ml/min/1.73 m seems to be a critical range below which the growth rate of infants tends to decline. The resultant uremia is one potential cause of growth failure. Electrolyte disturbances, acidosis, the need for excessive water intake interfering with food intake, and a variety of hormonal changes accompanying uremia, including insulin resistance or hyperglucagonemia, may be factors that contribute to the development of growth failure. The role of undernutrition in uremia has been studied in rats, and some studies show that inefficient energy use may also be a factor (15).

Undernutrition due to insufficient intake is probably a more common cause of growth failure in renal disease than has been realized. Children with chronic renal disease are often anorexic and have feeding difficulties. Anorexia may be a direct result of uremic toxins, but emotional depression must be ruled out. A negative energy balance also results from vomiting, intermittent fevers, and irritability, which are frequent accompaniments of renal disease. Calorie intake tends to be deficient in children on hemodialysis (16). A positive correlation between calorie intake and weight gain has been demonstrated in patients with chronic renal insufficiency (17), and in several studies improved growth rates and nitrogen balance were accomplished through calorie supplementation (18,19). Even marginal calorie intakes cause undernutrition in renal disease, because the catabolic rate tends to be increased.

Endocrine and metabolic abnormalities in chronic uremia are similar to those in protein-calorie malnutrition (PCM). For instance, fasting growth hormone levels of uremic subjects are usually elevated, and somatomedin, which mediates the effect of growth hormone on cartilage, is low in growth-retarded children with renal insufficiency (20,21). Following renal transplantation, somatomedin returns toward normal. Plasma amino acids are similar to PCM in that nonessential amino acids tend to be increased and the valine/glycine ratio is decreased.

Primordial and Small-for-Gestational-Age (SGA) Dwarfism

Primordial dwarfism and small-for-gestational-age (SGA) dwarfism are a heterogenous group of disorders with growth failure of prenatal onset due to diverse causes. Although the mechanism of growth failure has been well studied in experimental animals, most types seen in humans remain poorly understood. The term *primordial* indicates that growth potential is "inherently" deficient. Prenatal malnutrition is probably not a common cause of this type of short stature. Postnatal malnutrition may be an associated factor, although it is commonly blamed for growth failure, without proper foundation, in cases that do not have the physical stigma of a prenatal insult. Failure to diagnose the patient with a poor growth potential can have tragic consequences when a parent is falsely accused of having deprived the child. Conversely, failure to recognize postnatal malnutrition in these infants compounds the insult. Familiarity with this entity is therefore of paramount importance in the diagnosis of patients with growth failure.

Incidence

Lubchenco estimates that 30% of all LBW infants are small for gestational age at birth (22). If 10% is a reasonable estimate for the incidence of LBW infants in the United States, one arrives at a figure of about 3% for the incidence of SGA infants. In turn, 38% of these infants remain small after birth, according to Beargie (23), who followed 45 infants for up to 53 months. The incidence of SGA dwarfism is highest in lower socioeconomic populations. Although this has been attributed to protein-calorie malnutrition, other factors, such as harmful drugs, prenatal infection, and deficiency of single nutrients (e.g., folic acid), may be at fault. The fact that malnutrition is also common in this population group makes differentiation between primordial growth failure and postnatal growth failure even more important.

Description

A considerable number of primordial dwarfs are born small for gestational age. Others have a normal birth weight, but their growth decelerates soon after birth. Normal growth rates are resumed once the person's "growth channel" is reached. A large percentage of these infants have physical stigma, ranging from multiple gross deformities to minor and almost imperceptible abnormalities of external structures, such as earlobes, fingers, or palmar creases. The presence of minor abnormalities is diagnostically significant in the context of growth failure that cannot be linked to environmental factors and that does not respond to dietary manipulation, especially if the infant was SGA. All possible efforts must be made to diagnose recognized dysmorphology syndromes.

Primordial dwarfs tend to be underweight for height but are generally not below 85% of the normal mean weight for height, unless undernutrition is a complicating factor. Many have small features, a small frame, and slender limbs, which make their appearance contrast sharply with that of patients with growth failure due to growth hormone deficiency or psychosocial deprivation, who look more like normal children of a younger age (infantilism).

A variety of conditions that affect the pregnant woman cause intrauterine growth failure (Chapter 1). Only some of these are characteristically associated with continued growth failure after birth. They are exposure to radiation, viral infections such as rubella, and chromosomal abnormalities. These insults may affect linear growth in utero. Disproportionate intrauterine growth between body length and head circumference also tends to be associated with persistent growth failure after birth. By contrast, toxemia and late gestational insults, including maternal malnutrition, are not common causes of SGA dwarfism (24,25).

Diagnosis

The difficulties in recognizing a prenatal insult to growth and growth potential make it necessary to base the diagnosis mainly on the exclusion of postnatal causes (Chapter 5). Among these are malnutrition, environmental deprivation, and endocrine disorders. Since the growth failure of SGA dwarfism becomes apparent soon after birth and growth in infancy is not influenced by growth hormone deficiency, dietary and other environmental factors are usually suspected first. Determination of bone age may be helpful in the differential diagnosis. Bone maturation is consistent with chronological age in primordial dwarfism but decreased in chronic malnutrition. Although this seems to be a generally accepted rule, a number of cases with primordial dwarfism have a decreased bone age.

There is, unfortunately, no single test available for the diagnosis of this important entity. The basal metabolic rate could serve this purpose (26) if precise measurements were more readily available. This was shown in a study where the metabolic rate was measured in three groups of infants and small children at rest, 12 hours after a meal. The groups were as follows: (*1*) those with recognized dwarfing syndromes, (*2*) SGA dwarfs who had only minor external stigma, and (*3*) subjects with linear growth failure due to chronic undernutrition (Fig. 3-10). This approach was motivated by studies showing that DNA is decreased in major organs of patients with dwarfing syndromes (27). Since DNA is a measure of cell number, BMR measurements were expected to reflect these histologic changes (28). Infants with dwarfing syndromes and SGA dwarfs did indeed have lower BMR values than either age or height control subjects with growth failure due to undernutrition. Confusion arises when weight is used as a reference standard, because the BMR per unit of body weight in both primordial dwarfs and undernourished children is higher than in age control subjects. The practical usefulness of this tool is not enhanced by the fact that measurements must be made in the basal state in order to avoid the influence of growth on the specific dynamic action. Since undernourished infants are usually not growing at all prior to realimentation, their 3-hour postprandial metabolic rate is as low as the basal metabolic rate, while it is higher than the basal rate in primordial dwarfs. This erases the diagnostic difference that exists for measurements in the "truly" basal state. It is apparently not possible to distinguish BMR differences at birth. Differences at this early age are probably too small to be discernible through relatively crude techniques such as those used for measuring the BMR.

Occasionally, diagnosis may require hospital admission for a therapeutic trial (Chapter 5). Primordial dwarfs tend to be picky eaters with capricious appetites, and, like patients with psychogenic anorexia, will refuse to eat an amount of food sufficient for catch-up growth, but they eat enough to maintain a normal rate of growth. Consequently, height and weight remain in a channel below but parallel to the normal growth curve. These children eat poorly because of their decreased growth potential, whereas undernourished patients grow poorly because of their decreased intake. Psychogenic causes may coexist, since it is very likely that their parents have exerted undue pressures on eating for a long time.

TREATMENT

Objectives

Nutritional management of chronically ill children with growth failure due to undernutrition presents a challenge because they require more calories per kilogram body weight than children of similar age, but they frequently have poor appetites and are picky and capricious at mealtimes. The difficulties are greatest in infants, because they may not tolerate the volume necessary to supply the excess calories. Yet infancy is also the one period in life when the potential damage of malnutrition to growth and development is the greatest.

Whereas normal infants require between 95 to 115 kcal/kg, the malnourished infant requires upward of 130 and not infrequently as much as 180 or even 200 kcal/kg. It is advisable to aim first at an intake of 150 kcal/kg, using foods of high caloric density while avoiding foods disliked by the patient. Protein intake need not be tightly controlled, but at least 8% of total calories should be derived from protein. Protein intakes in excess of 4 g/kg, which are not uncommon in infants receiving meat products, should be avoided. Since high-calorie formulas tend to increase the renal solute load, osmolarity must be controlled, and it may be necessary in complicated cases to have the parents monitor urine specific gravity. Irrespective of the need for food of high caloric density, care must be taken to provide sufficient fluids, especially in those illnesses where excessive water loss occurs through evaporation, vomiting, or diarrhea.

Meal Schedules

The volume intake necessary to reach the caloric goal tends to be in excess of what the undergrown infant can accommodate comfortably, especially if a "diet for age" is prescribed and if this diet is given in three meals that are crowded into the 8 or 10 hours during which the infant is awake.

Unfortunately, this happens during hospitalization, because meals tend to be given at times that are convenient for personnel rather than for the patient. Small infants must be fed more often, sometimes every 3 hours, around the clock. Older infants and small children should be given four to five meals, spaced at least 4 hours apart, leaving 8 hours for uninterrupted sleep.

Food Choices

The type of food should be chosen after the volume capacity has been determined. Commercially prepared formulas (Table 2-5) are adequate as the sole source of nutrients as long as the infant's volume capacity is 1 l or less. These formulas are available in ready-to-feed form and greater than standard caloric density of 80 and 90 kcal/dl and a protein concentration of 2.2 and 2.45 g/dl, respectively. A caloric density of 80 kcal/dl can be prepared with less expense from the standard concentrate (134 kcal/dl), marketed as a "20 kcal/ounze" formula by diluting it 3 parts concentrate to 2 parts water. A hypothetical 9-month-old malnourished infant who weighs 6 kg and drinks 1 qt per day of an 80 kcal/dl formula thus can receive 135 kcal/kg and, of protein, 3.0 g/kg from milk alone, which is better accepted by the ill child than solid foods. To achieve an even higher caloric density of 90 kcal/dl, low electrolyte formulas are available in powdered form (Similac PM 60/40) which may be used in less than standard dilution to increase calories without the excessive increase in solute load and osmolality.

Infants, who require more than 800 to 900 kcal provided by a quart of one of these concentrated formulas, benefit from semisolid baby foods of high caloric density. Because of their high solute load, meat and egg should be omitted as long as the protein intake per kilogram derived from the formula is high. Baby foods with reasonably high caloric density are cereals, puddings, fruits, and selected vegetables (Table 2-8). Fat may be added to increase caloric density. MCT oil (115 kcal/tablespoon) is better tolerated than either butter or carbohydrates, which can cause diarrhea. Care should be taken to avoid protein dilution, because the percentage of calories derived from protein decreases after addition of these high-caloric low-protein baby foods. Meat and eggs should be added when protein calories decrease and approach 8% of total intake.

Psychological Factors of Treatment

In order to achieve the caloric goal, it is often necessary to use a variety of dietary manipulations. While it may be prudent to please the patient's food preferences, this may have psychological ramifications. Spoiling during early socialization deprives the child of the opportunity to build inner controls. On the other hand, it eases the burden on the chronically ill child who already has to suffer other restrictions, many of which may be construed as punishment. To get even, these children may learn to use eating behavior as a means to manipulate and frustrate the caretaker. Eating difficulties, which start out to be organic, thus may become psychogenic with time. It is therefore important to guard against these complications by creating a healthy mealtime atmosphere and by avoiding coaxing. To accomplish this in infants, it may help to place a few different varieties of baby foods in front of the patient for a choice. Older children should be treated like other members of the family at the dinner table. Special food preparations, such as calorie enrichment with butter or sweets, can be hidden from the patient, and food preferences can be shared by other family members to avoid the effect of "spoiling." These extra efforts during the early formative years will pay off later in the course of the chronic illness.

Congenital Heart Disease

It is especially important to feed the child with CHD frequently because patients with CHD of sufficient severity to cause FTT tend to tire easily, and if they are in respiratory distress, they have difficulty coordinating breathing and sucking. It is not wise to rely on demand feeding because sick infants with decreased vitality and a low activity level may not cry for food, but they may eat if food is offered.

Sodium balance is of particular concern in CHD because sodium excess jeopardizes water balance and precipitates heart failure. Foods therefore must be chosen carefully. Since some commercially prepared meats, dinners, vegetables, and soups contain considerable amounts of sodium, care must be taken that brands without added sodium are selected. Most high-caloric formulas (90 kcal/dl) are not recommended for infants at risk of developing heart failure for the same reason. For example, 1 l of such a formula supplies 150 kcal/kg/day for a 9-month-old, moderately nourished infant weighing 6 kg. On this regimen protein intake tends to be high (4 g/kg/day) and osmolality above a safe range of 360 to 400 mOsm/kg water. In order to increase the calorie concentration in these cases without increasing osmolality, low-sodium formulas (like Similac PM 60/40) are recommended, since they can be offered in below-standard dilutions without increasing osmolality excessively.

Chronic Renal Disease

The objectives in the treatment of chronic renal disease are (*1*) the decrease of waste products in cases with lowered glomerular filtration rate or (*2*) the substitution of nutrients that are lost at an excessive rate in tubular disorders. Efforts to accomplish this through dietary means should be made while maintaining adequate growth. Nutrients that may have to be restricted in certain cases are nitrogen, hydrogen, phosphate, potassium, and sodium. In tubular diseases, on the other hand sodium, potassium, and phosphorus may be lost, while hydrogen is in excess. Water intake must be limited in nephrotic syndrome but in renal conditions associated with hyposthenuria intake should cover urinary losses.

It is not feasible to correct sodium, phosphate, and potassium deficiency by dietary means, because appropriated diets would cause other imbalances. Correction is more easily accomplished through pharmacological measures. Recommended starting doses for electrolyte replacement, which must be adjusted empirically, are 0.2 g sodium chloride per kilogram; 1.5 mEq potassium per kilogram as potassium chloride or citrate.

A low-potassium diet may be indicated in renal failure. However, to lower potassium at a rapid rate, efforts must be made to establish a negative potassium balance by other than dietary means. Providing peritoneal dialysis is not indicated, this can be accomplished by use of ion exchange resin (Kayexalate, 1 g/day, in two divided doses, orally or as a retention enema). Reduction of dietary phosphorus may be considered in renal osteodystrophy. However, since a low-phosphorus diet requires restriction of milk and meat products, care should be taken to maintain minimum protein intake. Restriction of sodium chloride through special diets is rarely necessary except for the exclusion of added "salt to taste." This requires that attention be paid to the salt content of commercial baby food products. Hydrogen excess is corrected through alkali therapy in the form of sodium bicarbonate—1 to 3 mEq/kg/day, in four to six doses—or Shol's solution or Polycitra (Willen Drug Co.) The latter provides 1 mEq each of potassium and sodium per milliliter—equivalent to 2 mEq bicarbonate.

Nitrogenous waste restriction is of major concern in the treatment of uremia. This may be accomplished through low-protein diets consisting mainly of high-quality protein. However, necessary restriction may be greater than is compatible with normal growth. Restriction to less than minimum protein requirements and supplementation with essential amino acid mixtures (Amin-Aid, McGaw) may be attempted in such instances. In special cases and given adequate facilites for monitoring, supplementation with α-ketoacid analogs of essential amino acids may also be considered.

Minimum protein needs range from 1.8 g/kg/day for infants down to 0.9 to 0.75 g/kg/day for children. Milk and eggs are preferred as a source of high-quality protein. If this degree of restriction cannot reduce blood urea and does not maintain growth, calories should be increased in an attempt to minimize protein breakdown. If this is unsuccessful, one-third to one-half the protein may be replaced by essential amino acids. It has been demonstrated in infants with urea cycle enzyme defects that such a regimen can maintain growth. Since urea levels are elevated in renal failure and since urea serves as a nitrogen source in the de novo synthesis of nonessential amino acids, this form of therapy is potentially very useful in protein-depleted uremic patients (29). Aronson (30) reported growth and nitrogen retention in a 5-year-old girl who received 85 to 120 kcal/kg/day and 0.8 to 1.1 g/kg/day of half protein and amino acids. If the regimen maintains acceptable blood urea nitrogen levels but does not support growth, protein calories should be increased, because minimum recommendations (in grams per kilogram body weight) frequently provide only about 4% of total calories as protein if calorie intake is high. An adequate protein intake is especially important in uremic patients whose protein requirements are increased because of infection, proteinuria, altered amino acid absorption, and loss into dialysis fluid. Underestimation of calorie requirements is most often the cause of poor growth, since malnourished patients require more calories per body weight than normal patients.

Experience with α-ketoacid analogs in infants and children is insufficient. There are too few quantitative estimates of the efficiency of conversion of α-ketoacid analogs to amino acids to permit calculation of requirements. Available information suggests that the amount of ketoacid analogs required to replace amino acids is greater than the calculated value. Growth status and enzyme function are among the factors that influence efficiency of conversion. Knowledge gathered in studies of adults therefore cannot be applied to children. There is also a need for more experience with essential amino acid supplementation in infants.

Primordial and SGA Dwarfism

Therapy with high doses of human growth hormone (20 units per week) was attempted by several investigators and has produced varied results. Although some patients, who were generally less than 8 years old, responded, it was not shown that an accelerated rate of growth can be maintained. There is currently no sound basis for this costly form of therapy.

Teaching parents and the patient to accept the condition and to adjust to the realities of a short stature may be the best service a physican can render, providing the diagnosis of an inherently poor growth potential has been firmly established. Psychological support may be necessary intermittently during periods of emotional stress, such as entry into school and during puberty. Care must be individualized, as it depends on the associated presence of intellectual deficits and other anatomic abnormalities.

REFERENCES

1. Krieger I: Growth failure and congenital heart disease. *Am J Dis Child* 120:497, 1970.
2. Mehrizi A, Drash A: Growth disturbance in congenital heart disease. *J Pediatr* 61:418, 1962.
3. Miller RH, Schiebler GL, Grumbar P, et al: Relation of hemodynamics to height and weight percentiles in children with ventricular septal defects. *Am Heart J* 78:523, 1969.

4. Feldt RH, Stickler GB, Weidman WH: Growth of children with heart disease. *Am J Dis Child* 117:573, 1969.
5. Mitchell SC, Berendes HW, Clark WM Jr: The normal closure of the ventricular septum. *Am Heart J* 73:334, 1967.
6. Umansky R, Hauck AJ: Factors in the growth of children with patent ductus arteriosus. *Pediatrics* 30:540, 1962.
7. Naeye RL: Anatomic features of growth failure in congenital heart disease. *J Pediatr* 39:433, 1967.
8. Krieger I, Chen YC: Caloric requirements for weight in infants with growth failure due to maternal deprivation, undernutrition and congenital heart disease. *Pediatrics* 44:647, 1969.
9. Schärer K, Chantler C, Brunner FP, et al: Combined report on regular dialysis and transplantation of children in Europe, 1974. *Proc Eur Dial Transplant Assoc* 12:65, 1976.
10. West CD, Smith WC: An attempt to elucidate the cause of growth retardation in renal disease. *Am J Dis Child* 91:460, 1956.
11. Bergstrom WH, DeLeon AS, Van Gemund JJ, et al: Growth aberrations in renal disease. *Pediatr Clin North Am* 11:563, 1964.
12. Lilly JR, Giles G, Hurwitz R, et al: Renal homotransplantation in pediatric patients. *Pediatrics* 47:548, 1971.
13. Cooke RE, Boyden DG, Haller E: The relationship of acidosis and growth retardation. *J Pediatr* 57:326, 1960.
14. McSherry E, Sebastian A, Morris RC Jr: Correction of impaired growth in children with renal tubular acidosis (CRTA) by sustained correction of acidosis. *Clin Res* 21:700, 1973.
15. Chantler C, Lieberman E, Holliday MA: A rat model for the study of growth failure in uremia. *Pediatr Res* 8:109, 1974.
16. Simmons JM, Wilson CJ, Potter DE, et al: Relation of calorie deficiency to growth failure in children on hemodialysis and the growth responses to calorie supplementation. *N Engl J Med* 285:653, 1971.
17. Betts PR, Magrath G: Growth pattern and dietary intake of children with chronic renal insufficiency. *Br Med J* 2:189, 1974.
18. Abitbol CL, Holiday MA: Effect of energy and nitrogen intake upon urea production in children with uremia and undernutrition. *Clin Nephrol* 10:9, 1978.
19. Hyne BE, Fowell E, Lee HA: The effect of calorie intake on nitrogen balance in chronic renal failure. *Clin Sci* 43:679, 1972.
20. Saenger P, Wiedemann E, Schwartz E, et al: Somatomedin and growth after renal transplantation. *Pediatr Res* 8:163, 1974.
21. Schwalbe SL, Betts PR, Rayner PHW, et al: Somatomedin in growth disorders and chronic renal insufficiency in children. *Br Med J* 1:679, 1977.
22. Lubchenco LO: *The High Risk Infant.* Philadelphia, WB Saunders Co, 1976.
23. Beargie RA, Vernon LJ, Greene JW, Jr: Growth and development of small for date newborns. *Pediatr Clin North Am* 17:159, 1970.
24. Chamberlain R, Davey A: Physical growth in twins, post mature and small-for-dates children. *Arch Dis Child* 50:437, 1975.
25. Fitzhardinge PM, Steven EM: The small-for-dates infant: I. Later growth patterns. *Pediatrics* 49:671, 1972.
26. Krieger I, Woolley PV Jr: The basal metabolic rate in growth failure of prenatal onset. *Am J Dis Child* 127:340, 1971.
27. Naeye RL: Anatomic features of growth failure in congenital heart disease. *J Pediatr* 39:433, 1967.

28. Kricger I, Taqi Q: Metabolic rate and body composition in rats nutritionally deprived after weaning. *Pediatr Res* 11:796, 1977.
29. Giordano C: Use of exogenous and endogenous urea for protein synthesis in normal and uremic subjects. *Lab Clin Med* 62:231, 1963.
30. Aronson AS, Fürst P, Kuylenstierna B, et al: Essential amino acids in the treatment of advanced uremia: Twenty two months experience in a 5 year old girl. *Pediatrics* 56:538, 1975.

7
Nutrition and the Central Nervous System

EFFECT OF MALNUTRITION ON CNS GROWTH AND FUNCTION

Severe malnutrition during the first 2 years of life, especially if it occurs during the early months after birth, has a profound effect on brain growth (Chapter 1), evidenced by a reduction in head size (Figs. 7-1 and 7-2). Conversely, an expansion of the head circumference with spreading of the sutures may occur after refeeding of malnourished infants (1). Moreover, studies from the United States and developing countries have shown that malnutrition interferes with subsequent learning ability. It is unfortunate that many of the earlier studies were retrospective and suffered from lack of suitable control subjects, since environmental factors, which are known to affect intellectual function, were not comparable for malnourished infants and control subjects. Thus, malnourished infants often came from broken and poverty-stricken homes and were understimulated or grossly neglected, while control infants had lived in sanitary housing with less exposure to disease and were raised by better-educated parents. Subsequently, populations with a more uniform socioeconomic background were studied in several countries, notably Mexico and Guatemala, and earlier observations were by and large confirmed (2). In one study, performance of preschool youngsters and schoolchildren on Terman–Merrill, Gesell, and Goodenough draw-a-man tests (adapted to the study population) was positively correlated with body weights and heights (3). Perceptual deficits were also reported, as evidenced by difficulties in tracing shapes, differentiating by feeling the shape of blocks, fitting blocks into openings, and so on. It is thus apparent that through its effects on the CNS, nutrition has consequences that reach, individually by way of the pregnant mother, through the generations and touch on the health and economic stability of entire nations.

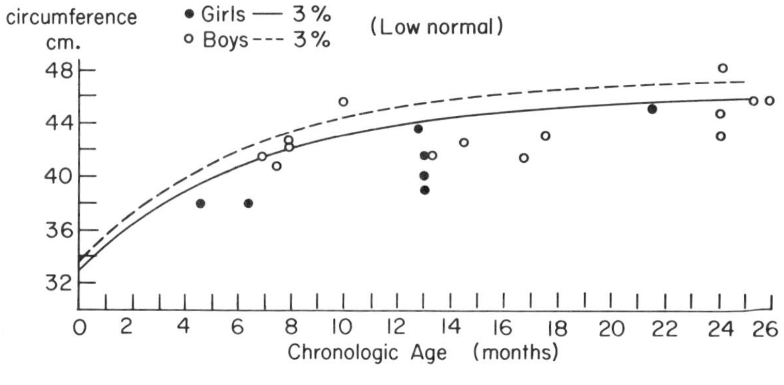

Figure 7-1. HEAD CIRCUMFERENCE OF 21 INFANTS WITH GROWTH FAILURE DUE TO MALNUTRITION, PLOTTED ON AGE AND COMPARED TO THE THIRD PERCENTILE OF NORMAL CONTROL SUBJECTS
By definition, 19 patients would be "microcephalic."

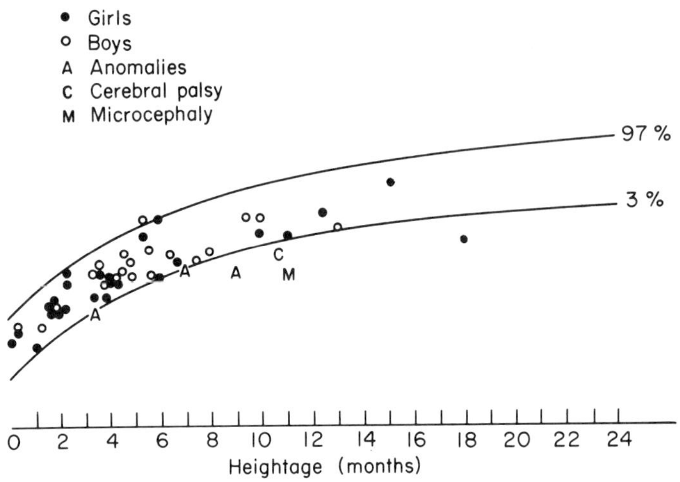

Figure 7-2. HEAD CIRCUMFERENCE OF 50 INFANTS AND CHILDREN WITH GROWTH FAILURE DUE TO MALNUTRITION, PLOTTED ON HEIGHT AGE
All but 5 patients had a head circumference proportionate for height. The 5 exceptions had mental retardation that did not improve after weight recovery and environmental stimulation and cerebral palsy (C) or evidence of prenatal injury, i.e. congenital anomalies (A), or grossly evident microcephaly (M).

NUTRITION IN PRIMARY CNS DISEASE

Whereas the effects of nutrition on the CNS appear to be subtle, the reverse relationship is more striking. A number of CNS diseases can cause malnutrition and affect nutrition in many different ways that require the attention of health care personnel in several disciplines. The question of whether CNS disease or malnutrition was primary rarely if ever arises, because these disorders are not difficult to diagnose. Notable among the diseases that cause nutritional problems are cerebral palsy, of both the spastic and athetoid varieties, and disorders that are associated with severe developmental delays.

In general, the mechanisms responsible for reduced food intake are neuromuscular dysfunction, delayed acquisition of feeding skills, and behavior problems. When mechanical feeding difficulties exist or when the sequential acquisition of feeding skills is delayed, parents may act inappropriately and either force-feed the child food he or she is not ready to accept or fail to encourage development of oral motor skills. Foods that are accepted by the handicapped child may be nutritionally inadequate. Because feeding the developmentally delayed child is a tedious process that interferes several times a day with other responsibilities, parents become overwhelmed. The caretaker may cease the feeding effort before the child has consumed the necessary amount, or the emotional tension may secondarily cause feeding problems. The defective child gives few clues concerning satiety, and sometimes the child's lack of response may not reinforce the parent to love, feed, and care for the child adequately.

Anxious, helpless, and disappointed parents tend to shop around for advice, which further adds to their confusion, as doctors tend to put different emphasis on causative factors that play but one role, and parents tend to look for simplistic answers. Thus, damage to the appetite center may be blamed by one physician, causing parents to reduce their efforts in finding solutions. Parents also may believe that growth failure is part of the primary disease rather than being intake related.

In the child with obvious neuromuscular disease, feeding difficulties are to be expected; however, it is generally not realized that the rather complex mechanism of sucking, swallowing, and coordinating the two with breathing may be disturbed in a variety of milder CNS disorders, some of which do not become evident until the patient is a few months old. In the meantime, mechanical feeding difficulties exist that may severely retard growth during a crucial phase of CNS development and thus add insult to injury. Histories of growth-retarded, mentally defective children commonly reveal vague feeding problems, vomiting, food refusal, and failure to gain during the early months of life.

These general types of problems that affect infants with CNS disorders do not cease after the child has reached sufficient maturity to function with regard to feeding, because behavioral problems tend to develop. Lack of stimulation and planned activity may result in boredom, causing these children to spend their days seeking and eating more food than they need. The sense of being different or of failure and inadequacy often causes inappropriate and even disruptive behavior. With regard to eating, this is furthered by parents who, in desperation, try different tactics—cajoling, bribing, and threatening—which then may have an effect opposite what was intended. Another cause of undereating occurs in hyperactive children, who are able to feed themselves but who—since they have a short attention span—stop eating early or play with the food.

In addition to these problems, which are of a general nature and are common in a variety of disorders, certain CNS diseases are associated with characteristic manifestations that predispose to unique nutritional problems. No attempt is made to cover the disease under discussion comprehensively.

Cerebral Palsy (CP)

The term *cerebral palsy* covers a group of syndromes of varying etiology that affect motor function and have their onset at birth or during the first few years of life (i.e., before full motor function is achieved). Three major types can be distinguished: spastic, dyskinetic, and ataxic. Subclassifications of spastic CP are based on the degree of involvement. Both extremities on the same side are affected in hemiplegia, four extremities in tetraplegia, legs only in paraplegia, and greater involvement of the lower limbs in diplegia. Patients with the dyskinetic form of CP display uncontrolled, purposeless movements, which tend to disappear during sleep. The most common of these are slow, wormlike, writhing movements, called *athetosis*, which involve the extremities, neck, and face, including the tongue. Some dyskinetics make violent, whipping motions that require considerable energy. Ataxic CP is not common in infancy. These patients are unsteady and have a wide-based gait and difficulties with fast, repetitious movements. Thus, they cannot turn rapidly and, in general, fall frequently. Mental handicaps are frequently associated with CP.

Nutritional studies show a general tendency of children with CP to be thin. Studies of body composition are also compatible with growth failure and malnutrition. Decreased body fat, increased extracellular water, decreased bone age, and decreased body cell mass have been decribed (4). Retardation in growth of height and weight is correlated with the degree of physical involvement and the presence of feeding difficulties. Although a correlation between growth retardation and calorie intake has been reported in some studies (5), failure to demonstrate a correlation in others is probably due to differences in activity between patients. It comes therefore as no surprise that the calories needed to maintain an ideal weight vary greatly (6). In patients with ataxia, activity is often limited because they choose not to move as much as normal patients for fear of falling. By contrast, the activity level of athetoid children is excessive.

Conversely, obesity may develop in adolescents who take as little as 1,461 kcal/day (6). Due to decreased activity, this is especially common in nonambulatory patients with spastic CP. Obesity must be avoided because it further handicaps the patient with neuromuscular disability and makes the use of braces and crutches difficult. In general, calorie requirements in spastic CP are roughly two-thirds the normal amount for height and age.

An analysis of the specific neuromuscular problem responsible for undernutrition is necessary in order to devise an effective treatment program. Examples are spastic infants who may have an exaggerated gag or bite reflex and hypotonic infants who have a poor suck and lip closure (see Chapter 4). The child with CP may only be capable of a vertical bite and not able to move the jaw sideways for molar grinding. Tongue motion may be abnormal and cause feeding difficulties because the bolus of food cannot be moved backward in swallowing or sideways in chewing. Chewing should therefore be analyzed in children with CP and mechanical feeding problems.

Treatment is aimed at preventing obesity or malnutrition. Ten kilocalories per centimeter of height is recommended for patients with restricted activity. Regardless of actual calorie intake, deficiency must be assumed if, at the onset of growth failure, weight increments are lower than height increments. Specific forms of therapy for neuromuscular feedings difficulties are discussed in Chapter 4.

Convulsive Disorders

Epilepsy is the term used for a variety of convulsive disorders of multiple etiologies. The common features are paroxysmal excessive neuronal discharges that cause either tonic–clonic muscle contractions, loss of tone, disturbances of consciousness and sensation, or autonomic nervous system abnormalities. Patients usually require long-term anticonvulsive drug treatment.

Nutritional deficiencies may be a cause of convulsions, but they comprise only a small percentage of the total. These causes include hypoglycemia, hypocalcemia, hypomagnesemia, hypertonic dehydration, pyridoxine deficiency, and inborn errors of protein and lipid metabolism. (These are discussed in detail in the appropriate sections.) Electrolyte and water imbalance may precipitate convulsions in epilepsy of other origin.

Nutritional disorders in association with convulsive disease occur mainly as a result of drug effects. Anticonvulsant drugs that cause loss of appetite are Diamox, Mysoline, and Phenurone. Other effects of anticonvulsant therapy involve vitamin D and folate metabolism. The literature contains many reports of cases with epilepsy and subnormal folate levels, generally less than 5 ng/ml. Megaloblastic anemia occurs in about 1% of cases or less (7), but the incidence of macrocytosis ranges as high as 40% in some surveys. The drugs most often responsible are phenytoin (Dilantin), primidone (Mysoline), and phenobarbital. Anticonvulsant drugs also seem to increase the need for vitamin D (8,9). Lifshitz and Maclaren (10) reported evidence of deficiency in 7% of institutionalized patients under 15 years of age, although they had received between 800 and 1,200 IU/day of vitamin D. The fact that they had been nonambulatory and infrequently exposed to sunlight may have been a factor. Low levels of serum phosphorus and elevated levels of alkaline phosphatase are the most common biochemical abnormalities reported. Anticonvulsive drugs appear to depress the activity of 25-hydroxylase in the liver. Epileptic children on long-term phenobarbital and phenytoin therapy therefore should receive larger doses than are ordinarily recommended.

Ketogenic Diet

Therapy with a ketogenic diet was first advocated in 1920 by Wilder (11) and was subsequently developed into a precisely calculated meal plan, low in carbohydrates and very high in fat (87% of total calories). This ratio of fat to nonfat calories leads to incomplete oxidation of fatty acids by the liver and results in the accumulation of ketone bodies. It was apparently necessary for the ratio to be the same for every meal. The diet is difficult to follow, unpalatable, and may cause hypercholesterolemia. As a result, it is either not attempted or is unsuccessful, because patients do not remain ketotic on partial compliance.

Given the precarious fluid and electrolyte imbalance of infants in general, it appears hazardous to maintain a young patient for prolonged periods on the verge of acidosis. Known side effects include abdominal cramps, nausea, vomiting, and diarrhea. Because of these considerations, this diet is recommended only as a last resort in otherwise unresponsive cases. It is thus sometimes used in hypsarrhythmia that is unresponsive to anticonvulsants and ACTH. It is possible that some patients reported in the literature with myoclonic seizures, who improved, may have had metabolic diseases, possibly of pyruvate breakdown. Ketone bodies provide an alternate source of energy and may circumvent a metabolic block like the one from pyruvate into the tricarboxylic acid cycle. Serum and CSF lactate and pyruvate, therefore, should be monitored before and during use of the ketogenic diet.

In recent years several reports have indicated that triglycerides of the medium chain fatty acids, octanoate and decanoate (MCT), are more ketogenic than long chain fatty acids. The MCT diet has an advantage over the traditional ketogenic diet in that the total fat required is less (about 20 or 15% of total calories from regular fat and 45 or 50% from MCT oil). Consequently, carbohydrate intake can be increased, leaving about 10% of total calories to be derived from protein, which is adequate for growth and safer than the 7% protein calories provided by the traditional ketogenic diet (Table 7-1). A constant ratio for fat to nonfat calories at every meal is maintained in infants on formulas but does not appear to be necessary (12). The diet has been recommended for intractable epilepsy (13) and may be of benefit in certain disorders of pyruvate metabolism (Chapter 13). The diet should be started in the hospital where

Table 7-1. Ketogenic Formula[a,b]

Formula	*Amount*	*Fat (kcal)*	*Protein (kcal)*	*Total calories*
MCT oil	13 ml	100	—	100
Standard "breast-milk-like" formula	150 ml	50	9	102
Casec (Mead Johnson)	1 level tbsp	—	17	17
Polycose (Ross)	8 ml			14
Water up to 350 ml				
Total		150	26	233

[a] Formula characteristics: 67 kcal/dl, protein 1.8 g/dl, fat calories 65% of total, protein 11%
[b] Supplemental vitamins are necessary.

the response can be tested and the parents can be taught the preparation of the diet and the necessary monitoring by daily urinalysis with a Ketostix. Induction of ketosis may be accelerated by having the infant fast for about 1 day, using only water to prevent dehydration. Growth and overall adequacy of the diet should be checked monthly. Supplementation with vitamins E and B, calcium, and iron is necessary. Although hypercholesterolemia is reported to be less common on this ketogenic diet, cholesterol and triglycerides should be checked occasionally.

Myelomeningocele

Neural tube defects are due to deficient closure of the vertebrae, meninges, and neural tube. Only the bony structures are involved in spina bifida, and the defect may not be visible externally (spina bifida occulta). A meningocele affects the vertebrae and meninges. Myelomeningoceles involve, in addition, neural tissue and cause neurological deficits ranging from weakness of the extremities to flaccid paralysis, loss of sensation, and bladder incontinence. Ninety percent of patients are born with or develop hydrocephalus. Mental retardation occurs either as an associated primary defect or as a result of poorly controlled hydrocephalus. Without multidisciplinary treatment, almost 90% of cases would succumb to such complications as meningitis, intracranial pressure, or kidney damage due to bladder paralysis. With early aggressive therapy, survival is possible in upward of 50% of cases.

Nutritional care is needed for several reasons. Foremost among these is the high incidence of obesity, which constitutes a serious additional handicap to the paralyzed patient. Aside from psychologically induced overeating, the development of obesity is facilitated because of decreased activity. Moreover, calorie requirements are probably less than normal, because a decrease in body cell mass is associated with muscle atrophy below the lesion. A decrease has been suggested by measurements of total body ^{40}K content (14). A calorie intake of 7 to 10 kcal/cm height has been recommended, as it has for other patients who are inactive because of neurological disease.

Vitamin C deficiency appears to be more frequent in patients with myelomeningocele, as evidenced by the finding of high urinary levels of tyrosine metabolites and the occurrence of spontaneous epiphyseal separation. Althought the reason for these observations is unclear, vitamin C supplementation is advisable (15).

An acid ash diet is sometimes prescribed for the prevention of urinary tract infections. Such a diet may lead to vitamin and mineral deficiency, because it restricts many fruits and vegetables as well as milk. Although it is possible to provide all essential nutrients with this diet, the limited choice of foods together with idiosyncrasies of the patient may cause deficiency if the diet is not supervised. Consequently, dietary records should be obtained intermittently.

Minimal Brain Syndrome (MBS)

Minimal brain syndrome (MBS) is known under several names, including hyperkinetic syndrome, functional hyperactivity, organic brain syndrome, and minimal brain damage. The meaning of these names reflects controversy concerning the cause of the syndrome.

Manifestations consist of (*1*) hyperactivity, (*2*) short attention span, (*3*) poor impulse control, and (*4*) swings in emotion. Because of these characteristics, patients have learning problems but may function adequately on intelligence tests. An organic origin may be assumed in patients who have, in addition to these manifestations, definite neurological impairment. It is, however, possible that MBS is psychogenic in diseases of proven organic origin, since psychological problems are common in organic disease. MBS occurs in children who have recovered from deprivation syndrome.

Nutritional disturbances in MBS consist predominantly of undernutrition. This complication may be drug related, since hyperactivity alone does not appear to be sufficiently severe and sustained to increase energy requirements to such a degree that the increase cannot be covered by additional food intake. These children are commonly treated with dextroamphetamine or methylphenidate (Ritalin), drugs that have a paradoxical calming effect but are also known appetite depressants. Safer et al. (16) noted that children receiving these drugs grew less in height than untreated children and that linear growth retardation was related to decreased weight gain. Dextroamphetamine, which is a commonly used specific appetite depressant, had the stronger effect of the two. Ritalin in doses of less than 20 mg/day appeared to be safe.

Growth retardation from these drugs does not appear to be severe. Therefore, if linear growth is markedly retarded, other causes should be suspected. The manifestations of MBS are also seen as sequelae of maternal deprivation in infancy after growth recovery. It is of considerable interest in this regard that Palmer mentions, in her description of children with MBS followed at Georgetown University between 1972 and 1974 (7), the "frequent observation of bizarre food habits" and refers to their "efforts to snack throughout the day." These are typical behavior deviations of children with psychosocial deprivation syndrome (Chapter 5).

In view of the uncertain etiology of MBS, it is not surprising that allergy is considered one of the possible causes. Shannon described in 1922 a condition similar to MBS (18), which the author attributes to an "anaphylactic reaction" to certain foods. Most recently, Feingold attributed hyperkinesis and learning disability to food additives, such as tartrazine and FD&C yellow #5 (19). Others (20–22) have also incriminated food allergy in MBS-like syndromes manifested by tension, fatigue, irritability, and depression. The foods that have been implicated include wheat, eggs, milk, chocolate, and a long list of fruits containing natural salicylates. Controlled studies investigating claims of the effectiveness of the Feingold diet are being conducted at various centers; early reports are conflicting.

If a group of children includes but a few who do respond to a specific diet, comparison with a control group may not show a significant difference. In view of the fact that any group of children with MBS is bound to be heterogeneous because of multiple etiologies, pediatricians may test patients individually and use them as their own control subjects. However, objectivity is of utmost importance to avoid unnecessary diet restrictions. Therefore, when the manifestations of MBS are not consistently present, testing with an elimination diet must be done for a sufficient length of time, and it should be followed by a challenge. As a first step, several of the foods commonly incriminated may be eliminated together. Identification of specific foods responsible for the symptoms may then be obtained by challenging the patient later with each food item separately. A teacher or other person in close contact and not cognizant of the changes in diet may be used as a "blind" observer. Records should be kept that list the frequency of the behaviors that were identified as "offensive."

Blindness

Congenital eye abnormalities or neurogenic blindness occur not infrequently in children with CNS disease. Since food is important to the normal infant as a link through which the first communication with the outside world is established, it is even more important to the blind child. Instead of learning about objects through touching, the normal child "mouths" them first. Moreover, food is one of the first objects that is "handled" by the normal infant with recognition and obvious delight. Food therefore can be exploited as a tool to teach the blind child nonvisual means of communication through tasting, touching, and smelling. Blind children should be encouraged to feel the texture of foods. This needs to be explained to the parents, who may consider the lack of neatness a stigma of blindness. Foods should be introduced one at a time and offered separately, so that the child can learn to associate the taste, smell, and feel of an object with its proper name. Blind children should be allowed to feed themselves at the same age as normal children and thus be allowed to develop a sense of autonomy. Use of a deep dish may help to avoid spillage. Spoon feeding by the caretaker should complement self-feeding efforts only to assure adequate nutrition.

Infantile Autism

Infantile autism deserves mention in the context of nutrition, first, because of its similarities to psychosocial deprivation syndrome and, second, because megadoses of vitamin C have been recommended for its treatment.

The term *autism* describes withdrawal from reality into a world of self-preoccupation. In adult medicine, autism is usually equated with schizophrenia. Infantile autism is different in that a variety of etiologies, including organic brain disease, are responsible for its manifestations.

The disorder develops gradually during infancy until, by $2\frac{1}{2}$ years of age, disease manifestations are obvious. This is also the time when the behavior abnormalities of psychosocial deprivation syndrome become diagnostic. Autistic children are usually placid and undemanding during infancy. This is also typical of those with maternal deprivation syndrome, which may be an antecedent of psychosocial deprivation dwarfism (PSD). Both autism and PSD share behavior abnormalities, such as bizarre food cravings, gorging, and temper tantrums. Language is defective in both, and there may be mutism. In PSD, food is at times used to express hostility. Autistic children are also noted for refusing food, gagging, or chewing without swallowing. When behavior modification is used to correct feeding abnormalities of autistic children, they tend to refuse the food at first, lose weight, and become lethargic; some develop ketosis due to starvation (23). This combination of growth failure and bizarre behavior is typical of PSD. Finally, gastrointestinal disturbances suggestive of malabsorption occur in both entities (24). Catatonialike posturing, considered typical of schizophrenia, is common in maternal deprivation syndrome (25). The response to a nurturing environment thus seems to be the major distinguishing feature. Children with maternal deprivation syndrome or PSD change readily, even in a hospital environment; they start to eat and gain weight, and gradually their behavior abnormalities disappear. By contrast, autistic children do not respond to people with recognition or affection when they are cuddled and held. Misdiagnosis of autism is therefore possible, especially if removal from the original environment is not used as a therapeutic trial.

Megavitamin therapy has been recommended for infantile autism as a result of Pauling's orthomolecular theory (26), which proposes the possibility of localized areas of vitamin deficiency in the brain due to genetic constitution, perhaps aggravated by dietary deficiency. The concept of genetic vitamin dependency is not a new one. Vitamins are precursors of cofactors that may be deficient because of genetic abnormalities in vitamin metabolism (see Chapters 11 and 13). Pyridoxine-dependent infantile convulsion is an example of a recognized entity, although the enzymatic basis is still unknown. However, in contrast to claims that have been made for the efficiency of vitamins in the treatment of autism or schizophrenia, the value of pyridoxine in the treatment of infantile convulsions can be tested objectively by observing EEG changes during vitamin infusion. There is no convincing proof yet that megadoses of vitamin C are helpful in infantile autism and objective tests are lacking. The recommendation to use megadoses of several vitamins in mental illnesses is potentially dangerous, because dependency can be created by this practice.

Down's Syndrome

Down's syndrome was also called *mongolism* in the past. The name *trisomy 21* characterizes the chromosomal disorder. The syndrome consists of several obligatory congenital abnormalities, notably of the face. Because the base of the skull is short, these patients have a flat profile and a depressed nose, undeveloped occiput with a low hairline, and a small oral cavity that causes the tongue to protrude. Oblique palpebral fissures cause the mongoloid appearance for which the disorder was originally named. Among other abnormalities of the musculoskeletal system, hypotonia and hyperextensibility of the joints are the most helpful diagnostic sign in infants, who normally have relatively stiff joints and a strong flexor tone. Mental retardation is present but usually causes no management problems.

There is an extensive literature on biochemical abnormalities, some with nutritional implications, but most are difficult to interpret in the context of the total picture. Thus, abnormal serum globulins (27) and impaired vitamin A absorption (28) were reported and have been linked with the susceptibility of these children to infections of the respiratory tract. There is also evidence for a disorder of pyridoxine metabolism (29). Decreased concentrations of pyridoxal phosphate in leukocytes and platelets have been reported (30,31). There are other reports suggestive of an abnormal tryptophan metabolism, including decreased serotonin levels in blood and platelets (32,33). Low plasma zinc levels were reported by Milunsky et al. (34), a finding which may have significance in view of the fact that picolinic acid is a tryptophan metabolite that improves zinc absorption (35). Pyridoxine is a cofactor in the enzymatic breakdown of tryptophan to picolinic acid. These findings should not be interpreted to indicate a potential for treatment of the mental retardation in Down's syndrome. It is unfortunate that such claims have been made for a number of treatment regimens, including vitamins and other dietary therapy.

Growth in infancy is normal, but the children become increasingly shorter relative to their peers as they grow older. The upper/lower segment ratio is increased. Head growth is also minimal after 3 years of age. Weight is not affected, and nutritional studies (36) indicate that calorie intake is generally appropriate for height. If failure to thrive develops in infancy, it may be caused by congenital heart disease. Endocardial cushion defects are common in Down's syndrome.

REFERENCES

1. Capitanio MA, Virkpatrick JA: Widening of the cranial sutures. *Radiology* 92:53, 1969.
2. Cravioto J, Nobles R: Evolution of adaptive and motor behavior during rehabilitation from kwashiorkor. *Am J Orthopsychiatry* 35:449, 1965.

3. Cravioto J: Nutrition growth and neurointegrative development: An experimental and ecologic study. *Pediatrics* 38(suppl):2, 1966.
4. Berg K, Isaksson B: Body composition and nutrition of school children with cerebral palsy. *Acta Paediatr Scand* 205:41, 1970.
5. Hammond MI, Lewis MN, Johnson EW: A nutrition study of cerebral palsied children. *J Am Diet Assoc* 49:196, 1966.
6. Eddy TP, Nickolson AL, Wheeler EF: Energy expenditure and dietary intakes in cerebral palsy. *Dev Med Child Neurol* 7:377, 1965.
7. Reynolds EH: Folate metabolism and anticonvulsant therapy. *Proc R Soc Med* 67:6, 1974.
8. Dent CE, Rickens A, Rowe DJF, et al: Osteomalacia with long-term anticonvulsant therapy in epilepsy. *Br Med J* 4:69, 1970.
9. Hahn TJ, Birge SJ, Scharp CR, et al: Phenobarbitol-induced alterations in vitamin D metabolism. *J Clin Invest* 51:741, 1972.
10. Lifshitz F, Maclaren NK: Vitamin D dependent rickets in institutionalized mentally retarded children receiving long-term anticonvulsant therapy: I. A survey of 288 patients. *J Pediatr* 83:612, 1973.
11. Wilder RM: The effects of ketonemia on course of epilepsy. *Mayo Clin Bull* 2:307, 1921.
12. Signore JM: Ketogenic diet containing medium chain triglycerides. *J Am Diet Assoc* 62:285, 1973.
13. Huttenlocher PR, Wilbourn AJ, Signore JM: Medium-chain triglycerides as treatment for intractable childhood epilepsy. *Neurology* 21:1097, 1971.
14. Grogan CB, Ekvall S: The body composition of spina bifida patients as determined by ^{40}K, urinary creatinine, and anthropometric measures. *Proc Xth Intl Congr Nutr*, Kyoto, Japan, 1975.
15. McKibben B, Toseland PA, Duckworth T: Abnormalities in vitamin C in spina bifida. *Dev Med Child neurol* 15(suppl):55, 1968.
16. Safer D, Allen R, Barr E: Depression of growth in hyperactive children on stimulant drugs. *N Engl J Med* 287:220, 1972.
17. Palmer S: Minimal brain dysfunction, in Palmer S, Ekval S (eds): *Pediatric nutrition in Developmental Disorders*. Springfield, Ill, Charles C Thomas, 1978, p 76.
18. Shannon R: Neuropathic manifestations in infancy and childhood as a result of anaphylactic reactions to foods contained in the dietary. *Am J Dis Child* 24:89, 1922.
19. Feingold B: Adverse reactions to food additives with special reference to hyperkinesis and learning disability. *Congressional Record* S-19738-42, 1973.
20. Kittler FJ, Baldwin DG: The role of allergic factors in the child with minimal brain syndrome. *Ann Allergy* 28:203, 1970.
21. Randolph TG: Allergy as a causative factor in fatigue, irritability and behavior problems in children. *J Pediatr* 31:560, 1947.
22. Crook W: The allergic tension-fatigue syndrome. *Pediatr Ann* 3:69, 1974.
23. Clancy H, Entch M, Rendle-Short J: Infantile autism: The correction of feeding abnormalities. *Dev Med Child Neurol* 11:569, 1969.
24. Goodwin MS, Cowen MA, Goodwin TC: Malabsorption and cerebral dysfunction: A multivariate and comparative study of autistic children. *J Autism Child Schizo* 1:48, 1971.
25. Krieger I, Sargent DA. A postural sign in the diagnosis of the sensory deprivation syndrome. *J Pediatr* 70:332, 1967.
26. Pauling L: Orthomolecular psychiatry. *Science* 160:265, 1968.
27. Griffiths AW, Sylvester PE, Bayles EM: Serum globulins and infections in mongolism. *J Clin Pathol* 22:76, 1969.

28. Sobel AE, Strazulla M, Sherman S, et al: Vitamin A absorption and other blood-composition studies in mongolism. *Am J Ment Defic* 62:642, 1958.

29. McCoy EE, Colombini C, Ebadi M: The metabolism of vitamin B_6 in Down's syndrome. *Ann NY Acad Sci* 166:116, 1969.

30. Mahuren JD, Coburn SP: Pyridoxal phosphatein lymphocytes, polymorphonuclear leukocytes and platelets in Down's syndrome. *Am J Clin Nutr* 27:521, 1974.

31. Coburn SP, Seidenburg M: Leucocyte pyridoxal-phosphate level in Down's syndrome and other retardates. *Fed Proc* 27:55, 1968.

32. McCoy EE, Rostafinsky MJ, Fishburn C: The concentration of serotonin by platelets in Down's syndrome. *J Ment Defic Res* 12:18, 1968.

33. Fallström SP, Liedholm M, Lundburg P: Evidence of altered cerebral serotonin in Down's syndrome from measurements of cerebrospinal fluid acids. *Pediatr Res* 7:52, 1973.

34. Milunsky A, Hackley BM, Hasted JA: Plasma erythrocyte and leucocyte zinc levels in Down's syndrome. *J Ment Defic Res* 14:99, 1970.

35. Cash R. Krieger I, Evans GW: Therapy of encrodermatitis with zinc picolinate. *Ped Res* 15:627, 1981.

36. Culley WJ, Goyal K, Jolly DH, et al: Caloric intake of children with Down's syndrome (mongolism). *J Pediatr* 66:772, 1965.

8
Nutritional Effects on the Immunodefense and Blood-Forming Systems

NUTRITION, INFECTION, AND IMMUNITY

The association of famine and pestilence has been recognized for centuries, but the causal relationships have been explored only in recent years. As awareness of the impact of malnutrition on public health increased, it became apparent that an understanding of these relationships was essential to the development of effective intervention strategies.

Certain aspects of the relation between nutrition and infection are quite obvious. Among these is the fact that infection causes depletion of body nutrient stores due to hypermetabolic losses that are not replenished during illness because of anorexia. It is also well known that factors operative in the poverty cycle along with poor nutrition predispose to infection. Important causes are substandard housing, crowding, and poor sanitation. A direct effect of malnutrition on immunodefense mechanisms has been recognized only in recent years as a prominent cause of infection. Most surprising was the finding that single nutrient deficiencies can modulate the immune response and thus alter susceptibility to infection. These observations were possible through the use of modern immunological techniques that allow an assessment of individual components of the host defense system.

Confusion may arise from conflicting observations. Some of the differences are attributable to the fact that malnutrition, as it presents itself in field studies, is extremely complex and observations are not comparable to animal experiments in which single nutrients are manipulated. For instance, it has been shown very recently that deficiency of zinc or pyridoxine has a specific effect on cell-mediated immunity that differs from the effect of protein-calorie malnutrition. The degree or acuteness of malnutrition also plays a role. For example, protein restriction of up to 5% in experimental animals enhances cell-mediated immunity and tumor cell killing and also retards development of the diseases of aging. Further restriction, on the other hand, has an adverse effect on the immune system. Acute starvation increases antibody production in experimental animals but may cause a minor decrease in the number of circulating lymphocytes. By contrast, chronic starvation impairs antibody-mediated immunity and increases cell-mediated immunity. No differences have been recognized between protein malnutrition or combined protein-calorie malnutrition.

Effects of Infection on Immunity

In contrast to animal experiments, human field studies of the immune response in malnutrition are influenced by many factors. Since infection stimulates a series of defense measures and also constitutes a drain on nutrition, a three-sided interrelationship exists, with nutrition-induced immunologic changes as the third facet. For instance, a severe generalized infection may stimulate immunodefense but may also cause anergy, and lymphocyte failure to respond in vitro to mitogens. Another example of altered reactivity induced by infection is an abnormal immune response to sheep red cells, which has been observed in mice who received at the time of stimulation a sublethal dose of an infectious organism.

Normally, when antigen is trapped by phagocytic cells in the reticuloendothelial system, immunocompetent cells react and initiate a series of cellular responses that culminate in humoral and cell-mediated immunity and trigger several nonspecific defense measures, including fever, mobilization of phagocytic cells, release of acute phase-reactant proteins, and the sequestration of iron and zinc. The removal of iron from plasma causes an increase of unsaturated transferrin that, in turn, withholds iron from microorganisms due to its affinity for iron and thus protects the host from infection. The humoral immune response begins with an increase in IgM and is followed by prolonged production of different species of IgG molecules with increasing antigen-specific binding affinities. Parasitic infections are potent stimulators of IgE, while infections that involve mucosal surfaces characteristically stimulate IgA. This requires production of secretory component by the mucosal cell which combines with IgA.

Effects of Malnutrition on Immunity

Reports from underdeveloped countries indicate that malnutrition mainly affects cell-mediated immunity. Humoral immunity and nonspecific host defense mechanisms are affected to a limited degree and inconsistently. As a consequence of their profound deficiency in cell-mediated immunity, children in underdeveloped countries frequently succumb to viral diseases, such as measles, that have a low mortality rate in the United States. Low resistance to infections with Gram-negative and intracellular organisms, including *Mycobacterium tuberculosis*, malaria, and *Pneumocystis carinii*, has been reported. In the developing countries, diagnosis of measles in a child with kwashiorkor is almost equivalent to a death sentence. Experience (1) in metropolitan areas of the United States is different, because malnourished children are often reported to be more resistant to colds than their better nourished siblings. Although this aspect has not been studied directly, data from animal experiments seem to offer an explanation for the discrepancy. These studies have shown (2,3) that chronic malnutrition improves cell-mediated immunity, which therefore could be responsible for the observed resistance to colds. Since deficiency of zinc (4) and pyridoxine (5) have the opposite effect, one must consider that malnutrition in underdeveloped countries is complicated by single-nutrient deficiency.

Cell-mediated immunity is assessed through tests that measure T-lymphocyte function, allograft rejection, and the memory response of the skin to ubiquitous antigen. Patients with protein-calorie malnutrition generally have a depressed response to trychophytin, mumps antigen, purified protein derivative (PPD), and ubiquitous recall antigens like candidin and streptokinase-streptodornase (SK-SD) (6,7). A number of studies have also shown impairment of the afferent or sensitizing arm of delayed hypersensitivity with skin tests using BCG vaccine; 2,4-dinitrochlorobenzene; or dinitrofluorobenzene. Studies of allograft rejection and graft-versus-host rejection have produced inconsistent results.

The thymus in malnourished children is shrunken, has lost its architectural organization, and shows degeneration of Hassall's corpuscles with lymphocyte depletion. Concomitant with these changes is a decrease in the number of circulating thymus-dependent T lymphocytes (8). By contrast, B lymphocytes are normal or even increased in number (9). "Null" cells, which are lymphocytes without a surface marker, are increased in malnutrition. If they are—as some observers believe—undifferentiated cells, an increase in "null" cells may be the result of the decrease in T

Table 8-1. Effects of Malnutrition on Immunodefense of the Human Host

Cutaneous delayed hypersensitivity	
	Decreased response to candidin, trichophytin, SK-SD, PPD, mumps vaccine
	Decreased sensitization with BCG vaccine, DNCB, DNFB
Thymus gland	
	Decreased size and corticomedullary differentiation
	Lymphocyte depletion
	Degeneration of Hassall's corpuscles
T lymphocytes	
	Decreased number of circulating thymus-dependent lymphocytes
	Increased number of "null" cells
	Decreased thymic hormone activity
	Decreased transformation in response to antigens and mitogens
Allograft rejection	
	Inconsistent results
B lymphocytes	
	Normal or increased in number
	IgG: normal
	IgM: increased
	IgE: often markedly increased
	IgA: normal or decreased
	S-IgA: decreased
Phagocytes	
	Normal number
	Normal bacteriostatic ability
Complement	
	Decreased C1q, C1s, C2, C3, C5, C6, C8
	Anticomplementary activity occasionally increased

lymphocytes that is characteristic of malnutrition. In line with this explanation is the observed (10) decrease in thymic hormone, which is thought to be responsible for lymphocyte differentiation. Lymphocyte transformation in response to antigens and mitogens is generally reduced. Lymphocytes seem to retain their ability to form migration-inhibitory factor. Other lymphocyte functions have not been systematically studied. Phagocyte number and bacteriostatic ability appear unaffected.

Corresponding to the finding of a normal or increased B-cell population are reports of normal or increased immunoglobulin levels (11). IgG levels tend to be normal. Levels of IgM and IgE are commonly elevated (12), whereas those of IgA may be decreased. Malnourished experimental animals do not demonstrate similar changes in humoral immunity. This difference suggests that the findings in human populations are a response to antigen exposure as a result of gastrointestinal, respiratory, or skin infections. The common finding of very high IgE levels supports this explanation, since intestinal infestation, which is not infrequent in the developing countries, stimulates IgE production. The response to specific antigens has been varied in different studies. Thus, decreased as well as increased antibody titers to measles, poliomyelitis, and cowpox virus have been reported. Diminished responses to typhoid, diphtheria, and yellow fever have been observed. It has been suggested that these discrepancies are due to the dose or route of injection, to the age of the patient, and to the severity of malnutrition.

Production of secretory component by the mucosal cells of the intestinal tract is deficient. This component must combine with IgA in order to make it resistant to digestion. The resultant S-IgA in duodenal and nasopharyngeal secretions is consequently decreased in malnutrition (13,14). S-IgA coats intestinal bacteria and blocks their entry into the intestinal wall. Decreased IgA levels therefore favor bacterial invasion and systemic infections. Failure of immunoexclusion of antigen by the intestines also predisposes to allergy, but an increased incidence has not been reported in malnutrition.

The complement system is usually also affected in malnutrition (15). Decreased complement components (C1q, C1s, C2, C3, C5, C6, and C8) have been reported, with C3 probably being the most sensitive indicator of malnutrition-induced changes in the complement system. Some data suggest increased anticomplementary activity in serum. Complement levels tend to be lower in kwashiorkor than in marasmus. Hemolytic complement activity is also low in kwashiorkor but normal in marasmus.

Provision of adequate nutrition results in rapid correction of the immunodeficiency, especially cell-mediated immunity. One of the earliest signs of beginning nutritional recovery appears to be an increase in T lymphocytes to normal numbers. While this occurs within a few days, normal lymphocyte function returns somewhat more slowly. If malnutrition was operative in utero during the critical stages of immunological development, recovery is much slower and may have long-lasting effects on cell-mediated immunity.

Specific nutrient deficiencies that impair the immunodefense system are iron, zinc, pyridoxine, and vitamin A deficiencies. Iron deficiency depresses some in vitro lymphocyte responses, mainly the production of leukocyte migration inhibition factor (16). Vitamin A, zinc, and pyridoxine deficiencies impair cell-mediated immunity. Deficiency of vitamin A may have this effect because it affects the surface membrane of the lymphocyte in such a way that antigen binding does not take place. The mechanism of action of zinc and pyridoxine deficiencies is not known. It may be similar, because pyridoxine is a cofactor in the pathway from tryptophan to picolinic acid, a ligand that enhances zinc absorption and that may have physiologic significance (17).

Plasma zinc is low in acrodermatitis enteropathica (AE) because of a genetic deficiency in zinc absorption. A similar abnormality seems to exist in the A-46 mutant of black-pied Danish cattle, because clinical manifestations are similar and include lowered resistance to infection, in addition to skin lesions, stunted growth, and CNS abnormalities. Zinc deficiency has been studied systematically in experimental animals, and it has been shown that its effects are similar to those encountered in human malnutrition, including decreased ability to form antibody-producing cells in response to thymus-dependent antigens (18), and deficiency of cytotoxic killer cells and thymic hormone (19). The role of zinc as a cause of the decrease in cell-mediated immunity in human malnutrition was tested in an ingenious manner by Golden et al., who applied skin tests with *Candida* antigen either with or without local zinc sulfate. They found a highly significant increase in the delayed hypersensitivity reaction at the site covered with zinc (20). The magnitude of the increase correlated negatively with plasma zinc concentrations. Malnourished infants given a zinc-deficient diet but adequate protein and calories show weight recovery but remain immunoincompetent.

NUTRITIONAL ANEMIAS

Diagnosis

Anemia is defined as a condition with low hemoglobin (Hgb) or hematocrit (Hct). In addition to a variety of other causes, anemia may result from nutritional deficiencies that interfere with heme synthesis, iron transport, nucleotide metabolism, or membrane stability. Iron deficiency is by far the most common of the six known nutritional anemias. The other five are anemias caused by deficiencies of folate, B_{12}, copper, vitamin E, and pyridoxine. The metabolism, function, source, and requirement of the individual nutrient, together with a description of the anemia and other deficiency symptoms, are described in Chapters 10 and 11. The clinical approach to the patient who has anemia or a history of inadequate nutrition requires further discussion.

The age of the patient and the history provide the most important clues to the diagnosis. Thus young infants, especially those who were born prematurely, are most prone to develop anemia. Iron-deficiency anemia may develop after birth when iron stores—contained mainly in the red cell mass—are used up and iron intake is insufficient to replenish the deficit. This occurs in full term infants between 4 and 6 months of age. Since premature infants develop the "physiologic low" for Hgb before full term infants, anemia tends to develop earlier too. Folate and B_{12} deficiencies are rare, but they do occur in infants of deficient mothers; and they are also more common in premature infants, because they exhaust their stores more rapidly during accelerated growth. Vitamin E-deficiency anemia occurs almost exclusively in premature infants, excluding cases of fat malabsorption. Dietary copper deficiency was first described in infants with severe combined nutritional deficiency and in very small premature infants who were fed cow's milk.

Diets that consist predominantly of a single type of food should always cause the physician to consider nutritional deficiencies. Cow's milk, unsupplemented by vitamins and minerals, predisposes to iron deficiency and, in rare cases, to copper deficiency. In several of the less common deficiency anemias, other predisposing conditions must exist in addition to the nutritional deficit. An example is the increased need for folate during pregnancy, during catch-up growth after prematurity or malnutrition, and with compensatory bone marrow hyperplasia associated with chronic hemolytic anemias. The diagnosis can be narrowed down during office examination by studying red cell morphology on a peripheral smear to determine cell size. Iron-deficient cells are microcytic and hypochromic, while folate- and B_{12}-deficient cells are macrocytic. Bone marrow examination is necessary in cases of macrocytosis. The mean corpuscular volume (MCV), which can be determined conveniently by electronic counter, is a useful aid in the diagnosis. Evaluation of MCV must take into account the developmental change that occurs with age; infants normally have smaller cells than older children and adults (upper limit 78 and $87\mu^3$ in infants and adults, respectively [Table 8-2]).

Red cells can be iron deficient in the absence of nutritional iron deficiency. For instance, ceruloplasmin, which has ferroxidase activity, decreases when copper is depleted, and this leads to failure of iron mobilization. Another example is B_6 deficiency, where iron is not utilized although serum iron and ferritin saturation are normal or increased. Consequently, this anemia is also characterized by the peripheral morphology of iron deficiency (i.e., microcytosis and hypochromasia). The same morphology, in conjunction with elevated serum iron levels, is seen in nonnutritional anemias where hemoglobin synthesis is deficient—mainly thalassemia and lead intoxication.

The routine complete blood count (CBC) and examination of a technically well-prepared blood smear provide enough information to narrow down the diagnosis so that only a few additional confirmatory steps are necessary. The smear in folate deficiency shows macrocytosis and hypersegmentation of neutrophilic nuclei. When iron and folate deficiency coexist, hypersegmentation is present, but MCV and other red cell indices are no longer reliable. If there is also leukopenia and if the smear shows thrombocytopenia, either folate or B_{12} deficiency is the most likely cause of the anemia, although orotic acidemia should be considered (see "Differential Diagnosis"). The routine workup of patients suspected of having anemia should include a reticulocyte count in areas where thalassemia and

Table 8-2. Differential Diagnosis of Nutritional Anemias

Deficiency	*Findings on Routine Workup*	*Confirmatory Diagnostic Workup*
Iron	Hypochromasia Microcytosis MCV < 70–78 μ^3[a]	FEP > 3 μg/g Hgb or > 100–200 μg/dl packed cells Transferrin saturation < 16%[b] Serum ferritin < 10 ng/ml[b] Serum iron, fasting < 40–60 μg/dl[b] Therapeutic trial: 3 mg/kg/day
Copper	Hypochromasia Microcytosis MCV < 70–78 μ^3[a]	Serum copper < 70 μg/dl, < 30 μg/dl at 0–3 months Therapeutic trial: 0.2 mg/kg/day
Pyridoxine	Hypochromasia Microcytosis	Therapeutic trial after exclusion of all other causes of microcytosis
Vitamin B_{12}	Macrocytosis Ovalocytes MCV > 77–87 μ^3[a] Neutropenia Thrombocytopenia	Megaloblastic bone marrow Serum B_{12} < 100 pg/ml Methylmalonic acid in urine Therapeutic trial: 1,000 μg IM per week
Folate	Macrocytosis MCV > 77–87 μ^3[a] Hypersegmented neutrophils Decreased Reticulocytes Neutropenia	Megaloblastic bone marrow with vacuolization Whole blood folate < 50 ng/ml, or Serum folate < 3 ng/ml[b] Therapeutic trial: 0.1 mg/day
Vitamin E	Normocytosis Normochromasia Acanthocytosis Increased Reticulocytes.	Serum α-tocopherol < 0.5 mg/dl

[a] Lower and upper limits are age dependent. The range of values is lower in infants.

[b] These confirmatory tests are not mandatory.

chronic hemolytic anemias are endemic. The reticulocyte count is low in iron deficiency and high in chronic hemolytic anemias.

The initial evaluation is not complete without consideration of physical findings. The B_{12}-deficient patient may show neurologic changes, including paresthesias, hyporeflexia, ataxia, a positive Babinski, and foot clonus; and there may be glossitis. Failure to thrive is not specific, although it is common in folate and B_{12} deficiency, whereas patients with iron deficiency are generally not underweight.

Once the diagnosis has been narrowed down sufficiently, only a few other tests are necessary to confirm the diagnosis (Table 8-2). Finally, it is advisable to demonstrate a positive therapeutic response, either by checking reticulocytes after 10 days or Hgb after 4 to 6 weeks of therapy. Changes in bone marrow morphology occur in folate and B_{12} deficiency within a few days. Since the reticulocyte response may be missed by a random examination on an outpatient basis, it is more practical to test the therapeutic response by following the Hgb value. Usually, one test after 4 weeks is necessary. A wrong diagnosis or lack of compliance should be suspected if there is no response to therapy.

Finally, there is one nutritional anemia that is the result of hemolysis although the degree is rarely severe enough to cause significant disease. This is the hemolysis caused by deficiency of vitamin E, which protects the lipids of the cell membrane against oxidative damage. In addition to nutritional vitamin deficiency, other factors are usually necessary to cause disease. These contributing factors coexist not uncommonly in premature infants: (*1*) decreased absorption; (*2*) deficient stores; (*3*) a high concentration of polyunsaturated fatty acids in many infant formulas, which increases vitamin E requirements; and (*4*) iron supplementation, which is frequently required in premature infants and has the undesirable side defect of donating unpaired electrons that may be used in the peroxidation of lipids in the cell membrane, thus increasing vitamin E requirements.

The red cells in vitamin E deficiency are normochromic and normocytic, and the reticulocyte count is increased, although rarely above 10%. Acanthocytes are commonly seen, but they are nonspecific. Diagnosis in infants is difficult because the physiologic low in Hgb concentration is reached at the same time that vitamin E deficiency is prevalent. Reticulocytosis is not a distinguishing feature, because the physiologic low is also followed by an increase in red cell mass. A serum concentration of alpha-tocopherol below 0.5 mg/dl is considered evidence of vitamin E deficiency. In view of premature infants' increased risk of developing vitamin E deficiency, prophylaxis is recommended.

Differential Diagnosis

The diagnosis of hypochromic microcytic anemias requires exclusion of lead intoxication in infants who have access to lead, mainly infants who eat loose plaster chips or chew on wood covered with paint containing lead. Thus, infants with pica or those with high levels of free erythroporphyrin (FEP) are suspect. An increased serum lead value confirms the diagnosis. Thalassemia should be ruled out if microcytic anemia is associated with reticulocytosis and does not respond to iron therapy, especially if the patient is of Mediterranean descent. Elevation of Hbg A_2 and Hgb F is diagnostic, but examination of the parents for microcytosis may be necessary in some cases. Idiopathic pulmonary hemosiderosis enters the differential diagnosis of iron-resistant microcytic anemia. These patients show reticulocytosis, typical lung lesions on x-ray, and sideroblasts in the sputum. Finally, a rare group of disorders are the sideroblastic anemias, which should be considered in cases of microcytic, hypochromic anemias that are unresponsive to iron. Characteristically, the bone marrow shows nucleated red cells with a perinuclear ring of coarse hemosiderin granules, called *sideroblasts*. Congenital absence of transferrin is another rare cause of microcytosis, which is, in these cases, the result of deficient iron transport rather than deficient intake.

Megaloblastic anemias due to nutritional deficiencies of folate or vitamin B_{12} should be distinguished from three genetic disorders with similar manifestations: (*1*) hereditary orotic aciduria, (*2*) dihydrofolate reductase deficiency, and (*3*) transcobalamine II deficiency. Congenital onset and retarded growth and development are typical of hereditary orotic aciduria and transcobalamin II deficiency. Patients with the latter disorder respond to high doses of B_{12} although their serum B_{12} levels are normal. Dihydrofolate reductase deficiency should be diagnosed in megaloblastic anemia resistent to both, folic acid and vitamin B_{12}. This is done by use of folinic acid which causes remission of the anemia.

Vitamin B_{12} responsive anemia may be the result of (*1*) dietary insufficiency, (*2*) an absorption defect due to lack of intrinsic factor (juvenile pernicious anemia), (*3*) defective ileal transport, or (*4*) transcobalamin II deficiency. In the juvenile form of pernicious anemia stomach histology and acid secretion are normal, and there are no serum antibodies against parietal cells or intrinsic factor. Consanguinity is common in parents of affected children.

The absorption of vitamin B_{12} is assessed by the Schilling test, using radiolabeled vitamin B_{12}. To induce urinary excretion of the label and thereby to prove that the vitamin was absorbed, the patient is given a flushing dose of 1,000 μg intramuscular (IM). Whereas normal patients excrete 10 to 30% of the label, patients with pernicious anemia excrete 2% or less. Intrinsic factor deficiency can be distinguished from other absorption defects by repeating an abnormal test along with the administration of a single dose (30 mg) of intrinsic factor. Distinction of B_{12} malabsorption from dietary deficiency is important, because the former requires parenteral vitamin B_{12}. An ileal transport defect should be considered in cases that are not dietary and that do not respond to intrinsic factor.

REFERENCES

1. Krieger I: Personal observations.
2. Kramer TR, Good RA: Increased in vitro cell-mediated immunity in protein-malnourished guinea pigs. *Clin Immunol Immunopathol* 11:212, 1978.
3. Cooper WC, Good RA, Mariani T: Effects of protein insufficiency on immune responsiveness. *Am J Clin Nutr* 27:647, 1974.
4. Chandra RK, Au B: Single nutrient deficiency and cell-mediated immune responses: I. Zinc. *Am J Clin Nutr* 33:736, 1980.
5. Willis-Carr JI, St Pierre RL: Effects of vitamin B_6 deficiency on thymic epithelial cells and T lymphocyte differentiation. *J Immunol* 120:1153, 1978.
6. Edelman R, Suskind R, Olson RE, et al: Mechanisms of defective delayed cutaneous hypersensitivity in children with protein-calorie malnutrition. *Lancet* 1:506, 1973.
7. Chandra RK: Immunocompetence in undernutrition. *J Pediatr* 81:1194, 1972.
8. Ferguson AC, Lawlor GJ Jr, Neumann CG, et al: Decreased rosette forming lymphocytes in malnutrition and intrauterine growth retardation. *J Pediatr* 85:717, 1974.
9. Bang BG, Mahalanabis D, Mukherjee KL, et al: T and B lymphocyte rosetting in undernourished children. *Proc Soc Exp Biol Med* 149:199, 1975.
10. Chandra RK: Serum thymic hormone activity in protein-energy malnutrition. *Clin Exp Immunol* 38:228, 1979.
11. Neumann CG, Lawlor GJ Jr, Stiehm ER, et al: Immunologic responses in malnourished children. *Am J Clin Nutr* 28:89, 1975.
12. Purtilo DT, Riggs RS, Evans R, et al: Humoral immunity of parasitized malnourished children. *Am J Trop Med Hyg* 25:229, 1976.
13. Sirisinha S, Suskind R, Edelman R, et al: Secretory and serum IgA in children with protein-calorie malnutrition. *Pediatrics* 55:166, 1975.
14. Reddy V, Raghuramulu N, Bhaskaram C: Secretory IgA in protein-calorie malnutrition. *Arch Dis Child* 51:871, 1976.
15. Sirisinha S, Suskind R, Edelman R, et al: Complement and C_3-proactivator levels in children with protein-calorie malnutrition and effect of dietary treatment. *Lancet* 1:1016, 1973.
16. MacDougall LG, Anderson R, McNab GM, et al: The immune response in iron-deficient children: Impaired cellular defense mechanisms with altered humoral components. *J Pediatr* 86:833, 1975.
17. Cash R, Krieger I, Evans GW: Therapy of acrodermatitis with zinc picolinate *Ped Res* 15:627, 1981.
18. Fernandes G, Nair M, Onoé K, et al: Impairment of cell-mediated immunity functions by dietary zinc deficiency in mice. *Proc Natl Acad Sci USA* 76:457, 1979.
19. Iwata T, Incefy GS, Tanaka T, et al: Circulating thymic hormone levels in zinc deficiency. *Cell Immunol* 47:100, 1979.
20. Golden MHN, Golden BE, Harland PSEG, et al: Zinc and immunocompetence in protein-energy malnutrition. *Lancet* 2:1226, 1978.

9
Nutrition in Gastrointestinal Disorders

SPECIFIC MALABSORPTION SYNDROMES
Diagnostic Approach
Laboratory Work-up
Carbohydrate Malabsorption
Lactose Intolerance
Sucrase-Isomaltase Deficiency
Glucose-Galactose Malabsorption
Fat and Protein Malabsorption/Maldigestion
Intraluminal Malabsorption Due to Pancreatic Disease
Intraluminal Malabsorption Due to Altered Bile Circulation
Treatment of Intraluminal Malabsorption
Mucosal Malabsorption (Including Gluten-Sensitive Enteropathy)
Mucosal Malabsorption Due to Surgical Conditions
Treatment of Mucosal Malabsorption
Disorders of Cellular Fat Transport
Protein Maldigestion and Protein-Losing Gastroenteropathies
Enterokinase Deficiency
Trypsinogen Deficiency
Exudative Protein-Losing Gastroenteropathies (EPLGE)

DIARRHEA
Acute Infectious Diarrhea
Etiology and Pathogenesis
Manifestations
Treatment
Chronic Nonspecific Diarrhea
Postgastroenteritis Syndrome with Malabsorption (Including "Intractable" Diarrhea)
Chronic Nonspecific Diarrhea Without Malabsorption

CHRONIC INFLAMMATORY BOWEL DISEASE
Crohn's Disease and Ulcerative Colitis
Comparison of the Two Disorders

SPECIFIC MALABSORPTION SYNDROMES

Most classifications of intestinal disorders are made according to the location of the anatomic defect or the type of biochemical abnormality. Unfortunately, patients do not present themselves for treatment in this fashion which makes the diagnostic process more difficult. A diagnostic workup that is not individualized is consequently exceedingly lengthy, uncomfortable for the patient, and time-consuming. During the investigations, patients are often placed on restrictive diets. Infants are usually switched from one formula to the other, often without making a substantive change, since only the proprietary name of the formula is different. These diets not only fail to cure the patient but may cause harm because malnutrition progresses while unnecessary tests are being performed, and this adds to the intestinal insult. Moreover, valuable time may be lost that could have been used for diagnosis by testing the effect of true dietary changes in the manner of a tolerance test.

Diagnostic Approach

The workup is determined by information that is obtainable from the patient in but a brief interview. This approach should be based on the type of stool abnormality, time of onset of diarrhea, and a classification of intestinal manifestations into acute and chronic disease. Bloody, mucoid stools and crampy pains prior to evacuation suggest large bowel disease, which is usually acquired after birth and may be infectious or nonspecific inflammatory. Watery stools, on the other hand, may be due to inflammatory small bowel disease or carbohydrate intolerance, which is either congenital or acquired. Large malodorous stools suggest fat and protein loss, which also develops either on a congenital or acquired basis (Tables 9-1 and 9-2).

A history of the diet and time of onset of diarrhea provide important diagnostic clues and help in the classification of the disorder into congenital and acquired defects. Since some congenital disorders do not become

Table 9-1. Causes of Watery Diarrhea (Diagnosis and Therapy)

Diagnosis	*Diagnostic Test*	*Therapy*
Lactase deficiency: Congenital, Developmental, Acquired.	Lactose tolerance	Restrict lactose
Glucose-galactose malabsorption: Congenital, Acquired.	Glucose and galactose tolerance	Restrict glucose, galactose, and lactose
Sucrase-isomaltase deficiency: Congenital, Acquired.	Sucrose tolerance	Restrict sucrose and starch
Congenital chloridorrhea	Stool electrolytes	Electrolyte replacement
Immunodeficiency	Immunologic workup	
Enterokinase deficiency	Duodenal trypsin activity, activated by enterokinase	Pancreatic enzymes
Trypsinogen deficiency	Duodenal trypsin activity, not activated by enterokinase	Pancreatic enzymes
Milk allergy	Milk elimination/ challenge	Restrict milk protein

manifest unless the specific digestive or absorptive function has been challenged, it is necessary to link the onset with the introduction of foods to the infant (Table 9-3). This requires not only a diet history but knowledge of the nutrient composition of infant foods and formulas. For example, congenital lactase deficiency and glucose-galactose malabsorption cause symptoms as soon as the newborn infant receives a milk-containing formula. Sucrase deficiency, on the other hand, may not cause symptoms until late in infancy although the defect is congenital, because infants frequently do not get foods sweetened with sugar until that time. Gluten-sensitive enteropathy develops when the infant is given wheat products, usually in the form of cereals at about 3 months of age.

Laboratory Workup

The initial workup (Table 9-4) includes tests to rule out infection and parasitic infestation as a cause of acquired diarrhea. In addition, the initial battery consists of a few simple screening tests, such as one for reducing substances (Clini-Test) indicative of unabsorbed sugars and a test of pH for the products of bacterial sugar fermentation, which cause the pH to drop to 6.0 or less. The xylose test assesses the intestinal absorbing surface

Table 9-2. Causes of Fat Malabsorption (Diagnosis and Therapy)

Diseases	*Diagnostic Tests*[a]	*Therapy*
Deficient pancreatic exocrine function		
Cystic fibrosis Schwachman syndrome (13) Hereditary pancreatitis (14) Adult relapsing pancreatitis	Sweat test. Duodenal enzymes[b].	Enzyme replacement[c] High caloric, high protein–low fat diet with MCT oil (15)
Altered bile circulation		
Biliary obstruction Ileal resection Cholestyramine therapy	Direct bilirubin. History. History.	MCT oil (16,17) and water-miscible vitamins A, D, E, and K
Gluten sensitivity:		
"Celiac disease" or Nontropical sprue	Elimination/challenge, xylose test, and intestinal biopsy.	Gluten restriction
Surgical conditions:		
Short bowel syndrome Stasis syndrome	History, GI-series, and culture of aspirate.	MCT oil (17), vitamins B_{12} and folate, and water-miscible vitamins A, D, E, and K
Deficient cellular fat transport	Intestinal biopsy.	MCT oil and water-miscible vitamins A, D, E, and K
A-betalipoproteinemia	LDL-cholesterol, blood smear.	
Wolman's disease	Bone marrow, and liver biopsy.	

[a] In all cases, 3-day stool collection for fat is indicated; normal < 5 g per day.

[b] Normal duodenal secretions, per kilogram body weight and per 50 minutes following stimulation: volume 3.9 ml; bicarbonate 0.19 mEq; trypsin 788 mcg; amylase 476 IU, lipase 1424 IU (11).

[c] Viokase, cotazyme, ilozyme, and pancrease (enteric coated), all of porcine origin; Viokase is available as bovine enzyme for patients with pork allergy. Dosage: Infants—15,000 units/meal; children—20,000–45 000 units/meal; adults—up to 90,000 units/meal, plus $\frac{1}{3}$ to $\frac{1}{2}$ the respective dose with each glass of milk or snack.

area. This sugar is carried across the intestinal absorptive cells by facilitated diffusion. Its rise in blood 1 hour after an oral load of 5 g has been standardized. An insufficient increase of less than 20 mg/dl suggests that the absorbing surface is decreased due to epithelial damage, as occurs, for instance, in gluten-sensitive enteropathy or other inflammatory small bowel diseases.

The further workup depends on the type of stool and the result of these screening tests. If unabsorbed sugars are present or if the watery part of the stool is acid because all sugars have been fermented, carbo-

Table 9-3. Diagnosis Based on Disease Onset

Disease	*Onset*
Food dependent onset:	Onset follows introduction of:
Congenital lactase deficiency	Milk and milk base formulas
Congenital glucose-galactose malabsorption	Milk and sucrose (in most hypoallergenic formulas)
Congenital sucrase-isomaltase deficiency	Sucrose; less after starch
Celiac disease	Gluten (gliadin)
Milk allergy	Milk
Allergic protein-losing gastroenteropathy	Food proteins
Food independent onset, genetic:	Onset is:
Cystic fibrosis	Variable
Acrodermatitis enteropathica	First month, unless breast-fed
Congenital chloridorrhea	Birth
Developmental lactase deficiency	Adolescence or later; earlier if precipitated by infection, or malnutrition
Enterokinase deficiency	Birth, improves after few months
Trypsinogen deficiency	Birth
Food independent onset, acquired:	Onset is associated with:
Disaccharidase deficiency	Diseases of mucosal lining, due to infection, severe malnutrition, ischemia, etc.
Monosaccharide malabsorption	
Enterokinase deficiency	
Lymphangiectasia	Cardiac failure, thoracic duct obstruction, granulomatous disease, etc.
Chronic, nonspecific diarrhea	Postgastroenteritis
Pancreatic insufficiency with bone marrow hypoplasia	Immunodeficiency (?)

hydrate tolerance tests are indicated. The choice is, again, guided by a history that attempts to match the onset of symptoms to the introduction of a specific carbohydrate. If the history does not provide clues, choosing the sequence of tolerance tests should be guided by the relative frequency of the different carbohydrate malabsorption syndromes, starting with a lactose load and followed by sucrose and then glucose if both are positive. Occasionally, these tolerance tests are abnormal because gastric emptying is delayed. If an inaccurate result is suspected, it may be necessary to repeat the test by giving the carbohydrate load via a nasoduodenal tube. The dosage used is generally 2 g/kg body weight.

Stools that are bulky and greasy and that float on water are suggestive of fat malabsorption. Fatty stools may be the result of defective intraluminal

Table 9-4. Basic Laboratory Workup

Stool inspection (watery? greasy? floating? malodorous?)
Stool pH and reducing substances (check liquid stool)
Stool culture (rotavirus, *Salmonella, Shigella, Klebsiella, Proteus*, enteropathic or enteroinvasive *E. coli*)
Stool for ova and parasites, including *Giardia lamblia*
Xylose test (1-hour blood level)
Serum carotene (diet must contain carotene)
Serum folate
Sweat chloride
If stool quality suggests fat malabsorption:
 3-day stool for fat, stool weight,
 Gastrointestinal x-ray series and
 Duodenal aspiration for pancreatic enzymes (if sweat test normal)
If stool quality, pH, and reducing substances suggest carbohydrate malabsorption:
 Specific carbohydrate withdrawal/challenge, followed by specific tolerance tests
If gluten withdrawal/challenge suggests gluten sensitivity:
 Intestinal (capsule) biopsy

digestion of dietary triglycerides by pancreatic lipase or poor absorption of the products of digestion (i.e., fatty acids and monoglycerides). A rough distinction between the two causes of fatty stools can be made by use of the xylose absorption test. If it is abnormal, defective intraluminal digestion is an unlikely cause. Rather, stools are bulky because fatty acids, which form calcium soaps, are not absorbed due to injury to the absorptive cells. Fat malabsorption is usually associated with protein malabsorption, which accounts for the putrid odor of the bulky stools. Abnormally low serum folate levels corroborate a diagnosis of malabsorption at the mucosal level. Low serum carotene, on the other hand, suggests fat malabsorption in general, providing insufficient carotene intake is not the cause of hypocarotenemia. Thus, carotene malabsorption, normal serum folate, and a normal xylose absorption test are indicative of defective intraluminal fat digestion. In these cases, aspiration of duodenal juice for enzyme analysis is recommended. However, pancreatic enzyme analysis is not necessary if the sweat test is abnormal (sweat chloride above 60 mEq/dl), since this test is by itself diagnostic of pancreatic insufficiency due to cystic fibrosis.

Capsule biopsy of intestinal mucosa is indicated if certain diseases (Table 9-2) are suspected at this point in the workup. Biopsy is not necessary if carbohydrate tolerance tests are compatible with a specific disorder and if the patient improves upon the withdrawal of the offending carbohydrate. Quantitative analysis of brush border disaccharidases (lactase, sucrase, maltase, and isomaltase) does not consistently correspond with clinical evidence provided by challenge/withdrawal testing. Therapy should be guided by tolerance tests and the response to withdrawal of the offending carbohydrate.

Carbohydrate Malabsorption

Lactose Intolerance

A high incidence of lactose intolerance due to decreased intestinal lactase activity has been observed in several racial groups. The term *lactose intolerance* refers to the presence of watery diarrhea, abdominal pain, bloating, and flatulence following ingestion of lactose in persons with proven lactose malabsorption. Diagnosis of lactose malabsorption is made by use of a lactose tolerance test (2g/kg, given orally) (Table 9-5). As a consequence of low lactase activity, undigested lactose remains in the gut and draws in fluid from the tissues. Some or all lactose is metabolized by bacteria to lactic acid, which contributes to the osmotic force and also tends to create an acid environment that acts as an irritant to the gut.

Three forms of lactase deficiency have been described: (*1*) congenital; (*2*) primary, late onset, or "developmental"; and (*3*) secondary hypolactasia. The congenital form is extremely rare. Infants with this inborn error of metabolism develop symptoms as soon as they receive milk. The enzyme is deficient, but the intestinal mucosa is histologically normal. The majority of infants with lactase deficiency have acquired the deficiency as a result of mucosal damage. Consequently, other functions may be affected, including absorption of fat and amino acids (1). The acquired disorder is usually reversible. However, on occasion, full lactase activity is not achieved after recovery from the primary disease (2). It is obvious that such cases could later in life be diagnosed as primary, developmental. The etiology of primary developmental lactase deficiency has been the subject of considerable study and debate. The most convincing observations to date suggest that it is a hereditary enzyme defect with late expression and varying frequency among racial groups. While the incidence is less than 15% in individuals of Northern European descent, Africans, American Indians, Arabs, Ashkenazi Jews, and Orientals have an incidence of 80 to 90%. The time of onset has varied in different population studies. Since

Table 9-5. Intestinal Carbohydrate Digestion

Carbohydrate	*Brush Border Enzyme*	*Product*	*Transport Mechanism*
starch ↓			
maltose and α-dextrins	maltase and isomaltase	glucose	active
lactose	lactase	galactose and glucose	active
sucrose	sucrase	glucose and fructose	active passive

it is unlikely that this difference in onset is genetically determined, it has been suggested that early expression of the defect can be induced by a variety of intestinal insults, including malnutrition or infection (3). Other observers consider these types of insults the major cause of developmental lactase deficiency. Failure of induction of lactase activity by food is not a cause, because lactose activity remains intact in individuals who, for medical reasons, have been on a completely lactose-free diet—for instance, patients with galactosemia.

Lactase is measured in the duodenal mucosa, obtained by capsule biopsy, but this test is not necessary for confirmation of the diagnosis. Inconsistencies between the enzyme test and the clinical response to the lactose tolerance test (LTT) are common. A number of explanations have been

Table 9-6. Galactose-Free Diet[a,b]

Food Group	*Foods to Avoid*	*Foods Allowed*
Milk and beverages	Milk, milk drinks, filled milks, whey, milk curds, milk solids	Formulas without lactose: casein hydrolysate, soy or meat base formulas; all fruit drinks, carbonated beverages, coffee, and tea
Breads and baked goods	Bread products containing milk or lactose	Crackers, homemade bread, and baked goods without milk or butter added
Cereals	Cream of wheat and any cereal containing milk or lactose	All others
Sweets and Desserts	Ice cream, sherbet, cake, cookies, candy, etc. containing lactose, milk, milk products, chocolate or butterscotch	Baked goods, candy, marmelade and puddings made without milk, lactose or chocolate; gelatin, fruit ices, carob, marshmallows
Eggs	None	All
Fats	Butter, cream, cream cheese, dressing, and margarine containing milk or milk products	Margarine without milk solids; salad oils, shortening, mayonnaise, bacon, lard
Fruits	Prepared fruits and juices containing lactose or glutamates	All fresh, canned, or frozen fruits that are not processed with lactose
Meat, fish, and cheese	Creamed or breaded meat, cold cuts, weiners and meat containing glutamates, lactose, or milk; all organ meats, cheeses, shell fish	Beef, fish, fowl, lamb, poultry, pork, veal, and fish not listed to avoid

suggested, including the site of the biopsy (4). To circumvent this problem, it is recommended that lactase activity be expressed as the ratio between sucrase and lactase activity (5). Other causes for inconsistencies between LTT and enzyme tests are related to the technique and variable gastric emptying.

Differences between the results of LTT and milk tolerance tests are also not uncommon. There is no consensus yet concerning the significance of these differences. The issue is of practical importance to the practitioner who must advise the lactose-intolerant patient on a diet. The amount of lactose used for the LTT in adolescents exceeds the amount of lactose ingested ordinarily at any one time. Thus, only about half of a small group of lactose-intolerant, black adolescents, examined by Mitchell et al. (6), were also intolerant to 250 ml of milk. Other investigators (7) have also claimed that black children who are lactose "malabsorbers" according to standard tests of the blood glucose response can tolerate 1 cup of milk but

Table 9-6. (Continued)

Food Group	*Foods to Avoid*	*Foods Allowed*
Potatoes and other starchy foods	Mashed potatoes and other foods containing milk, milk products or lactose: dehydrated potato products, frozen french fries, potato chips, creamed, escalloped, or buttered foods	White and sweet potatoes, hominy, macaroni, noodles, rice, spaghetti
Soups	Consomme and soups containing milk or lactose	Broth, vegetable soups that do not contain peas or lima beans
Vegetables	Beans, peas, lentils, legumes, creamed vegetables, sugar beets, and any prepared vegetable to which lactose has been added	All others
Miscellaneous	Chewing gum, cocoa, instant coffee, cream sauces, milk gravy, monosodium glutamate, imitation coffee cream	Nuts, peanut butter, catsup, mustard, olives, pickles, plain popcorn, salt, vinegar, spices, and flavoring not containing lactose or glutamate

[a] For patients with galactosemia. (Note: Lactose is hydrolyzed to galactose and glucose.)
[b] A lactose-free diet is prescribed for lactase deficiency; foods that contain galactose but no lactose are allowed; (i.e., peas, lentils, legumes, beans, sugar beets, chocolate made without milk, cocoa, gum, glutamate are allowed): The diet is otherwise like the galactose-free diet.

tend to become symptomatic when drinking more than that at a time. Not infrequently, patients with an abnormal lactose tolerance test do not develop watery diarrhea or pain and flatulence (8). It appears logical, therefore, to distinguish between *lactose malabsorption, lactose intolerance,* and *milk intolerance*. However, use of the latter term may cause confusion with *milk protein allergy*, a distinctly different entity.

These observations indicate that treatment of lactase deficiency must be individualized. Strict adherence to a milk-free diet may not be necessary. Prepared foods containing small amounts of milk solids often are tolerated, as are milk products, such as cheese, with a low lactose content per serving. Growth must be carefully monitored in growing children with lactase deficiency who continue to drink some milk, because calories may be lost even in the absence of intestinal symptoms. Lactase-deficient infants should be placed on a lactose-free formula (Table 9-6). Soy formulas or Nutramigen are suitable milk substitutes.

Sucrase-Isomaltase Deficiency

This disorder is either congenital in onset or acquired. The congenital form is a rare autosomal recessive disease which becomes symptomatic when sweetened foods like puddings, sugared cereals, or cookies are first introduced. The disorder is not associated with abnormal mucosal histology. The manifestations of carbohydrate malabsorption may be severe, with profuse watery diarrhea, or there is only bloating and some abdominal discomfort after ingestion of sweets. The defective enzyme hydrolyzes both sucrose and the branched oligosaccharides, called α-dextrins, apparently because the enzyme protein has two active sites. Maltase activity may be slightly decreased, since the enzyme has also some activity toward maltose. Only certain starches form α-dextrins after being acted upon by pancreatic amylase. Since these branched oligosaccharides are relatively large molecules, they have little osmotic effect and contribute insignificantly to the watery diarrhea. As a result, affected patients can tolerate starch although it is not completely absorbed. The disorder should be distinguished from acquired disaccharidase deficiency.

Treatment requires complete elimination of sucrose from the diet and moderate restriction of starch. After adolescence, these patients may be able to tolerate some sucrose, although enzyme activity per unit of brush border remains deficient. This has been attributed to an increase in total sucrase activity with growth of the small intestine. Infants tolerate all milk base formulas, breast milk, and cow's milk. Glucose and fructose may be used as sugar substitutes (Table 9-7).

Glucose-Galactose Malabsorption

This is a specific defect of monosaccharide transport that causes symptoms like those seen in defects of carbohydrate digestion. Although extremely rare, this disorder must be considered in the differential diagnosis of

Table 9-7. Sucrose- and Starch-Free Diet[a]

Food Group	*Foods to Avoid*	*Foods Allowed*
Milk and beverages	Milk drinks with sugar, condensed milk	All others
Breads and baked goods	Bread of any kind, crackers, flour, pancakes, waffles, cornbread, pretzels, biscuits, muffins, bread crumbs, rolls	None
Cereals	All	None
Sweets and desserts	White sugar, brown sugar, powdered sugar, candy, jam, marmalade, preserves, jelly, syrup, gum, sweetened baked goods, ice cream, sherbet, puddings	Honey, glucose
Eggs	None	All
Fats	Salad dressing with added sugar	All others
Fruits	Sweetened fruits and fruit juices (Check labels on can; use only those which say "unsweetened" or "no sugar added.")	All fresh, dried, canned, or frozen fruits or fruit juices without sugar
Meat, fish, and cheese	Lunch meats, weiners, bread dressings	Beef, pork, veal, lamb, poultry, cheese
Potatoes and starchy foods	White potatoes, sweet potatoes, rice, noodles, spaghetti, potato chips, popcorn, macaroni, cornstarch	None
Vegetables	All others	Asparagus, Green beans, Wax beans, Broccoli, Brussels sprouts, Cabbage, Cauliflower, Celery, Chard, Collards, Cucumbers, Eggplant, Kale, Kohlrabi, Lettuce, Mushrooms, Okra, Peppers, Parsley, Spinach, Tomato, Watercress
Miscellaneous	Carbonated beverages, food or drinks with flour or sugar added	Tea, salt, pepper, herbs, spices, vanilla, lemon, unflavored gelatin, broth, unsweetened pickles

[a] For patients with sucrase-isomaltase deficiency.

congenital disorders of carbohydrate tolerance. Inheritance is autosomal recessive. Infants are intolerant to starch and all sugars except fructose. They do not tolerate milk, and as a result, serious nutritional problems are common. Blood glucose does not rise after the ingestion of either lactose, sucrose, or glucose. Moderate amounts of sucrose are better tolerated than comparable amounts of lactose because one of its monosaccharide constituents is fructose.

The biochemical defect involves the active, energy-dependent transport site in the intestinal mucosal cell. Fructose, which is taken up by passive diffusion, is consequently tolerated. By contrast, fructose is also poorly absorbed in acquired disorders of mucosal transport following severe mucosal cell injury ("intractable" diarrhea).

Therapy of the genetic disease is extremely difficult because it requires lifelong restriction of milk and starchy foods, which are major nutrients in our diet (Tables 9-6 and 9-7). Fruits, fat, and meats are tolerated. Vegetables that should be restricted because they contain substantial amounts of galactose and glucose are beans, peas, lentils, beets, sweet potatoes, squash, and the like. Fructose is the only tolerated sugar substitute.

Fat and Protein Malabsorption/Maldigestion

Intraluminal Malabsorption Due to Pancreatic Disease

The gross appearance of the stool is diagnostic of intraluminal fat malabsorption when an oily film is noted on the surface of the water that contains the stool. The oil and a greasy coating of the stools reflect undigested neutral fats that occur in lipase deficiency due to disorders of exocrine pancreatic function. In the majority of disorders, all pancreatic enzymes are involved. However, fat "maldigestion" is the major abnormality because starch and protein digestion do not depend entirely on pancreatic excretions. Protein digestion is only decreased to about 80% of normal. Breakdown of unabsorbed protein by intestinal bacteria is responsible for the putrid odor of the stools.

Deficiencies of isolated pancreatic enzymes appear to be exceedingly rare. A few cases of lipase deficiency have been reported in the literature, but the data suggest that both amylase and/or trypsin were not entirely normal. The basic defect in cases with intraluminal fat and protein malabsorption thus appears most commonly to be one that affects the entire secretory activity of the pancreatic acinar cells—for instance, in Schwachman syndrome and familial hereditary or adult relapsing pancreatitis (Table 9-2). The only well-documented genetic deficiency of a single pancreatic enzyme appears to be a case with trypsinogen deficiency, described by Townes (9). This syndrome is clinically different from other pancreatic enzyme disorders in that hypoproteinemic edema is the major feature and the diarrhea tends to be more watery.

By far the most common disorder of intraluminal fat and protein malabsorption is cystic fibrosis. It is also one of the most common genetic diseases in general, with an incidence of about 1 in 1500 (10). The basic biochemical defect is not known. The disorder affects multiple systems and is characterized by abnormalities in the secretions of many organ systems, including pancreas, lung, liver, and sweat glands. The most reliable diagnostic abnormality is an increased concentration of sodium and chloride in sweat of over 60 mEq/l. Increased viscosity is a feature common to all of the affected secretions. In addition, multiple other biochemical abnormalities have been described.

The increased viscosity explains many of the disease manifestations of this disorder, which was originally called *mucoviscoidosis.* The water content of pancreatic secretions is measurably decreased, a feature that distinguishes cystic fibrosis from other disorders of pancreatic exocrine dysfunction (11). Ductal obstruction caused by the increased viscosity leads to dilation of the pancreatic ducts with flattening of the epithelium and, ultimately, fibrosis. This feature of mucous secretions is also responsible for meconium ileus, which occurs in about 15% of affected newborns. The ratio of wet weight to dry weight is 4.3 in normal meconium and 2.2 in the meconium of infants with ileus (10). In the liver there is excess mucus in bile duct radicles with periportal cirrhotic changes (12). Focal liver cirrhosis is evident histologically in about 25% of cases, but the cirrhotic process in the majority is not progressive, because clinically evident liver cirrhosis occurs only in 4 to 6% of the cases (10). The most serious complications of viscous secretions develop in the lung, where obstructive emphysema is an early manifestation, visible on x-ray as increased radiolucency. Frequent infections are the result of poor bronchial toilet. Fibrosis develops, and pulmonary insufficiency is the cause of the ultimate demise in most cases. At the time of diagnosis, pulmonary manifestations are pronounced in about 20% of cases, but by age 2 years more than 75% have pulmonary symptoms. (Clinical manifestations are listed in Table 9-8.)

The Schwachman syndrome is the second most common disorder of pancreatic exocrine function, but compared to cystic fibrosis, it is rare. The major features of the syndrome are linear growth failure, eczema, susceptibility to infection, neutropenia or pancytopenia, metaphyseal dysostosis, and diabetes mellitus. A familial incidence has been observed. Current immunological concepts are compatible with the theory that a hereditary immunologic deficiency makes these patients susceptible to pancreatic injury, possibly as a result of viral infections. Histologically, one finds only scattered clusters of acinar tissue, widely separated by fat. The condition has been described as "congenital hypoplasia with lipomatosis", "pancreatic insufficiency with bone marrow hypoplasia" or "pancreatic insufficiency with metaphyseal dysostosis." The pancreozymin-secretin test (11) shows decreased secretion of enzymes but a normal

Table 9-8. Manifestations of Cystic Fibrosis (10)

Pancreatic insufficiency	85%
Pulmonary disease	75%–100%
Meconium ileus or equivalent	15%
Rectal prolapse	22% (less if
Growth retardation	needed)
Glucose intolerance	40–60%
Liver Cirrhosis	>10%
Vitamin deficiency (2° fat malabsorption)	4%
Lactase deficiency	2–10%
Clinical diabetes mellitus	16%[a]
Intussusception, volvulus	2–10%
Recurrent acute pancreatitis	1%
Cholelithiasis and cholecystitis	<2%
Hypoproteinemia (in infancy)	<2%
	<2%

[a] High incidence is probably in part due to inclusion of patients with developmental lactase deficiency.

volume output, a feature that distinguishes this syndrome from cystic fibrosis.

Intraluminal Malabsorption Due to Altered Bile Circulation

Long chain triglycerides, the major portion of dietary fat, are insoluble in water and therefore must be dispersed in the intraluminal water of the intestines before pancreatic lipase can be effective. This is accomplished by bile salts, which are secreted by the liver into the duodenum. Bile salts also solubilize the end products of digestion (i.e., long chain saturated fatty acids, monoglycerides, and cholesterol). Bile salt deficiency consequently causes fecal losses of both neutral fats and fatty acids.

Major causes of bile salt deficiency in the gut are congenital biliary atresia and acquired bile duct obstruction due to infection, choledochal cysts, or other tumors. Bile salt depletion results from cholestyramine therapy and ileal resection. Bile acid deficiency contributes to the diarrhea in short bowel syndrome if the resection includes a significant portion of the terminal ileum where bile acids are reabsorbed. A new syndrome of bile acid deficiency without obstruction, which is thought to be caused by a synthetic defect, has been described (18). The stools in these disorders contain both neutral fats and the products of lipolysis.

Treatment of Intraluminal Malabsorption

Pancreatic enzyme replacement therapy and dietary management control the symptoms of fat malabsorption in most cases of pancreatic exocrine deficiency. There is, however, no effective therapy for the pulmonary disease in cystic fibrosis. A variety of pancreatic extracts are available (see footnote of Table 9-2). The initial dose is based on age, but it should be increased if the quality of the stools does not improve. Three-day stool collections for fat analysis may be necessary to monitor effectiveness. A well-balanced normal diet with vitamin supplements is usually sufficient early in the course of the disease. However, as the disease progresses, patients may develop growth failure despite seemingly adequate pancreatic replacement therapy and diet. The cause is generally related to the energy burden imposed by repeated pulmonary infections and respiratory insufficiency. Anorexia often plays a role as well. It is necessary in these cases to check the adequacy of the diet intermittently through 24-hour recalls.

Several causes of growth failure must be considered if the nutritional assessment indicates a normal intake per body weight. The patient's energy requirements may be abnormally high because of the pulmonary disease. Consequently, calorie and protein supplements should be prescribed. Easily absorbed protein hydrolysates are available for this purpose as flavored drinks, including Vital (Ross) and Vivionex "standard" or "high-nitrogen" (Norwich-Eaton). Flexical (Mead Johnson) provides in addition 18% of the fat calories as MCT oil.

Another possible cause of growth failure is ineffectiveness of pancreatic enzyme replacement. In cases where maximum amounts are given, enzymes may be inactivated. Postprandial depression of duodenal pH below 4, which causes degradation of lipase, does occur in adults with chronic pancreatitis. Since patients with cystic fibrosis have decreased secretions of bicarbonate, a similar mechanism is possible. The use of cimetidine to maintain an alkaline pH has been effective in adults with pancreatitis and may be useful in children with exocrine pancreatic deficiency. Enteric-coated enzyme preparations also may be tried (Pancrease). Use of MCT oil as the major dietary fat is the treatment of choice if lipase deficiency is indeed the only reason for growth failure in patients on replacement therapy. Portagen, which provides 85% of fat calories as MCT oil, may be used as infant formula or milk substitute in such cases.

Medium chain fatty acids are water soluble and can be absorbed without the intervention of bile salts. Moreover, some medium chain triglycerides are absorbed without being first hydrolyzed by pancreatic lipase. MCT oil is thus ideally suited for treatment of pancreatic insufficiency and biliary obstruction. Since medium chain fatty acids are absorbed directly into the portal circulation, they are also extremely useful in the dietary treatment of patients with disorders associated with lymphatic obstruction (see following).

Mucosal Malabsorption (Including Gluten-Sensitive Enteropathy)

Mucosal damage affects all absorptive functions if the damage is severe. Carbohydrate absorption and digestion by brush border enzymes is deficient only if the entire length of the small intestine is involved.

Malabsorption of fat and protein is therefore the major abnormality in gluten sensitivity, because usually only the upper small intestine is diseased. Coexistence of fat and protein malabsorption is also a characteristic of pancreatic insufficiency, but protein malabsorption is comparatively more severe in mucosal malabsorption syndromes. Moreover, absorption of protein is more deficient than absorption of amino acids. This suggests that the lack of peptide hydrolysis by damaged epithelial cells is a major factor in disorders of mucosal absorption.

Mucosal damage may be the result of infection, allergy, and nonspecific inflammatory changes as well as gluten sensitivity. Massive infestation with *Giardia lamblia* has a similar effect, because this parasite burrows into the crypts between the villi and blocks absorption. The upper intestine is predominantly involved, a feature shared with gluten sensitivity. The stools are foul smelling, and there is steatorrhea in all these disorders.

Gluten-sensitive enteropathy was described as "celiac disease" in 1950 by Dicke (19), who attributed it to the "harmful effects of certain types of cereal." The term *nontropical sprue* has been used to describe the disorder in adults. A flattened mucosa with villous atrophy and deep crypts is characteristic of the disease. The decrease in total absorbing surface is variable, since the lesions vary in severity and extent, possibly as a result of differences in gluten exposure.

Clinical manifestations range from severe involvement with so-called celiac crises to mild, late onset disease. Stools are loose, bulky, and malodorous, and the abdomen is distended. Some patients become edematous. Malnutrition develops in severe cases. The protruding abdomen over thin legs and wasted buttocks has been described by the French as "marrons sur deux alumettes." Since anorexia is ordinarily not present, the patient may be successful in compensating for the caloric loss by overeating. Lack of malnutrition consequently does not rule out gluten-sensitive enteropathy.

Diagnosis rests upon the demonstration of characteristic mucosal lesions and a dramatic response to a strict gluten-free diet. Biopsy is necessary. It is important that the patient receives gluten and is symptomatic when the biopsy is obtained. Although often described as the most common malabsorption syndrome, the incidence of gluten sensitivity is probably less than original estimates, because strict diagnostic criteria often were not used in the past.

The mechanism by which gluten or its breakdown product, gliadin, damage the intestinal mucosa is not known. An inborn error of an enzyme, resulting in the accumulation of a toxic gluten peptide, as well as immune deficiency have been considered, but there is no conclusive data yet in support of either hypothesis.

Mucosal Malabsorption Due to Surgical Conditions

Several postsurgical conditions are known to cause malnutrition due to chronic malabsorption if appropriate prophylactic steps are not taken.

Foremost among them is the short bowel syndrome. Several congenital anomalies or acquired conditions may necessitate massive bowel resection that would not have been attempted in former times when total parenteral nutrition was unavailable. Since survival of the immediate postoperative period is now possible, infants with as little as 40 cm remaining small intestine, who have chronic malabsorption problems, will have to be managed on a lifelong basis. These patients tend to have an increase in the rate of acid production for months after surgery (20). Since pancreatic enzymes are inactivated if the postprandial pH in the lower duodenum is less than 5.0, malabsorption develops. Fat absorption of patients with terminal ileal resection is compromised by bile acid depletion due to deficient reabsorption. If the resection includes the mid and distal jejunum and part of the ileum, fluid balance will be disturbed. Malabsorption of calcium, magnesium, and zinc also may result (21). Thus, three factors contribute to the malabsorption in short bowel syndrome: increased acidity, bile acid depletion, and the decrease in absorbing surface due to the resection itself.

The mechanism of malabsorption is different in the so-called stasis syndrome, which is uncommon in the pediatric age group. It results from chronic, relatively mild partial bowel obstruction, which is a rare complication of volvulus, malrotation with obstructing bands across the gut, or partial intraluminal diaphragms. These conditions usually cause symptoms of acute obstruction, including vomiting and pain. However, if there is chronic diarrhea associated with these or other anatomic abnormalities, stasis syndrome should be considered. Side-to-side or end-to-side anastomoses also create stasis in a blind loop (22). The steatorrhea in stasis or blind loop syndrome has been attributed to bacterial overgrowth, but the mechanism remains uncertain. Degenerative changes are usually not visible by light microscopy, but abnormalities in the absorptive cells have been recognized with the electron microscope (23).

Treatment of Mucosal Malabsorption

Restriction of gluten-containing grains is required for celiac disease and should be lifelong (Table 9-9). The following grains, common to the American diet, contain gluten: wheat, alfalfa, barley, rye, and oats. Some (hydrolyzed) vegetable proteins, vegetable gums, food starches, and malt flavoring also may contain gluten. All are commonly used additives in prepared foods and should be avoided. Substitute flour for cooking and baking is available from soybeans, corn, potatoes, rice, and lima beans. Some relaxation of dietary restrictions is possible in older children and adults, using subjective symptoms as a guide. Patients should be directed toward recipe books, which assist them in devising a varied and appetizing diet (24).

Treatment of other mucosal diseases and surgical conditions should be aimed at the correction of underlying causes, including therapy for infestation, infection, or surgery, as indicated. Stasis due to inoperable

Table 9-9. Gluten-Free Diet

Food Group	*Foods to Avoid*	*Foods Allowed*
Milk and beverages	Ovaltine, prepared drinks that contain malt, wheat, or rye flour	Milk, cocoa, carbonated beverages, coffee, tea
Breads and baked goods	Biscuits, breads, waffles, pancakes, crackers, bread crumbs, rolls, pretzels, Zwieback, rusks, melba toast, and other foods made with wheat, oats, rye, or barley	Breads made with cornmeal, gluten-free wheat starch, soy, potato, or rice flour
Cereals	All others	Cooked cereals made from rice or cornmeal; cornflakes, puffed rice, Rice Krispies
Sweets and desserts	Any pudding thickened with wheat or rye flour	Gelatin, sherbet, ice cream, homemade custard, rice pudding, tapioca, jelly, jam, honey, syrups
Eggs	Eggs thickened with flour	All
Fats	Commercial salad dressings	Butter, margarine, salad oil, shortening, lard, pure mayonnaise, peanut butter, cream, homemade salad dressings thickened with cornstarch
Fruits	Stewed fruits if thickened with flour, commercial fruit pie fillings	All pure fruits

conditions may be treated intermittently for 1 to 2 weeks with antibiotics. In short bowel syndrome, antacids may be tried in addition to MCT oil. Some benefit may be derived from the use of MCT oil in disorders associated with widespread mucosal damage. This has been attributed to the fact that exudation of lymph is diminished, because MCT oil is absorbed directly into the portal system, thus relieving the load on lymphatic fat absorption. Supplemental vitamins, especially vitamin B_{12}, should be given. Bile salt replacement is not recommended for short bowel syndrome because excess may cause diarrhea.

Disorders of Cellular Fat Transport

A few rare genetic disorders have in common a defect in fat transport from the mucosa to the lymphatics, although the mechanism is not the

Table 9-9. (Continued)

Food Group	*Foods to Avoid*	*Foods Allowed*
Meat, fish, and cheese	Breaded or creamed products, luncheon meats, frankfurters, sausage unless pure meat; cheese sauces or spreads unless known to be wheat-free	All plain meat, fish, poultry, and cheese
Potatoes and other starchy foods	Spaghetti, noodles, and macaroni (unless made with potato or rice flour), creamed or scalloped potato (unless thickened with cornstarch)	Potato, rice
Soups	Soups containing commercially prepared noodles, macaroni, spaghetti	Broth, homemade cream soups if thickened with cornstarch, rice or potato flours
Vegetable	Creamed or escalloped vegetables if thickened with flour or topped with bread crumbs	All
Miscellaneous	Commercially prepared gravies and sauces containing wheat flour	Gravies and sauces thickened with rice or potato flours, gluten-free wheat starch, cornstarch

same. They include A-betalipoproteinemia and Wolman's disease. Fatty acids and monoglycerides are absorbed normally in A-betalipoproteinemia. They are reesterified back into triglycerides but are not incorporated into chylomicron. Histologic examination shows normally structured villi, but they contain an excess of lipid droplets. Diarrhea with bulky stools due to steatorrhea starts soon after birth. Protein malabsorption is also present. Serum lipids and cholesterol are decreased. This deficiency causes secondary red cell, central nervous system, and retinal changes resembling retinitis pigmentosa. Acanthocytosis and low levels of LDL-cholesterol are diagnostic. Presence of ataxia, neuropathy, and mental retardation in patients with steatorrhea should suggest the diagnosis.

Wolman's disease, a genetic defect associated with lysosomal storage in liver, lung, spleen, adrenals, and intestines, also starts in early infancy. Lipid-filled histiocytes infiltrate the lamina propria, and there may be loss of normal villous structure. Foamy histiocytes are found in bone marrow aspirates. The stored fat contains up to 20 times the normal amount of cholesterol. The disease has been attributed to deficiency of acid lipase. It causes steatorrhea and inanition, and it is usually rapidly fatal.

Protein Maldigestion and Protein-Losing Gastroenteropathies

Only a few intestinal diseases are associated with edema due to protein maldigestion and absorption. Although protein and fat loss generally coexist in disorders of intestinal absorption, fat losses are usually more severe, especially in intraluminal malabsorption syndromes like cystic fibrosis. Occasionally, protein malabsorption is severe enough in mucosal malabasorption syndromes to cause hypoproteinemic edema. By contrast, edema is a major feature of two rare genetic disorders of protein digestion: enterokinase deficiency and trypsinogen deficiency. In addition, it is the most impressive and occasionally the sole manifestation of protein-losing enteropathies.

Enterokinase Deficiency (25)

This disorder is marked by watery diarrhea and occasional vomiting, with onset soon after birth. The lack of protein digestion causes hypoproteinemia, failure to thrive, and, ultimately, hypoproteinemic edema. Normal activity of amylase and lipase in duodenal aspirates is a feature that distinguishes this disease from Schwachman syndrome or cystic fibrosis. Tryptic activity is absent in duodenal juice, but is restored upon addition of enterokinase. The dagnosis may be confirmed by demonstrating decreased enzyme activity in biopsy specimen of small intestinal mucosa.

Trypsinogen Deficiency (26)

The clinical manifestations, which are due to an isolated deficiency of tryptic activity, are similar to enterokinase deficiency. However, the inability of enterokinase to restore tryptic activity in duodenal aspirates distinguishes this disorder from enterokinase deficiency. Failure to thrive and edema may be the only sign of abnormality in occasional cases that do not manifest diarrhea. Hair depigmentation, reminiscent of kwashiorkor, has been reported.

Treatment of both disorders consists of pancreatic enzyme replacement. Doses similar to those for cystic fibrosis are suggested. In trypsinogen deficiency bovine trypsin is able to activate the patient's own intestinal procarboxypeptidases and chymotrypsin. Edematous infants benefit from the use of protein hydrolysate formulas.

Exudative Protein-losing Gastroenteropathies (EPLGE)

Normally, serum proteins are lost into the gastrointestinal tract, digested, and then partly reabsorbed. Hypoproteinemia and edema develop when the rate of protein catabolism exceeds the body's protein-synthetic capacity. EPLGE is thus not a malabsorption syndrome, but rather an imbalance between excretion and reabsorption. However, since EPLGE can cause secondarly fat malabsorption and clinically resembles disorders of protein digestion, discussion of this entity in this context appears justified.

Exudative protein loss has been demonstrated in over 40 disorders (27). Diagnosis is established by use of intravenously administered radioactive proteins, including ^{131}I-albumin, ^{51}Cr-albumin, ^{131}I-polyvinylpyrrolidone, and ^{67}Cu-ceruloplasmin. It has been shown by these techniques that some protein exudation occurs also in gluten-sensitive enteropathy (28,29), cystic fibrosis, milk allergy, diarrhea of immunodeficiency diseases, and chronic inflammatory bowel disease (27). EPLGE has been described in adults with gastric polyps and carcinomas, intestinal granulamatous disease, and amyloidosis. It is a major feature of two other disorders, seen mainly in adults, Whipple's disease and giant hypertrophy of the gastric mucosa. Disorders of the lymphatic system are the most common cause of EPLGE in the pediatric age group.

EPLGE occurs in congestive right heart failure and has been described in children with constrictive pericarditis (30). High venous pressure, which increases lymph production and causes partial obstruction to the entry of lymph into the central vein, is thought to be responsible. All serum proteins are decreased, including immunoglobulins. The loss of lymph into the gut causes lymphocyte depletion, resulting in multiple deficiences of the immunodefense system. This mechanism must be distinguished from primary immunodeficiency diseases, which may be associated with chronic diarrhea and protein loss. In EPLGE due to right heart failure, correction of the lesion will reverse the immunodeficiency (31). Roentgenograms of the small intestine are either normal or show mucosal edema. Dilation of submucosal lymphatics can usually be recognized on capsule biopsy specimen.

Intestinal lymphangiectasia is often familial and becomes symptomatic in the majority of cases during the early teens (32). A congenital malformation is the most likely cause, but acquired lymphatic obstructions must be ruled out. Hypoproteinemia is due to rupture of dilated lymph vessels. Chylous effusions have been described (33). Patients tend to have more severe reductions of serum proteins, including transferrin and ceruloplasmin, than patients with other types of EPLGE. Lymphocytopenia is always present. The edema is usually generalized, although it may be asymmetrical or even focal. A majority have intermittent diarrhea, but EPLGE without gastrointestinal symptoms has been observed. Absorption of fat is occasionally decreased. The xylose test is normal. Diagnosis can be confirmed by demonstration of lymph (34) in intestinal aspirates or by lymphangiography. The diagnosis cannot be made by quantitative determination of fecal nitrogen.

Finally, EPLGE may be present in infancy as a result of allergy, mainly to milk proteins (32). Gastrointestinal symptoms are generally mild. Vomiting may occur after milk ingestion. Occult intestinal blood loss, which does not disappear after iron therapy, is considered typical. Allergy is suggested by the presence of other allergic manifestations, a family history of allergy, and the finding of eosinophils in the intestinal submucosa, the peripheral blood, and the stools (Charcot–Leyden crystals). The triad of hypoproteinemic edema, hypocupremia, and hypoferremia should suggest EPLGE due to milk allergy (35).

Treatment of EPLGE depends on the cause of the disorder. Thus, it may require ligation of a lymphatic fistula, resection of a granulomatous or ulcerative portion of the intestinal tract, or correction of cardiac disease. Corticosteroids may be tried in ulcerative colitis. Dietary measures are the only form of therapy available for widespread inoperable lesions, such as lymphangiectasia. Low-fat diets, using mainly fats with a high content of unsaturated fatty acids, have been successful in the past. Therapy has been greatly facilitated since the introduction of MCT oil and increased understanding of the mechanism of its action. It is believed that MCT oil decreases the flow of lymph because it is absorbed directly into the portal system. As a result, pressure in the chronic duct decreases, and protein loss is diminished although the primary defect is not altered (36,37).

DIARRHEA

Acute Infectious Diarrhea

Acute diarrhea due to infectious gastroenteritis is a potentially fatal disease in young infants unless dehydration and electrolyte imbalance are adequately treated. It accounts for most of the deaths of preschool children in the developing countries. Prompt attention to fluids and electrolytes through dietary management could prevent complications and obviate the need for intravenous therapy in many cases. Dietary management is also important during the recovery phase of acute diarrhea after weaning from intravenous therapy. This requires an understanding of the mechanism of diarrhea and the anticipated electrolyte imbalance.

Etiology and Pathogenesis

Causes of infectious gastroenteritis vary in different areas of the world Thus viral infections are a more common cause of infectious diarrhea in the United States, while *Salmonella, Shigella,* cholera, and *E. coli* predominate in the developing countries (38). However, small outbreaks of diarrhea due to these agents do occur in the United States. *E. Coli* causes disease either through enteroinvasion and inflammatory destruction of epithelium, mainly in the lower intestine and colon, or through toxin production. The latter is the more common mechanism. Enterotoxins increase AMP production, which leads to increased secretion and decreased absorption of fluid. Prostaglandins may play a role in the pathogenesis of this type of secretory diarrhea. Other organisms that cause watery diarrhea are *Klebsiella pneumoniae, Pseudomonas aeruginosa,* and *Yersinia enterocolitica.*

Viruses are a common cause of gastroenteritis in the United States. Since they spread fast and are highly contagious, they are responsible for many institutional outbreaks. Among them is a rheovirus-like agent, also called rota virus, which is an important cause of infantile diarrhea throughout the world. Although it is transmitted to adults, who respond by seroconversion, they rarely develop symptoms, apparently because of previously acquired immunity. Virus invasion causes villous cell destruction and a cryptlike appearance in the intestinal mucosa. Salt and water absorption diminish, and intestinal brush border enzymes, mainly lactase, may decrease.

Manifestations

Two types of infectious diarrhea can be distinguished on clinical grounds, depending on the site of involvement. When the colon is affected by *Shigella dysenteriae, Salmonella,* or enteroinvasive *E. coli,* stools are mucoid and sometimes bloody and may contain leukocytes. Water loss is not significant, and fever is usually present. By contrast, infection of the small bowel by enterotoxic *E. coli,* cholera, and other organisms causes profuse watery diarrhea and dehydration. Electrolyte loss is variable. Mild fever may be present but is usually absent in diarrhea due to enterotoxic *E. coli.* Duration varies from 9 to 7 days.

Five percent dehydration is not clinically recognizable except for the presence of thirst. Dehydration of 5 to 10% causes a decrease in skin turgor, dry mucosa, sunken eyes and fontanels and, gradually, the urine volume decreases. Body weight may reflect the amount of water loss. Shock may be a complication in 10 to 15% dehydration. Diarrhea stools are usually isotonic, with sodium concentrations ranging from 30 to 60 and potassium from 20 to 50 mEq/l. Both lower and higher extremes are observed, especially in cholera, where sodium concentration may range up to 120 mEq/l. Hypotonic dehydration results when stools have a high electrolyte content and solute-poor solutions are taken orally. Hypertonic dehydration is usually the result of inappropriate oral fluids, mainly the use of undiluted skim milk. Hypertonic dehydration is especially dangerous because of CNS complications (Chapter 10) and because the degree of dehydration tends to be masked, thus delaying intervention. Changes in skin turgor and blood pressure develop slowly in the presence of hypertonicity, because water moves from the cells to the extracellular compartment and vascular space.

Treatment

It is current practice to withhold food and offer only fluids during the first 24 to 48 hours. Ideally, these fluids should be designed to replace the electrolytes lost in the stools and other excretions. However, since the exact deficit is rarely known, it is advisable to offer electrolytes in the lower range of losses generally encountered during diarrhea (i.e., 30 mEq/l sodium and 20 to 25 mEq/l potassium). This will allow the kidney to make the remaining adjustments. Commercially available electrolyte solutions such as Lytren (Mead Johnson) and Pedialyte (Ross) fulfill these requirements. They may be given full strength or perferably diluted, 1:1 with water, to decrease the osmolar load. Unsweetened orange juice may be given as a source of electrolytes. In addition, calories should be provided to slow down the rate of catabolism until feeding can be resumed. Since commercial electrolyte solutions contain only 30 to 20 kcal/dl, addition of glucose would be desirable. However, higher glucose concentrations constitute an excessive osmolar load that may aggravate the diarrhea. Polycose (Ross) is therefore preferred as an added calorie source, since the osmolality is only one-fifth that of glucose solutions with equal caloric density. Refeeding should be resumed as soon as possible to prevent malnutrition. Since acute infections may cause transient deficiency of disaccharidases, mainly lactase, feeding of milk or milk base formulas is not advisable during the recovery phase. Lactose free formulas are made with soy protein or casein hydrolysate. They should be used initially in one-quarter strength, and the concentration should be rapidly increased if the stool quality remains improved. Fruit juices should be given liberally since they provide caloric energy (50 kcal/dl) in the form of fructose, which does not require enzyme hydrolysis and is passively absorbed.

Chronic Nonspecific Diarrhea

Postgastroenteritis Syndrome with Malabsorption (Including "Intractable" Diarrhea

Protracted diarrhea, which follows an acute gastroenteritis, is probably the most common malabsorption syndrome in infancy. In contrast to genetic enzyme deficiencies, intestinal biopsy specimen reveal histologic alterations in these cases, mainly inflammatory infiltration of the lamina propria and blunting of the villi that affects brush border enzymes. Consequently, deficiency of disaccharidases, mainly lactase, should be suspected in any case of acute gastroenteritis that does not improve within 1 week of onset. Prolonged restriction of milk is advised. Sucrose is often tolerated better than lactose.

Some cases do not respond despite adequate dietary therapy, and they will have diarrhea even though a "predigested" formula is given. Even glucose solutions and "modular" formula combinations cause diarrhea when the mucosal transport of multiple nutrients is defective. Parenteral nutrition is the only lifesaving measure in these challenging cases. Although this should allow the intestinal mucosa to heal, diarrhea may continue, and repeated trials of food introduction may be followed by exacerbations for months after onset. Cases of watery diarrhea not associated with reducing substances may be due to excessive spillage of bile acids into the colon, which induces secretion of water and electrolytes. The excess is a result of accquired malabsorption of bile acids and may respond to cholestyramine therapy (39,40). Prolonged malabsorption of bile acids that is not compensated for by a corresponding overproduction can ultimately produce bile acid depletion and fat malabsorption as a further complication of the intractable diarrhea syndrome.

Treatment consists of total parenteral nutrition and gradual introduction of formulas that contain no disaccharides. A carbohydrate-free formula may be tried initially, adding either fructose or glucose if the formula base is tolerated. It is important to continue partial parenteral nutrition during the gradual introduction of oral feeding in order to avoid malnutrition that further complicates the intestinal injury. Cholestyramine should be tried in patients who have persistent watery diarrhea while receiving total parenteral nutrition. Cholestyramine has the advantage of also binding other substances, including toxins. If fat malabsorption develops, patients will usually respond to the partial provision of fat calories as MCT oil. Therapy with bile acids should not be contemplated in cases with suspected bile acid malabsorption because substitution in amounts matching the losses is not possible and excess bile may be irritative.

Chronic Nonspecific Diarrhea without Malabsorption

This disorder has been given several nonspecific names, such as "irritable colon" or "sloppy stool syndrome." It is a relatively benign, self-limited disorder with unknown pathogenesis. Rapid transit, possibly related to emotional stimuli, is one explanation. Stools are loose to watery and often explosive, but there may be intermittent constipation. Diarrhea begins usually after 4 months of age and is not associated with malnutrition. Problems rarely continue past 4 years of age. There is often a family history of similar problems in siblings or one parent.

Pressured by the parents' concern, these patients are usually placed on multiple dietary regimens that are ineffective and may cause iatrogenic malnutrition if the diets are low caloric. This complication makes it difficult to determine cause-and-effect relationships, since malnutrition alone can cause digestive disorders. Diarrhea without malabsorption is also a manifestation of the psychosocial deprivation syndrome. In that disorder malnutrition and growth failure improve if the patient is given a full diet.

Management calls for a basic diarrhea workup, which may be used in conjunction with a normal growth record to demonstrate to the parents conclusively that a serious problem does not exist. Dietary modifications that lead to a decreased calorie intake should be avoided. If changes are attempted, they should be done systematically, each for a period of 2 to 3 weeks, and the parents should keep a record of stool quality and quantity. The changes should represent true elimination of potentially pathogenic nutrients rather than changes in formula names. If the parents are not kept apprised of the goal of the "diagnostic process by elimination" and of the benign nature of the disorder, any change tends to heighten the anxiety and complicate management. Use of a name for the syndrome helps in reassuring the parents, providing the benign, self-limited nature of the disorder has been pointed out. Caution must be exercised when interpreting the response to elimination of a specific nutrient, because the disorder is intermittent and a beneficial response may be coincidental. For this reason, rechallenge and repeat elimination trials are necessary. In the typical nonspecific diarrhea, no diet regimen has a lasting effect. Consequently, treatment of the parents becomes more important than treatment of the patient. Recent observations in three patients with nonspecific diarrhea indicate that judicious use of a trial with zinc therapy is justified, especially in cases with familial nonspecific diarrhea (41).

CHRONIC INFLAMMATORY BOWEL DISEASE

Crohn's Disease and Ulcerative Colitis

Comparison of the Two Disorders

Crohn's disease and ulcerative colitis are two chronic disorders of unknown pathogenesis that have similar clinical manifestations. Onset is usually after 20 years of age, but about 20% begin during adolescence. Ulcerative colitis has been described in infants. The distribution of cases is about equal between males and females. Both the familial occurrence and a higher incidence in Jews suggest that genetic factors are operative. Behavior disorders have been described, but they are now considered to be the result rather than the cause of chronic bowel disease. There is also no evidence to implicate any constituent of the diet. Whereas both disorders affect the colon, only Crohn's disease extends into the ileum, which may be the sole site of involvement in some cases (regional ileitis). The inflammatory process in ulcerative colitis involves the mucosa with infiltrates and abscesses and tends to be widespread. By contrast, Crohn's disease is a transmural inflammatory process, occasionally localized and consisting of noncaseating granulomas that involve only segments of the gut. These distinctions are not clear when the disorder begins in childhood, and there is uncertainty whether they represent different pathologic processes or extremes of a single spectrum of pathologic involvement.

Manifestations

A number of signs and symptoms are shared by the two disorders. They consist of mucoid or bloody diarrhea, abdominal pain, anorexia, fever, weight loss, growth failure, and delayed puberty. Gastrointestinal protein loss is common, although varying in degree. Joint pain is seen in severe cases. Finger clubbing develops in long-standing cases.

Biochemical studies are of limited value in the diagnosis but are helpful in guiding and evaluating therapy. Abnormalities like a low hemoglobin, elevated sedimentation rate, and hypoalbuminemia are not consistently present, and they seem to reflect the presence of complications (i.e., blood loss, secondary infections, and protein-losing enteropathy).

Treatment

The role of diet in the treatment of chronic inflammatory bowel disease has been the subject of controversy. It is the current consensus that specific restrictions, like a low-roughage or a bland diet, are not necessary and may be counterproductive if they are not palatable. Instead, emphasis should be placed on offering a balanced and nutritious diet, using high-caloric supplements, but only to the extent that they are accepted by the patient. Some cases with ileal involvement may have an acquired lactase deficiency that requires milk restriction. Milk protein allergy is not considered a cause of the disease by most observers. Consequently, milk restriction is not necessary, although it may be tried on a temporary basis. Patients with ileal involvement should receive monthly B_{12} injections.

Necrotizing Enterocolitis

This disorder usually strikes disabled or premature infants weighing less than 1,500 g, generally during the first 2 months of life. Both colon and ileum may be involved, and the process affects the entire bowel wall. The disease has never been reported in an infant who has not been fed, although the onset may be as early as the second day of life. Onset is either slow, with gradually increasing diarrhea, or it progresses rapidly, causing bloody diarrhea, acute abdominal distension, perforation, and shock. Radiologic exam may show dissection of the inner layer of the gut with entry of air.

The etiology remains obscure. Several theories have been advanced, but no single one explains all features of the disease. Epidemiologic studies have not been very helpful. The disorder was rare before 1960, suggesting that a component of medical management, which has become more aggressive in recent decades, could play a role. The following mechanisms have been considered: stress-induced reflex vasoconstriction, infections, and feeding-induced mucosal damage. However, the ischemia theory fails to explain the common delay in onset following perinatal stress and the absence of abnormality in other parts of intestine. An infectious agent or toxin has not been identified. Claims have been made that breast milk protects against the still unknown noxious agent by virtue of its immunoprotective properties, but this has not been proven either. The feeding of formulas with high osmolality has also been implicated, especially in cases where the formula was introduced directly into the gut through a nasoduodenal feeding tube. These practices have changed, but there is no evidence to date, that the incidence of necrotizing enterocolitis is on the decline. However, a contributory role of high osmolality must be seriously considered. Increased osmolality of intestinal contents may cause hypovolemia of the splanchnic vessels, mucosal ischemia, malabsorption, further injury by unabsorbed foods or products of digestion, and toxic insults.

Treatment and Prevention

In view of the possible etiologic role of feeding practices, care should be taken to increase the feeding of small premature infants gradually and, if necessary, complemented by partial parenteral nutrition. Tube feeding should be done by nasogastric tube, using formulas with an osmolality of about 300. Premature infant formulas are available that deliver a high caloric density (80 kcal/dl) while staying within the limits of osmolality that are considered safe. They are Enfamil Premature Formula (Mead Johnson) and Similac 24 LBW (Ross). The combination of high caloric density and relatively low osmolality (Table 2-5) is accomplished by using larger oligosaccharides in place of mono- or disaccharides as an energy source.

There is no specific treatment for the disease other than allowing the process to heal while withholding all food and feeding the infant through total parenteral nutrition.

MILK ALLERGY

The term *milk allergy* describes a sensitivity to milk proteins that manifests itself in disturbances that disappear following removal of milk from the diet. The most common clinical manifestations are a variety of gastrointestinal disturbances, eczematous or urticarial rashes, and, less commonly, respiratory symptoms like rhinitis, coughing, wheezing, or symptoms comparable to idiopathic pulmonary hemosiderosis. The term *allergy* implies an antigen–antibody reaction. Newborn infants appear to be most vulnerable to antigen–antibody responses because secretory immunoglobin levels (S-IgA) are low during the early weeks of life, allowing direct absorption of macromolecules. Demonstration of antibodies to a specific protein does not imply that the characteristic clinical manifestations are due to an immune response. Thus, children with a normal immune system will make some antibodies against cow's milk proteins, but most will not be sensitive to cow's milk consumed in customary quantities. Consequently, diagnosis must be made by demonstrating a causal relationship between antigen challenge and the specific immune response.

Manifestations

The diarrhea in milk allergy is watery, but it may be mucoid and occasionally bloody (42). It is usually associated with abdominal pain. Vomiting, which starts within an hour of ingestion, occurs in about half the cases. Although the gastrointestinal tract is the major target organ of the antigen–antibody response, other allergic symptoms coexist in a small percentage of cases (i.e., rhinitis, urticaria, atopic dermatitis, and wheezing). The presence of these recognized allergic manifestations is a helpful diagnostic sign. The duration of symptoms ranges from $\frac{1}{2}$ hour to several days. In addition to secretory diarrhea, other gastrointestinal disorders have been attributed to protein sensitivity, including protein-losing gastroenteropathy (27) with or without iron and copper deficiency, ulcerative colitis or proctitis (43), and chronic occult blood loss of sufficient severity to cause iron deficiency anemia (44).

Diagnosis

The patient with milk protein allergy is sensitive to any one or several of the cow's milk antigens: β-lactoglobulin, casein, α-lactalbumin, serum globulin, and serum albumin. The most antigenic in this group is β-lactoglobulin, followed by casein. Diagnosis may be made by observing the response to challenge with the individual protein, but this is rarely done. Improvement following withdrawal of milk protein is observed first. A casein hydrolysate formula is given, which is preferable to soy protein formulas, because patients with an atopic constitution may be sensitive to both milk and soy protein (45). Following improvement, the patient should be given sufficient time to recover, both from malnutrition and possible secondary lactase deficiency. A lactose tolerance test (2 g lactose per kilogram body weight, given orally) may be the next step unless there is doubt about the cause-and-effect relationship, in which case rechallenge with milk protein is conducted first. Infants with a history of severe diarrhea and dehydration should be challenged initially with only 15 ml, followed after 2 days of milk-free diet by rechallenge with larger amounts. Providing lactase deficiency has been ruled out by a normal lactose tolerance test, a patient who responds to milk challenge with diarrhea should be challenged at least twice with the same dose. Some investigators advise a total of three challenges (46). Symptoms following repeat challenge are usually similar with regard to cause, type of response and duration.

Diagnosis by response to treatment is bound to cause misdiagnosis in this disorder, because gastrointestinal symptoms are alike in milk protein allergy and lactose intolerance. An unfortunate choice of terms by the Protein Advisory Group (PAG) of the United Nations System (47) has not corrected the potential for confusion. "Milk intolerance" was defined as "clinical signs [i.e., abdominal pain, diarrhea, bloating, and flatulence] consistently following a few hours after ingestion of milk or milk containing products in usual amounts in a person with proven lactose malabsorption." Since both milk and all currently marketed milk base formulas contain milk protein as well as lactose, and since milk protein-free formulas are also free of lactose, confusion between "milk intolerance" and "milk protein intolerance," or allergy, is bound to arise.

Treatment and Prophylaxis

Complete elimination of milk and milk products from the diet is necessary for at least 1 year (Table 9-6). Casein hydrolysate should be tried first. Soy, or meat base formulas are well-accepted substitutes for infant feeding, except in cases with associated allergy to other proteins. Since a considerable number of milk-sensitive infants will tolerate some milk by the end of the first year, gradual introduction of small amounts may be tried at that time. By the end of the second year, most infants will tolerate customary quantities of milk. The exception are patients with late onset disease, which if often permanent. The degree of restriction should be individualized in these cases.

Prophylaxis is advised in infants from atopic families, who should be breast-fed for 6 weeks after birth and preferably longer. Since the intestinal mucosal barrier is deficient during the early weeks of life, the protection from protein penetration afforded by human milk during this crucial time may prevent sensitization (Chapter 2).

DIARRHEA IN IMMUNODEFICIENCY DISEASES

The gut, which has an abundance of lymphoid tissue in the intestinal wall, plays an important role in immunodeficiency diseases. Secretory IgA, the major immunoglobin in intestinal secretions, protects against the invasion of antigens. While gastrointestinal diseases may cause a breakdown of the immunoprotective barrier, the reverse causality also exists. Thus, immunodeficiency diseases are not uncommonly associated with chronic diarrhea. The mechanism of the intestinal disorder is not known, although food has been implicated because entry of dietary macromolecules is to be anticipated in the absence of secretory IgA.

Viral or fungal infections and infestation are other possible causes of chronic diarrhea in immunodeficiency diseases. This diarrhea may be associated with malabsorption for several reasons. Mucosal fat malabsorption is seen in *Giardia lamblia* infestation and may be anticipated if immunodeficiency causes colonization of the proximal small bowel. Chronic mucocutaneous candidiasis should be ruled out as a cause of diarrhea in disorders of T-cell immunity.

Protein sensitivity is suspected as a cause of some of the symptoms in Wiskott-Aldrich syndrome, which consists of eczema, bloody diarrhea, frequent infection, and thrombocytopenia. A defect in specific immunoresponsiveness exists, although there is no decrease in humoral immunity, plasma cells, or B and T lymphocytes.

Gluten-sensitive enteropathy has been described in association with hypo-γ-globulinemia (48). Coexistence of the typical histologic changes and immunoglobulin deficiency requires exclusion of primary gluten sensitivity, which is occasionally associated with exudative protein-losing enteropathy leading to loss of immunoglobulins. However, histologic changes similar to gluten sensitivity may be secondary to immunodeficiency diseases in which case the patients do not respond to gluten restriction.

Trial therapy with gluten restriction or protein elimination is warranted in diarrhea that is associated with immunodeficiency diseases, providing infection has been ruled out. There is also a theoretical basis for the use of casein hydrolysate formulas as prophylactic therapy, especially when considering the seriousness of the underlying disorder and the deleterious effects of complicating gastrointestinal disease due to protein allergy. Breast feeding is advised for infants with immunodeficiency diseases.

REFERENCES

1. Paige DM, Graham GG: Nutritional implications of lactose malabsorption. *Pediatr Res* 6:329, 1972.
2. Dahlquist A, Lindquist B: Lactose intolerance and protein malnutrition. *Acta Paediatr Scand* 60:488, 1971.
3. Brasseur D, Mandelbaum I, Vis HL: Effect of an episode of severe malnutrition and age on lactose absorption by recovered infants and children. *Am J Clin Nutr* 33:177, 1980.
4. Newcomer AD, McGill DB: Distribution of disaccharidase activity in the small bowel of normal and lactase-deficient subjects. *Gastroenterology* 51:481, 1966.
5. Bolin TD, Davis AE, Seah CS, et al: Lactose intolerance in Singapore. *Gastroenterology* 59:76, 1970.
6. Mitchell KJ, Bayless TM, Paige DM, et al: Intolerance of eight ounces of milk in healthy lactose-intolerant teenagers. *Pediatrics* 56:718, 1975.
7. Garza C, Scrimshaw NS: Relationship of lactose intolerance to milk intolerance in young children. *Am J Clin Nutr* 29:192, 1976.
8. Paige DM, Bayless TM, Dellinger WS Jr, et al: Relationship of milk consumption to blood glucose rise in lactose intolerant individuals. *Am J Clin Nutr* 28:677, 1975.
9. Townes PL, Bryson M, Miller G: Further observations on trypsinogen deficiency disease: Report of a second case. *J Pediatr* 71:220, 1967.
10. Shwachman H: Gastrointestinal manifestations of cystic fibrosis. *Pediatr Clin North Am* 22:787, 1975.
11. Hadorn B, Zoppi G, Shmerling DH, et al: Quantitative assessment of exocrine pancreatic function in infants and children. *J Pediatr* 73:39, 1968.
12. Oppenheimer EH, Esterly JR: Hepatic changes in young infants with cystic fibrosis: Possible relation to focal biliary cirrhosis. *J Pediatr* 86:683, 1975.
13. Schwachman H, Diamond LK, Oski FA, et al: The syndrome of pancreatic insufficiency and bone marrow dysfunction. *Pediatrics* 65:645, 1964.
14. Comfort MW, Steinberg AG: Pedigree of a family with hereditary chronic relapsing pancreatitis. *Gastroenterology* 21:54, 1952.
15. Hashim SA, Roholt HB, Van Itallie TB: Pancreatogenous steatorrhea treated with medium-chain triglyceride. *Clin Res* 10:394, 1962.
16. Zurier RB, Hashim SA, Van Itallie TB: Effect of medium-chain triglyceride on cholestyramine-induced steatorrhea in man. *Gastroenterology* 49:490, 1965.

17. Zurier RB, Campbell RG, Hashim SA, et al: Use of medium-chain triglycerides in management of patients with massive resection of the small intestine. *N Engl J Med* 274:490, 1966.
18. Powell G, Jones A, Richardson J: A new syndrome of bile acid deficiency—a possible synthetic defect. *J Pediatr* 83:758, 1973.
19. Dicke WK: Coeliac disease: Investigation of harmful effects of certain types of cereal on patients with coeliac disease. *Thesis*, Netherlands, University of Utrecht, 1950.
20. Avery GB, Randolph JG, Weaver T: Gastric response to specific disease in infancy. *Pediatrics* 38:874, 1966.
21. Ladefoged K, Nicolaidow P, Jarnum S: Calcium, phosphorus, magnesium, zinc, and nitrogen balance in patients with severe short bowel syndrome. *Am J Clin Nutr* 33:2137, 1980.
22. Bayes BJ, Hamilton JR: Blind loop syndrome in children. *Arch Dis Child* 44:76, 1969.
23. Ament ME: Malabsorption syndromes in infancy and childhood: Part II. *J Pediatr* 81:867, 1972.
24. Baum Sheedy C, Kaifetz N: *Cooking for Your Celiac Child.* New York, Dial Press, Inc, 1969.
25. Hadorn B, Tarlow MJ, Lloyd JK, et al: Intestinal enterokinase deficiency. *Lancet* 1:812, 1969.
26. Townes PL: Trypsinogen deficiency disease. *J Pediatr* 66:275, 1965.
27. Waldmann TA: Protein-losing enteropathy. *Gastroenterology* 50:422, 1966.
28. Huizenga KA, Wollaeger EE, Green PA, et al: Serum globulin deficiencies in non-tropical sprue, with report of two cases of acquired agammaglobulinemia. *Am J Med* 31:572, 1961.
29. Swift PN: Hypogammaglobulinaemia, steatorrhea and megaloblastic anaemia. Response to gluten-free diet and folic acid. *Postgrad Med J* 38:633, 1962.
30. Plauth WH Jr, Waldmann TA, Wochner RD, et al: Protein-losing enteropathy secondary to constrictive pericarditis in childhood. *Pediatrics* 34:636, 1964.
31. Nelson DL, Blaese RM, Strober W: Constrictive pericarditis, intestinal lymphangiectasia, and reversible immunologic deficiency. *J Pediatr* 86:548, 1975.
32. Waldmann TA, Gordon RS Jr, Dutcher TF, et al: Syndromes of gastrointestinal protein loss, in: *Plasma Proteins and Gastrointestinal Tract in Health and Disease*, Copenhagen, Ejnar Munskgaards Forlag, 1962, p 150.
33. Rosen FS, Smith DH, Earle R Jr, et al: The etiology of hypopro[illegible]inemia in a patient with congenital chylous ascites. *Pediatrics* 30:696, 1962.
34. Stoelinga GBA, Van Muenster PJJ, Sloof JP: Chylous effusions into the intestine in a patient with protein-losing gastroenteropathy. *Pediatrics* 31:1010, 1963.
35. Wilson JF, Lahey ME: A unifying concept for the pathogenesis of the syndrome of iron deficiency anemia, hypocupremia and hypoproteinemia in infants. *J Clin Invest* 44:1112, 1965.
36. Jeffries GH, Chapman A, Sleisenger MH: Low-fat diet in intestinal lymphangiectasia: Its effect on albumin metabolism. *New Engl J Med* 270:761, 1964.
37. Holt P: Dietary treatment of protein loss in intestinal lymphangiectasia. *Pediatrics* 34:629, 1964.
38. Moffett ML, Shulenberger MK, Burkholder ER: Epidemiology and etiology of severe infantile diarrhea. *J Pediatr* 72:1, 1968.
39. Tamer MA, Santora TR, Sandberg DH: Cholestyramine therapy for intractable diarrhea. *Pediatrics* 53:217, 1974.

40. Berant M, Wagner Y, Cohen N: Cholestyramine in the management of infantile diarrhea. *J Pediatr* 88:153, 1976.

41. Krieger I, Evans GW, Zelkowitz, P: Zinc dependency as a cause of chronic diarrhea in variant acrodermatitis enteropathica. *J Pediatr* (in press).

42. Wilson JF, Lahey ME, Heiner DC: Studies on iron metabolism: V. Further observations on cow's milk-induced gastrointestinal bleeding in infants with iron deficiency anemia. *J Pediatr* 84:335, 1974.

43. Gryborski JD, Burkle F, Hillman R: Milk-induced colitis in the infant. *Pediatrics* 38:299, 1966.

44. Heiner DC, Sears JW, Kniker WT: Multiple precipitins to cow's milk in chronic respiratory disease. *Am J Dis Child* 103:634, 1962.

45. Ament ME, Rublin CE: Soy protein—another cause of flat intestinal lesion. *Gastroenterology* 62:227, 1972.

46. Goldman AS, Anderson DW Jr, Sellers WA, et al: Milk allergy: I. Oral challenge with milk and isolated milk proteins in allergic children. *Pediatrics* 32:425, 1963.

47. PAG Ad Hoc Working Group on Milk Intolerance: Nutritional implications. *PAG Bull* 2:7, 1972.

48. Swift PM: Hypogammaglobulinaemia, steatorrhea and megaloblastic anaemia: Response to gluten-free diet and folic acid. *Postgrad Med J* 38:633, 1962.

10
Vitamin Deficiencies

NUTRITIONAL VS. GENETIC COFACTOR DEFICIENCY

Nutritient deficiencies develop whenever there is inadequate use of a nutrient by the respective intracellular system. According to this rather broad definition, an inability to use the nutrient, although it is delivered in adequate amounts, causes symptoms of nutritional deficiency. This occurs in some genetic disorders of vitamin metabolism or as a consequence of drug interaction. Other causes of nutritional deficiency are inadequate delivery to the tissue because of deficient intake, decreased absorption or transport, and increased inactivation or excretion. The term *nutritional vitamin deficiency* is restricted in this discussion to the latter groups of causes, and these are distinguished from genetic disorders of vitamin metabolism that cause deficiency symptoms.

Dietary vitamin deficiencies are not common in the United States. This was demonstrated by several recent nutrition surveys. Although calorie deficency that causes growth failure is fairly common in select ethnic groups, these populations do not show a comparable incidence of vitamin deficiencies, most probably because the American diet usually has an

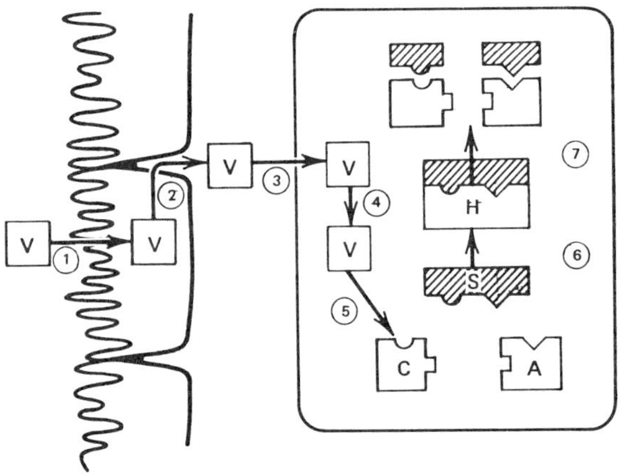

Figure 10-1. SCHEMATIC REPRESENTATION OF STEPS IN VITAMIN METABOLISM AND TRANSPORT EACH STEP MAY BE AFFECTED BY MUTATIONS, THUS CAUSING GENETIC DISEASES THAT SIMULATE NUTRITIONAL VITAMIN DEFICIENCY.

(*1*) Absorption of vitamin (V) into the intestinal villus cell. (*2*) Transport across the basolateral membrane into the extracellular fluid space and on into the blood stream. (*3*) Transport into the peripheral tissue cell. (*4*) Transport within the cell; (may involve transport into mitochondria). (*5*) Conversion into coenzyme (C). (*6*) Complex formation with apoenzyme (A) into holoenzyme (H), which combines with substrate (S) and thus facilitates the metabolic breakdown of substrate. (Any one of the indicated steps may consist of several steps, as in the case of vitamin B_{12} conversion into coenzyme.)

Table 10-1. Causes of Vitamin Deficiency, Other Than Dietary

Thiamine
- Increased requirement: alcoholism
- Decreased absorption: liver and intestinal disease
- Genetic: Leigh's disease (?)

Riboflavin
- Deficiency uncommon

Niacin
- Increased requirement: neoplasia, hyperthyroidism, febrile illness
- Drug interaction: isoniazid
- Genetic intestinal transport defect: Hartnup disease

Pyridoxine
- Drug interaction: isoniazid, penicillamine, hydralazine, cycloserine, levodopa, oral contraceptives
- Dependency after megavitamin therapy (includes effect on fetus)
- Genetic cofactor abnormality, causing deficient function of:
  - glutamic acid decarboxylase (B_6-dependent infantile convulsions); unknown enzyme (B_6-responsive anemia); cystathionine synthase (homocystinuria); cystathioninase (cystathioninuria); kynureninase (xanthurenic aciduria)

Vitamin B_{12}
- Deficient transplacental nutrition: vegetarian mothers
- Decreased absorption: intrinsic factor deficiency, defective ileal transport, short gut, blind loop syndrome, gastric resection, fish tapeworm infestation
- Genetic deficiency of:
  - synthesis of adenosylcobalamin (methylmalonic acidemia); synthesis of methyl- and adenosylcobalamin (homocystinuria with methylmalonic acidemia); transcobalamine II (megaloblastic anemia with normal serum B_{12})

Folate
- Increased requirement: pregnancy, growth recovery after malnutrition or premature birth, hemolytic anemias, malignancy, chronic infection
- Decreased absorption: short gut, blind loop syndrome
- Drug interaction: methotrexate, pyrimethamine, triamterene, trimethoprim
- Genetic deficiency of:
  - N^5, N^{10} methylene THF reductase (homocystinuria); dihydrofolate reductase (congenital megaloblastic anemia), and others (see text)

Biotin
- Genetic deficiency of:
  - holocarboxylase synthetase (multiple carboxylase deficiency); cofactor interaction with propionyl-CoA carboxylase; biotin absorption

Vitamin C
- Increased requirement: lactation, surgery, other stress
- Drug interaction: dilantin, oral contraceptives

Vitamin A
- Decreased absorption: lack of fat intake or fat malabsorption
- Deficient conversion of carotene: liver disease
- Deficient retinol binding: protein deficiency
- Genetic: familial, follicular hyperkeratosis

Table 10-1. (*Continued*)

Vitamin D
Decreased absorption: fat malabsorption
Drug interaction: dilantin, phenobarbital
Decreased activation: liver or kidney diseases, dilantin, phenobarbital
Genetic deficiency of: renal hydroxylase ("vitamin D dependent rickets")
Vitamin E
Deficient stores at birth
Decreased absorption: fat malabsorption
Vitamin K
Deficient stores at birth
Decreased absorption: fat malabsorption, prolonged antibiotic use
Drug interaction: coumarin, phenobarbital, dilantin

adequate nutrient composition so that children who consume low quantities get enough specific nutrients for the level of growth they can achieve. Therefore, in cases with symptoms of vitamin deficiency inadequate intake should be considered last and other causes should be ruled out, including the use of drugs that affect vitamin metabolism, and organic diseases and genetic abnormalities that prevent absorption or peripheral utilization of vitamins (Table 10-1).

The metabolism of vitamins involves several steps, starting with ingestion of the vitamin and ending at its final utilization as a coenzyme (cofactor) in metabolic reactions. The absorption and subsequent conversion of the vitamin into a coenzyme often requires proteins as carriers or catalysts. The coenzyme then forms a complex with the respective apoenzyme. The resultant holoenzyme functions by combining with a substrate that must be metabolized (Fig. 10-1). A block in the metabolic chain can be the cause of either faulty apoenzyme or coenzyme formation and may lead to deficiency of a metabolic product beyond the block, or to the accumulation of substrate, if alternate pathways of breakdown are not available.

Genetic defects of vitamin metabolism, caused by the mutation of genes that code for a carrier protein or a catalyst, are well documented. They are usually transmitted as autosomal recessive traits. Because of the increasing importance of differentiating these disorders from dietary vitamin deficiencies, discussions of known genetic cofactor deficiencies are included in this chapter.

WATER-SOLUBLE VITAMINS AND DEFICIENCY STATES

Thiamine

Biochemistry and Function

Thiamine pyrophosphate functions as a coenzyme in pathways of carbohydrate metabolism, mainly the oxidative decarboxylation of pyruvate, α-ketoglutarate, and branched chain α-ketoacids. As the coenzyme in transketolation, it participates in the hexose monophosphate shunt with generation of NADPH; it is also required for the synthesis of acetylcholine. Considering the importance of acetylcholine in nerve conduction and of glucose as a source of energy, it is not surprising that the deficiency of this vitamin causes dysfunction of the nervous system.

Source and Requirements

The highest concentrations of thiamine are found in milk, meats, and legumes, while cereals, fruits, and eggs are only fair sources of this vitamin. Polishing of cereals reduces the content of vitamins because they are located predominantly in the covering of the grain. Thiamine requirements are related to carbohydrate metabolism. They are usually expressed as a function of calorie intake, based on the assumption that carbohydrate calories make up a fairly constant percentage of total calories. Judged by the average thiamine intake of infants without signs of deficiency, it has been estimated that the requirement is 0.2 mg/1,000 kcal. The recommended dietary allowance (RDA) is 0.3 mg/day from birth to 6 months, 0.5 mg/day from 6 to 12 months, and 0.7 mg/day from 1 to 3 years of age. The mean intake of U.S. population groups studied in the Ten-State Nutrition Survey (Center for Disease Control, 1972) was above this dietary requirement. Breast milk supplies 0.16 mg/l, while cow's milk provides 0.44 mg/l. The intake of a 6-month-old breast-fed infant is therefore about 0.16 mg/day, less than the RDA; but deficiency is unlikely, because the RDA values are intended to be liberal.

Manifestations of Deficiency

The deficiency state, generally called beriberi, causes edema and fatty degeneration of heart muscle with subsequent dilation of the heart. Effusions into serosal cavities and enlargement of viscera occur. There is degeneration of myelin and axon cylinders of peripheral nerves, and the brain shows vascular dilation, hemorrhages, and proliferation surrounding the third ventricle (Wernicke's hemorrhagic polioencephalitis). The clinical correlates of these anatomic lesions are congestive heart failure, psychic disturbances, and signs of neuritis. The manifestations of neuritis include ptosis, atrophy of the optic nerve, absent knee and ankle jerks, hoarseness due to paralysis of the laryngeal nerve, and paresthesia or hyperesthesia. The nerve trunks are tender, and atrophy of the muscles develops secondary to the neuritis. There may be signs of increased intracranial pressure, including convulsions. Ataxia, loss of deep sensation, lethargy, and ultimately coma occur in severe cases.

Causes

Nutritional deficiency generally results from dietary lack of meats, milk, legumes, and other thiamine-rich staples. Diets consisting principally of polished grains produce thiamine deficiency. Cooking in hot water decreases the thiamine content of many foods if the water is discarded. Poor absorption is the cause of deficiency symptoms in gastrointestinal and liver diseases. Patients with chronic diseases and alcoholism may exhibit thiamine deficiencies due to insufficient intakes in relation to their increased need for thiamine.

Genetic Deficiency

Leigh's disease is a genetic disorder with certain manifestations similar to thiamine deficiency. These are typical histological CNS changes, increased serum lactate and pyruvate, and elevation of alanine, the gluconeogenic precursor of pyruvate. The disease usually starts during infancy, although onset of chronic cases may be as late as 7 years. Clinical symptoms are those of progressive CNS degeneration. Neurogenic respiratory disturbances, marked by episodic hyperventilation, apnea, or sobbing ventilation are common. These episodes are precipitated by startling stimuli and, contrary to the apnea of "sudden infant death syndrome," do not occur during sleep. There may be ataxia, hemiplegia, convulsions, and nystagmus. In addition to CNS involvement, patients exhibit signs of peripheral neuropathy, such as hypotonia and loss of reflexes. Several enzyme deficiencies have been described in cases thought to be Leigh's disease, including pyruvate carboxylase deficiency. However, thiamine is not a coenzyme for this reaction. Brunette et al. (1) described a patient who improved on large doses of up to 20 mg thiamine and speculated that the vitamin facilitates the removal of pyruvate and lactate by an alternate pathway that requires thiamine as a coenzyme (i.e., the formation of acetyl-CoA by pyruvate dehydrogenase).

Deficiency of thiamine triphosphate in the brains of children with Leigh's disease was reported by Cooper et al. (2). The demonstration by the same group of investigators of an enzyme-inhibiting factor in urine (3) was thought to provide a convenient means for early diagnosis. Unfortunately, this test has not proven to be specific. These investigators suggest that thiamine triphosphate is the active coenzyme in the brain and that its formation is inhibited in Leigh's disease.

Patients with deficiency of each of the components of the pyruvate dehydrogenase complex have been described who had clinical findings of variable severity, some not unlike those seen in Leigh's disease. However, anatomical lesions resembling thiamine deficiency were not described in these patients.

One patient with maple sugar urine disease (MSUD) was described who improved on 10 mg thiamine (4). The deficient enzyme in this disease is a branched chain ketoacid decarboxylase that requires thiamine as a coenzyme. However, the dependency on thiamine was not borne out by in vitro studies. Thiamine can be expected to raise residual enzyme activity in patients with intermediate MSUD due to partial decarboxylase deficiency and thus cause some clinical improvement. Although the manifestations of MSUD do not resemble nutritional thiamine deficiency clinically, this disorder is one example of the potential benefit to be derived from high doses of vitamins for inborn errors involving a metabolic step where the vitamin is a coenzyme.

Diagnosis

Nutritional thiamine deficiency may be diagnosed by observing the clinical response to therapy and monitoring serum pyruvate. Laboratory measures (Table 3-6), such as red cell transketolase activity and urinary thiamine excretion, do not correlate well with clinical symptoms (5). Diagnostic levels of urinary thiamine for five pediatric age groups were suggested by the Ten-State Nutrion Survey. Leigh's disease must be differentiated from nutritional thiamine deficiency by the diet history. The heart is not affected in Leigh's disease and CNS manifestations are relentlessly progressive. A characteristic distribution of CNS lesions is diagnostic.

Treatment

Nutritional thiamine deficiency in children is usually treated with 10 mg thiamine per day. It may be given orally or, in cases of poor absorption, intramuscularly. In Leigh's disease, pyruvate dehydrogenase deficiency, and other congenital lactic acidoses trial therapy with thiamine, 50 to 100 mg/day is justified. Lower doses may be effective in MSUD.

Riboflavin

Biochemistry and Function

Vitamin B_2 is the precursor of the coenzymes flavin mononucleotide and flavin adenine dinucleotide, which function in amino acid, xanthine, and aldehye oxidation and which are coenzymes for succinic dehydrogenase.

Source and Requirements

The vitamin is abundant in liver, kidney, yeast, milk products, leafy vegetables, and whole grains. Deficiency is hardly ever seen without deficiency of other B vitamins. The amount of breast milk ingested by the average 6-month-old infant provides about 0.36 mg/day while cow's milk provides 1.75 mg/day. The RDA has been set at 0.4 mg/day from birth to 6 months, 0.6 mg/day from 6 to 12 months, and 0.8 mg/day from 1 to 3 years of age.

Manifestations of Deficiency

The symptoms of riboflavin deficiency are largely confined to the mouth, face, and eyes. There is keratitis, conjunctivitis, corneal vascularization, photophobia, and increased lacrimation. Cheilosis or perlèche, which is a fissure at the angle of the mouth, is frequently seen. The tongue is smooth, sometimes red, and shows loss of papillary structures. Seborrheic dermatitis of the face and trunk may occur. In pregnant animals riboflavin deficiency is teratogenic and produces abnormalities similar to those of thalidomide.

Causes

Nutritional causes of riboflavin deficiency are similar to those of thiamine deficiency. Hepatic disease is often a contributing factor. In the Ten-State Nutrition Survey, 5% of infants from low-income families had insufficient riboflavin intake but no clinical signs of deficiency. Drug-induced riboflavin deficiency has been observed in experimental animals fed boric acid, which forms a complex with the vitamin that is readily excreted by the kidney. Whether this also occurs in humans is unknown. There are, to date, no known genetic causes of riboflavin deficiency.

Diagnosis

The most reliable diagnostic method is the determination of erythrocyte glutathione reductase activity. Urinary riboflavin excretion is sometimes used, but it reflects current intake and is not a reliable indicator of deficiency. Diagnostic levels for four pediatric age groups were suggested by the Ten-State Nutrition Survey (Table 3-6).

Treatment

Oral administration of 3 to 10 mg riboflavin per day is advised. If no response is obtained, intramuscular injections of 3 mg twice daily should be given.

Niacin

Biochemistry and Function

Niacin or one of its derivatives, nicotinic acid and nicotinamide, is an essential component of NAD and NADP, the coenzymes I and II, which play an important role in many biochemical reactions, most importantly in the generation of ATP through oxidative phosphorylation. The urinary metabolites are 2-pyridone and N-1 methylnicotinamide.

Source and Requirements

Because niacin plays an important role in the generation of ATP, its requirements are a function of the need for energy through oxidative phosphorylation. When the calories derived from food are used to cover energy requirements and none are stored, food intake must be matched by an appropriate amount of niacin. The requirement of niacin is therefore a function of the caloric intake and is expressed as such. Niacin can be synthesized from trytophan and is, by strict definition, consequently not a vitamin. The intake of proteins that supply tryptophan modifies the niacin requirement. It is therefore useful to express the vitamin content as niacin equivalents, where 60 mg of tryptophan is taken to represent 1 mg of the vitamin. The niacin content of human milk is roughly equivalent to 5 mg/l, but only 1.47 mg is preformed vitamin. The RDA for infants is set high because of uncertainty over their capacity for conversion of tryptophan to niacin. Thus, 6 mg/day (niacin equivalents) is advised for infants under 6 months, but only 8 to 9 mg/day for older infants and children.

Manifestations of Deficiency

Anorexia, irritability, insomnia, and lassitude are early signs of deficiency in the pediatric age group. The full-blown deficiency state is known as pellagra. At the height of the disease, patients develop symptoms referred to as the "three D's": dermatitis, diarrhea, and dementia. The dementia is due to patchy demyelinization and degeneration of nerve cell bodies in the brain and spinal cord, mainly the posterior and lateral columns. Early neurologic signs consist of numbness, dizziness, and burning sensations. Depression, disorientation, and delirium follow. Skin manifestations may be provoked by a variety of irritants, especially sunlight. The dermatitis begins with a sharply demarcated erythema, which has been called pellagrous boot or glove when it covers the distal portion of the extremities. When the swelling and erythema disappear, desquamation follows, and small vesicles and bullae may appear that leave pigment changes upon healing. Some patients may only have a dry, scaly skin. Gastrointestinal symptoms include stomatitis, glossitis, and diarrhea alternating with constipation. Either the margin or the entire tongue and sometimes only the lips are bright red, with swollen papillae and ulcerations.

Causes

Niacin deficiency is rare in the United States because the dietary tryptophan intake alone is usually sufficient for the formation of niacin. Nutritional deficiency occurs when the diet consists predominately of corn (maize) and is devoid of milk. It is otherwise seen in patients with chronic liver disease and in stressful conditions such as prolonged febrile illness, neoplasm, and hyperthyroidism. Occasionally, tuberculosis patients on prolonged isoniazid therapy develop deficiency, which is probably due to the pyridoxine antagonism of the drug, since pyridoxine is necessary in the conversion of tryptophan to niacin. Only poorly nourished patients on isoniazid therapy are in jeopardy.

Genetic Deficiency

Hartnup's disease is a genetic disorder of the intestinal and renal transport of neutral amino acids, including tryptophan. It is the only genetic disorder of vitamin metabolism that is due to a mutation that produces deficiency of a vitamin precursor. Patients with this disorder develop dermatitis and dementia and may demonstrate ataxia.

Diagnosis

Nutritional deficiency is diagnosed by observing the response to therapy, which is generally quite rapid, and by the finding of decreased urinary levels of N-methylnicotinamide (Table 3-6).

Treatment

The customary dose ranges between 50 and 300 mg niacin per day. This amount should be given in divided doses since flushing, dizziness, and hypotension are unpleasant side effects of high doses.

Pyridoxine

Biochemistry and Function

The B_6 vitamins, found in animal products, are pyridoxal, pyridoxamine, and pyridoxine. These compounds are converted in the cell by a specific kinase into the physiologically active form, pyridoxal-5-phosphate (PLP). Heat converts the vitamin into an inactive disulfide of PLP. Pyridoxine hydrochloride, which is added to many commercial products, is more heat stable. An oxidation product of the vitamin, 4-pyridoxic acid, is excreted in the urine. The active form functions in reactions involving nonoxidative degradation of amino acids (i.e., transaminations, deaminations, decarboxylations, racemations, and electron shifts).

Source and Requirements

The B_6 vitamins are present in milk, grain, and animal products like eggs, meat, and liver. Requirements appear to be related to protein intake. Most protein-rich foods are also rich in vitamin B_6. The RDA is 0.3 to 0.6 mg/day for infants and children up to 3 years of age. Human milk contains 0.1 mg/l or 9 μg/g protein, while cow's milk contains 0.64 mg/l or 18 μg/g protein. Infants on breast milk rarely develop deficiency, although the average intake of a 6-month-old infant is only about 0.1 mg/day or one-third the RDA.

Manifestations of Deficiency

The major manifestations of deficiency are convulsions and sideroblastic anemia. Convulsions were reported in the early 1950s in infants who were receiving a commercially prepared formula deficient in B_6 because of a new type of heat processing. The mechanism of the convulsions is not known. Theoretical considerations suggest that they are caused by the reduced formation of gamma-aminobutyric acid (GABA) from glutamic acid, since this is a pyridoxine-requiring step and GABA is a known inhibitory neurotransmitter. The peripheral blood smear is similar to that of iron-deficiency anemia, although iron stores are abundant and iron therapy is of no avail. Other manifestations include cheilosis, glossitis, seborrhea, lymphopenia, decreased antibody formation, oxaluria, and hyperglycemia.

Causes

Breast milk contains less than the RDA for infants less than 6 months old. It is thus not surprising that B_6-responsive convulsions have been observed in infants on breast milk. Peripheral neuropathy develops after prolonged antituberculosis therapy with isoniazid, which is a pyridoxine antagonist. Penicillamine, hydralazine, and contraceptives are other pyridoxine antagonists that may cause vitamin-deficiency symptoms. Dependency on high doses of B_6 has been produced experimentally in adult volunteers who received 200 mg B_6 daily for 1 month. Newborns of mothers receiving large doses of B_6 for hyperemesis gravidarum have been observed to develop pyridoxine-dependent convulsions, probably due to a transient decrease in binding of vitamin B_6 to the apoenzyme, glutamate decarboxylase. Reduced formation of GABA on this basis imitates genetic dependency on high doses of vitamin and is an example of the need for caution with regard to the indications for megavitamin therapy.

Genetic Deficiencies

Genetic disorders of apoenzyme–coenzyme interaction exist that have clinical manifestations in common with nutritional B_6 deficiency. Among them is a condition called B_6-"dependent" infantile convulsions, starting anywhere from a few hours to several weeks after birth and responding to high doses of B_6. Deficiency in the function of glutamate decarboxylase was demonstrated in one patient with this disorder (6). Addition of an excess of pyridoxal phosphate to the in vitro enzyme assay corrected the deficiency. This suggested indeed that the mutation affected, not the apoenzyme, but rather the vitamin-derived coenzyme, presumably leading to defective interaction with glutamate decarboxylase and nonfunctioning of the holoenzyme. Not infrequently these deficiencies can be overcome by treatment with high doses of vitamin B_6.

A second genetic disorder that shares clinical features with nutritional B_6 deficiency is called B_6-responsive (better, B_6-dependent) anemia. The apoenzyme, which requires B_6 as coenzyme, is not known.

Two other genetic conditions have been recognized that can be corrected by saturating amounts of B_6. They are cystathioninuria and xanthurenic aciduria. It appears doubtful, at present, that these conditions are harmful. Moreover, they do not constitute disorders that enter into the differential diagnosis of nutritional B_6 deficiency.

A fifth condition that responds to very high doses of B_6 is homocystinuria due to cystathionine synthase deficiency. This defect prevents the metabolic breakdown of homocysteine and causes accumulation of homocystine, which is excreted in the urine (Fig. 10-2). The disorder is associated with

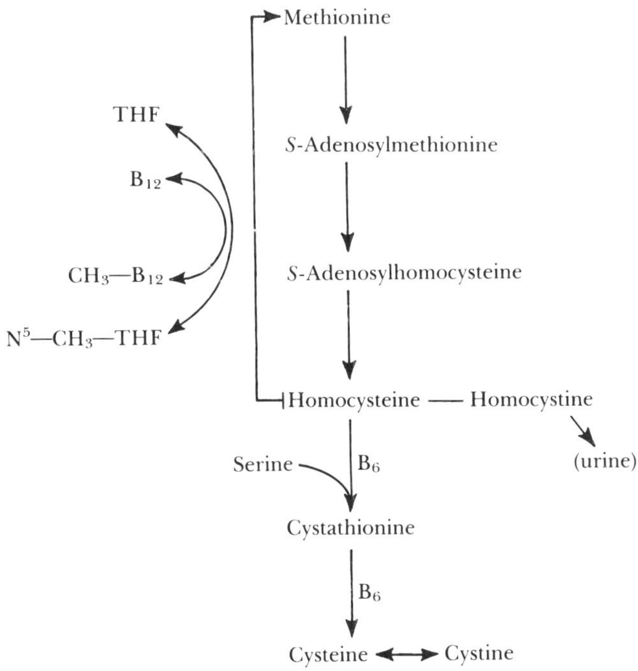

Figure 10-2. ROLE OF VITAMINS IN METABOLIC PATHWAYS
Example of the role of coenzymes, derived from vitamins B_6, B_{12}, and folic acid (THF), in methionine metabolism. Defective vitamin metabolism causes homocystinuria.

abnormalities of the vessel walls that lead to thromboses, mottled skin, and telangiectasias. There are also skeletal changes, including osteoporosis, arachnodactyly, scoliosis, and pectus deformities, as well as growth failure and lens dislocation. Neurological manifestations include mental retardation, nervousness, impaired reasoning, schizophrenic phenomena, and convulsions. B_6-dependent infantile convulsions should be differentiated from those seen in cystathionine synthase deficiency by testing the urine for homocystine. (see Chapter 13).

Diagnosis
Nutritional deficiency is diagnosed by fluorometric determination of the major urinary metabolite, 4-pyridoxic acid (7); and by measurement of RBC glutamic pyruvic acid transaminase and RBC oxaloacetic acid transaminase. Diagnostic urinary pyridoxine levels were suggested for six pediatric age groups by the Ten-State Nutrition Survey (Table 3-6). The diagnosis of B_6-dependent infantile convulsions is based on the EEG response to B_6. The urinary excretion of kynurenic and xanthurenic acid after tryptophan loading may be used in the diagnosis of nutritional deficiency, but is not diagnostic of B_6-dependent infantile convulsions.

Treatment

Nutritional or drug-induced deficiency is treated with 3 to 10 mg/day. Patients with B_6-dependent infantile convulsions should be given a test dose of 100 mg intramuscularly while the EEG response is monitored. Chronic treatment of this disorder consists of 50 to 100 mg daily by the oral route. Homocystinuria may require doses as high as 500 mg/day.

Vitamin B_{12}

Biochemistry and Function

Vitamin B_{12} was originally called the antipernicious anemia factor. It has a complex chemical structure with a central cobalt nucleus. The commercially available vitamin is cyanocobalamin. It carries a cyanide radical attached to the cobalt atom, which is an artifact of isolation. Cyanocobalamin is converted to hydroxycobalamin and carried to the tissue cell where the active coenzymes are formed (Fig. 10-3).

B_{12} functions in transmethylation reactions, including the conversion of homocysteine to methionine. It is also important in DNA synthesis and in the metabolism of pyrimidines and purines; it is a coenzyme for methylmalonyl-CoA mutase, an important enzyme in the catabolism of branched chain amino acids, fatty acids, and cholesterol.

Absorption and Transport

Vitamin B_{12} metabolism involves a complex mechanism of absorption and coenzyme synthesis. Thus, absorption requires a glycoprotein, called the "intrinsic factor," which is formed in the stomach and binds the ingested vitamin, or "extrinsic factor." The two form a complex that acts at a receptor site in the intestinal wall in order to be transported into the cell. There, B_{12} combines with a receptor protein until it is released to cross the cell wall into the blood stream. Further transport of B_{12} requires special globin molecules, transcobalamin I and II. The amount of transcobalamin II in serum is relatively small, but since deficiency causes megaloblastic anemia, it is presumed that it functions mainly in transport into bone marrow. It is possible that other transport mechanisms are necessary to carry transcobalamin into peripheral cells, through cytoplasma and into mitochondria where cofactor synthesis takes place. Any one of these steps may be affected by a mutation, thus causing vitamin dependency (Figure 10-1).

In order to convert hydroxycobalamin into the active cofactor, several steps are necessary, including three reductions of the cobalt atom and, finally, either a methyl or an adenosyl transfer, which forms either methylcobalamin or adenosylcobalamin. Each may be affected by mutations that lead to defective cofactor synthesis. As a result holoenzyme is unable to bind with substrate at maximum rate and capacity or is destroyed at an excessive rate.

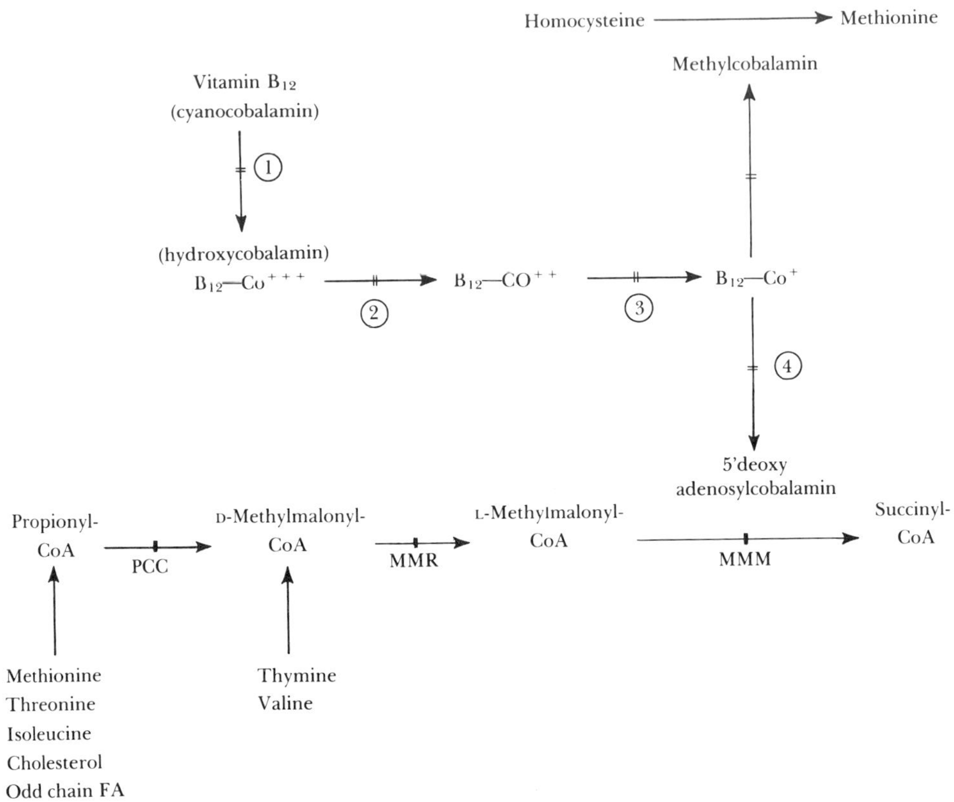

Figure 10-3. VITAMIN B_{12} METABOLISM, REQUIRING MULTIPLE STEPS UNTIL TWO ACTIVE COENZYMES, ADENOSYLCOBALAMIN AND METHYLCOBALAMIN, ARE FORMED
Defects of four steps in B_{12} metabolism are known (double bars). Heavy bars indicate known enzyme defects, which are responsible for propionic acidemia (PCC) or methylmalonic acidemia (MMR and MMM). PCC: Propionyl CoA carboxylase; MMR: methylmalonyl racemase; MMM: methylmalonyl mutase.

Source and Requirements
Vitamin B_{12} is found almost exclusively in animal tissues. It is synthesized by microorganisms in the intestines of animals, as well as in soil and water. The RDA is 0.5 μg/day for infants below 1 year of age and 1.5 μg/day for 1- to 3-year-olds. Breast milk, which contains 0.3 μg/l, barely supplies the RDA for infants. Cow's milk provides an excess of vitamin B_{12}—4.0 μg/l.

Manifestations of Deficiency
Megaloblastic anemia is a major manifestation of nutritional vitamin B_{12} deficiency, B_{12} malabsorption, and of transcobalamin II deficiency. Severe cases show irritability, listlessness, glossitis, leukopenia, and thrombocy-

topenia. Manifestations of spinocerebellar dysfunction are ataxia, paresthesias with decreased vibratory and position sense, hyporeflexia, and positive Babinski reflex. Serum concentrations of B_{12} are decreased, and urinary methylmalonate and homocystine are increased in deficiencies due to inadequate intake or absorption. A number of other metabolites that may be found in urine are cystathionine, glycine, methylcitrate, 3-hydroxypropionate, and formate.

Causes

B_{12} deficiency is on the increase in the United States because of the popularity of vegetarian diets. It has been observed in a 24-month-old breast-fed infant of a vegetarian mother. The infant had severe anemia, coma, and hyperpigmentation of the extremities. Absorption of B_{12} is defective after ileal resection, in intestinal diseases that involve the ileum or cause rapid passage, in blind loop syndome, fish tape worm infestation, and in inherited or acquired intrinsic factor deficiency. A genetic deficiency of ileal B_{12} absorption has been described.

Genetic Deficiencies

Two inborn errors of vitamin B_{12} metabolism are known that cause coenzyme deficiency and are associated with increased urinary excretion of methylmalonic acid, a feature they share with nutritional B_{12} deficiency. One of these inborn errors is called B_{12}-responsive methylmalonic acidemia (MMAemia). Synthesis of 5'deoxyadenosylcobalamin, which is the coenzyme of methylmalonyl mutase, is defective in this disorder. The other inborn error of B_{12} metabolism is a form of homocystinuria. The abnormality affects an earlier step in B_{12} metabolism because both 5'deoxyadenosylcobalamin and methylcobalamin are deficient. These patients excrete methylmalonate, homocystine, and cystathionine and have low serum levels of methionine. Associated megaloblastic anemia has been seen in a single case (8). The disorder appears to be rare (Fig. 10-2).

MMAemia is one of the more common genetic organic acidemias. Both, the vitamin B_{12}-responsive and the unresponsive form of MMAemia are characterized by vomiting, episodic ketoacidosis, and coma. In addition to abnormal fatty acid metabolism, there is elevation of lactate and pyruvate and hypoglycemia. These changes appear to be due to inhibition of gluconeogenic enzymes. Pancytopenia, which develops during severe acidotic episodes, is due to the inhibitory effect of MMA on marrow cell growth (9). MMA excretion is usually higher than in nutritional B_{12} deficiency, and it may reach levels of up to 5 g/day. Late onset and a relatively mild course appear to be characteristic of B_{12}-responsive MMA-emia. Patients with the unresponsive form develop severe, often fatal, illness in the newborn period. Episodes of ketoacidosis are precipitated by stress and high protein loads. Repeated episodes cause cumulative brain damage (see Chapter 13).

Diagnosis

Nutritional B_{12} deficiency is diagnosed on the basis of clinical manifestations—mainly megaloblastic anemia, determination of serum B_{12} by radioimmunoassay, and urinary methylmalonic acid excretion. Serum levels below 100 pg/ml are abnormal.

Treatment

Anemia due to inadequate absorption of vitamin B_{12} requires weekly intramuscular injections of 100 μg until the anemia is corrected, followed by monthly injections of 1,000 μg as maintenance therapy. Much lower oral doses (1 μg/day) suffice in deficiency due to inadequate intake. Biweekly injections of 500 to 1000 μg are necessary in B_{12}-responsive MMAemia, although, initially, injections should be given daily or every other day until acidosis is corrected.

Folic Acid

Biochemistry and Function

Folic acid is a complex molecule composed of a pterin ring, *p*-aminobenzoic acid and glutamic acid. Dihydrofolate is reduced to tetrahydrofolate (THF). As the precursor of five coenzymes, it becomes the carrier of methyl or formyl groups at different linkages. There are five known conversions of THF to coenzyme, each requiring the catalytic action of an enzyme. These enzyme proteins are subject to mutations that may affect the conversion of THF and thus cause peripheral tissue deficiency of the respective folate derivative. Folate coenzymes are required in the synthesis of methionine, glutamate, serine, purines, as well as thymine.

Absorption

Dietary folates exist primarily in the form of polyglutamates, which cannot be absorbed directly. Conversion into the monoglutamate takes place in the intestinal tract with the help of a conjugase enzyme, which is found in the intestinal mucosa, the stomach, and the pancreas. The monoglutamate is absorbed in the duodenum and jejunum by an active transport process and is stored mainly in the liver. Compared with vitamin B_{12}, storage capacity is limited.

Source and Requirements

The vitamin is contained in leafy green vegetables, fruits, meats, and milk. Between 30 and 45 μg/day has been recommended for full term infants, 100 to 300 for children, and approximately 400 μg/day for adults. The content of human milk and cow's milk is 52 to 55 μg/l. Goat's milk, which was used in the past for allergic disorders caused by cow's milk, contains only one-tenth that amount.

Manifestations of Deficiency

Signs of deficiency appear in distinct order with the following sequence: (*1*) decreased serum folic acid levels, (*2*) appearance of hypersegmented neutrophils in the peripheral blood, (*3*) increased urinary excretion of formiminoglutamic acid (FIGLU) after histidine loading, and (*4*) megaloblastic bone marrow changes with anemia and thrombocytopenia. Infants may have skin rashes, chronic diarrhea, and failure to thrive. It is not certain whether folate deficiency can cause mental retardation and neurological dysfunction.

In developing countries, where deficiency in pregnant women is common, the condition may be a contributing factor in the incidence of mental deficit and of congenital and developmental abnormalities.

Causes

Infants fed goat's milk are at risk of developing folate deficiency because its folate content is low (6 μg/l) compared with cow's milk and human milk (55 μg/l). Heat treatment lowers the folate content, a fact that is responsible for the low concentration of evaporated milk—about 20 μg/l or less. Other causes of nutritional deficiency are conditions that are associated with increased requirements for folate as a result of rapid growth or increased cell turnover. This is the case after premature birth; during catch-up growth from malnutrition; in hemolytic anemia, including sickle cell diseases; and in other illnesses, such as diarrhea, chronic infection, and malignancy. Inadequate absorption is a cause of folate deficiency in diseases of the small bowel. Megaloblastic anemia and mental retardation due to congenital folate malabsorption, which seems to be caused by a genetic transport defect, has been described.

Premature infants are at risk of developing folate deficiency because their liver stores are low and during the early months of life, they are not consuming the liter of milk that supplies the folate they need. However, premature infants with megaloblastic anemia generally have had associated predisposing illnesses, like bacterial infections or diarrhea. Patients with cardiac disease are also susceptible to folate deficiency. Requirements are increased in children with genetic diseases receiving chronic glycine therapy and in disorders of purine and pyrimidine metabolism, including Lesch–Nyhan syndrome and orotic aciduria. Pregnant or lactating women are at risk of developing folate deficiency because their requirements are increased—600 to 800 μg/day. Low values have been observed in several U.S. surveys in low-income pregnant women.

Anticonvulsants (phenytoin, primidone, and phenobarbitone), antifolic cytotoxic agents (methotrexate, aminopterin), antimalarial drugs (pyrimethamine), and oral contraceptives cause folate deficiency. Thus, folate deficiency may be the cause of dysmorphic syndromes commonly seen in offspring of mothers receiving anticonvulsants during pregnancy.

Genetic Deficiences

Deficient function of each of the five coenzymes of folic acid has been recognized. However, not many cases have been reported, a fact that may be due to difficulties in diagnosis. Central nervous system dysfunction is a common but nonspecific feature of these disorders. Megaloblastic anemia, which is easy to recognize, occurs in only one type, dihydrofolate reductase deficiency. The anemia responds to treatment with N^5-formyltetrahydrofolic acid (folinic acid) but not to folic acid (9a). The activation of folic acid requires a complex of other interconversion reactions, which may be deficient due to genetic mutations. A specific aminoaciduria that allows easy diagnosis exists in another type—N^5,N^{10}-methylene THF reductase deficiency. In this disorder synthesis of N^5-methyl THF is impaired, and homocystinuria occurs due to failure of remethylation of homocysteine and conversion to methionine, causing hypomethioninemia. Homocystinuria is detected by simple urine screening tests (Fig. 10-2). This defect is only one of three types of homocystinuria that respond to high doses of a vitamin.

Diagnosis

Nutritional folate deficiency is diagnosed through measurement of serum and RBC folate levels by a radioimmunoassay method. Normal serum levels are above 6 ng/ml, and RBC folate should be above 160 ng/ml (Ten-State Nutrition Survey). Levels below 3 and 140 ng/ml, respectively, reflect deficiency. Premature infants usually have low levels during early infancy but rarely show evidence of megaloblastic anemia. Serum folate levels are normal in genetic cofactor deficiencies.

Treatment

Nutritional deficiency is treated by oral administration of 2 to 5 mg folic acid daily for 2 to 3 weeks. Addition of ascorbic acid has been recommended. Anemia that is unassociated with megaloblastic changes will not respond to treatment with folic acid. Since vitamin B_{12} deficiency is also a cause of megaloblastic anemia, physicians commonly prescribe both folate and B_{12}. This approach can be justified by the increased need for folic acid in B_{12} deficiency. Folate supplementation of 1 mg/day over 1 to 3 months is recommended for low birth weight infants.

Biotin

Function

Biotin plays a role in carboxylation reactions, most importantly in fatty acid synthesis as the coenzyme for pyruvate carboxylase, propionyl-CoA carboxylase, and 3-methylcrotonyl-CoA carboxylase. Amino acid incorporation into protein is decreased in biotin deficiency.

Source and Requirements

Biotin is present in soil and most foods. It is synthesized by bacteria, including the intestinal microflora. Because of this unique situation, no spontaneously occurring biotin deficiency has ever been reported. No RDA has been determined, but "adequate and safe" intake values for different age groups were estimated by the Food and Nutrition Board in 1980 (Table 1-3).

Manifestations of Deficiency

The only knowledge of nutritional biotin deficiency stems from experiments with volunteers who were fed a diet containing a biotin inhibitor, raw egg white, and little additional biotin. Manifestations include dermatitis, grey pallor, anemia, somnolence, hyperesthesia, and muscle pain.

Genetic Deficiency

Biotin responsive propionyl-CoA carboxylase deficiency has been described. Multiple carboxylase deficiency appears to be more common, as evidenced by reports of more than 10 cases in the past decade. The disorder causes alopecia, erythematous dermatitis, ketoacidosis, and failure to thrive. Biotin responsiveness can be explained by deficiency of holocarboxylase synthetase which attaches biotin to the inactive apoenzymes (Chapter 13, Table 13-6). These patients show a dramatic response to biotin, 5–10 mg/day.

Pantothenic Acid, Choline, and Inositol

Pantothenic acid is now considered a vitamin, but there is controversy over the role of choline and inositol in human metabolism. All three are widely distributed in most foods; no deficiency states in humans have been reported, and no RDA has been determined.

Choline can be synthesized by the human body, but appears to be an essential nutrient for some animal species. Pantothenic acid is a component of coenzyme A, an important cofactor in carbohydrate, fat, and protein metabolism. The Food and Nutrition Board estimated "adequate and safe" intake values for pantothenic acid, which were published in 1980 (Table 1-3).

Inositol is present in substantial amounts in human and cow's milk and is a critical constituent of brain, heart, and skeletal muscle phospholipids. The Committee on Nutrition recommends that 2.6 mg/100 ml be incorporated into artificial formulas. This is less than the amount found in human milk, 16 mg/100 ml.

Vitamin C

Biochemistry and Function

Vitamin C, also called antiscorbutic factor, is the popular name for l-ascorbic acid and its oxidized form, dehydroascorbic acid. The vitamin's chief function is the maintenance of connective tissue integrity, possibly through its role in the hydroxylation of proline and/or the reduction of hydroxylysine. It also functions as a coenzyme in both the oxidation of tyrosine and the hydroxylation of tryptophan, and it appears to play a role in several important reduction reactions, such as that of ferric to ferrous iron in the gut and the reduction of folic acid into its active form, tetrahydrofolate.

Source and Requirements

Lemon and orange pulp are considered the major sources of vitamin C in the American diet, although certain vegetables offer a higher concentration than either lemon or orange. These include broccoli, brussels sprouts, collard and turnip greens, kale, and black currants. The RDA for infants and children is 35 to 40 mg/day. This is far in excess of the estimated 5 to 10 mg/day required for the prevention of scurvy. The liberal recommendations of the Food and Nutrition Board allow for higher needs during periods of infection and other stressful situations, such as cold exposure, protein depletion, surgery, and lactation. Fresh cow's milk provides an average of about 20 mg/l. However, after processing and storage, the content may be as low as 2 or 3 mg/l. Human breast milk is an adequate source of vitamin C if the mother's intake is adequate. Requirements are higher during pregnancy and lactation. Consequently, a seemingly healthy mother on marginal intakes will pass on a deficiency of vitamin C to the infant.

Manifestations of Deficiency

Scurvy is the manifestation of vitamin C deficiency. In this disorder, osteoblasts are unable to form osteoid, and tooth dentin becomes defective. There is decreased perivascular collagen and vacuolar degeneration of the capillary endothelial cells. Bony trabeculae become brittle, and hemorrhages cause elevation of the periosteum and palpable purplish swellings over the shafts of the legs. The earliest clinical manifestations of scurvy are irritability, anorexia, and tenderness of the extremities, which frequently causes infants to hold their legs in a froglike position. Advanced cases may develop epiphyseal separation along the costochondral junction of the ribs, causing a depression of the sternum. It feels like a ridge that has been called "scorbutic rosary" in analogy to the "rachitic rosary," although it does not resemble a row of beads. Petechial hemorrhages occur in the skin, mucous membranes, and eyes. Subdural hematomas develop, giving rise to increased intracranial pressure.

X-rays are characteristic. The lack of trabeculation gives the long bones a ground-glass appearance, with the cortex and the epiphyseal border contrasting as a thin, sharply drawn line. The zone of preparatory calcification is dense and has a zone of rarefaction just under it, a finding of particular diagnostic value. This rarefaction may progress inward from the cortex to produce a linear break parallel to the dense zone of preparatory calcification. Epiphyseal separation occurs along this line. Subperiosteal hemorrhages are not visible on x-ray until they begin to heal and show up as calcifications. This appearance may suggest an inflammatory process and should not be confused with the x-ray appearance of periosteal changes in syphilis.

Causes

During the latter part of the first year, scurvy is occasionally seen in breast-fed infants of vitamin C-deficient mothers, or in infants on a diet of cow's milk without supplementation with fresh fruits, vegetables, or vitamin C-fortified processed foods. Dietary surveys, including the Ten-State Nutrition Survey, have shown that up to 30% of infants receive less than the recommended dose, although deficiency is rare. Heating and storage are responsible for the low vitamin C content of home-prepared fruits and vegetables. Pregnant mothers may become deficient because the fetus acts parasitically, taking what it needs irrespective of the mother's requirement. Oral contraceptives reduce tissue levels of vitamin C. Hypertrophy of the gum, which is often seen in patients on chronic dilantin therapy, is probably in part caused by vitamin C deficiency due to drug interaction. Newborns, especially premature infants, commonly have transient tyrosinemia. The associated excretion of tyrosine metabolites is called tyrosyluria. This disorder is due to impairment of *p*-hydroxyphenylpyruvic acid oxidase and responds to vitamin C.

Diagnosis

In the absence of overt clinical manifestations, diagnosis is difficult. Urine concentrations of ascorbate reflect the vitamin C intake prior to the test. Low serum concentrations are also more indicative of the intake during the preceding days or weeks than of actual vitamin stores. However, levels of 0.3 mg/dl or higher seem to rule out deficiency in most instances. The vitamin concentration in leukocytes appears to be a more reliable indicator of vitamin C deficiency, because scurvy does not develop until tissues, including leukocytes, become depleted of vitamin C. Urinary excretion of tyrosine metabolites that are detectable through a simple color reaction, the nitrosonaphthol test, should suggest vitamin C deficiency. However, this test is positive only when the C-deficient patient receives a high-protein diet, rich in tyrosine.

Treatment

Active scurvy is treated with 100 mg of vitamin C two to three times per day for about 1 week. Follow-up is necessary to assure reversal of all manifestations and institution of sound dietary habits. Newborns with neonatal tyrosinemia should receive 50 to 100 mg/day. Longterm therapy with vitamin C may be tried in osteogenesis imperfecta (50 mg/day), the Chédiak–Higashi syndrome (200 mg/day), and lysyl hydroxylase deficiency of Ehlers–Danlos syndrome type VI (4 g/day) (11).

FAT-SOLUBLE VITAMINS AND DEFICIENCY STATES

Vitamin A

Biochemistry and Function

The term *vitamin A* is used to designate a group of compounds: retinal, retinoic acid, and retinyl ester. Only retinal, which is an oxidation product of retinol, is active in vision. It is formed in the intestines from dietary retinyl esters or carotene. Rhodopsin, the photosensitive pigment in the retina, is a combination product of retinal and a protein called *opsin*. Retinoic acid has no function in vision, but supports growth and epithelial differentiation. Carotene is found in animal and plant tissues as alpha-, beta-, and gamma-carotene. Beta-carotene appears to play the major role as a provitamin for utilization by humans. The dietary carotenes are partly absorbed in the upper intestinal tract. Most are enzymatically cleaved in the mucosal cell into two molecules of retinol. Dietary and synthesized retinol are then esterified with long chain fatty acids and incorporated into lymph chylomicrons. Absorption of carotene is not as efficient as absorption of vitamin A. Consequently, biological activity of carotene is only about half that of vitamin A. Vitamin A compounds are stored as retinyl esters in the liver. They are hydrolyzed prior to mobilization from liver stores and are transported while bound to a protein called retinol-binding protein. Vitamin E facilitates storage of vitamin A. Carotene is not stored in significant amounts in the body. Consequently, circulating carotene levels are a better measure of intake and absorption than of vitamin A sufficiency. Conversion of carotene to retinol is stimulated by thyroxin.

Source and Requirements

Vitamin A occurs only in animal tissues, with highest concentrations in liver, eggs, dairy products, and meat. Carotenes are present in both yellow and green vegetables. The outer green leaves may contain up to 20 times as much as the inner white ones.

Requirements can be expressed in international units (IU) of vitamin A or as retinol equivalents (RE). One IU equals 0.3 μg retinol or 0.6 μg beta-carotene. The conversion factor takes in account the variable absorption and conversion rates of the carotenoids. The RDA for infants under 3 years is 1400 IU or 400 RE. This amount is easily ingested by infants receiving any type of milk and the ordinary variety of baby foods offered after 6 months of age.

Manifestations of Deficiency

The earliest sign of vitamin A deficiency is night blindness, caused by deficient formation of the photosensitive pigment in the retina, rhodopsin. Clinical manifestations are reversible at this stage. If untreated, there is progression of the eye signs with degeneration of the epithelium of the eye, drying of the cornea (xerosis), with silvery grey plaques on the bulbar aspect of the conjunctiva (Bitot's spots), and hyperkeratosis. Ultimately, the cornea becomes wrinkled and then ulcerated. At this stage perforations may occur. The skin is dry and scaly. At times follicular hyperkeratosis develops over the extensor surfaces of the extremities and the buttocks. Infants manifest failure to thrive, mental retardation, and increased susceptibility to infection.

Causes

In underdeveloped countries, deficiency is usually due to lack of dietary fat and protein, since vegetable sources of vitamin are not scarce. When protein intake is low, retinol-binding protein becomes deficient, so that vitamin A cannot be mobilized, even though it is stored in the liver. In developed countries, vitamin A deficiency is more common in abnormalities of fat absorption. Protein deficiency also plays a role in these disorders, because fat malabsorption is frequently associated with protein malabsorption. Conversion of carotene to vitamin A is limited in hypothyroidism and liver disease. The resulting carotenemia is characterized by an orange-yellow pigmentation of the skin. Lack of pigmentation of the sclera distinguishes carotenemia from jaundice. Although the clinical manifestations of carotenemia are common in hypothyroidism, vitamin A deficiency is rarely observed. Vitamin A metabolism is abnormal in Down's syndrome (12).

Genetic Deficiency

The report of a large family with an unusually high incidence of follicular keratosis over three generations suggests that genetics may play a role in disorders of vitamin A metabolism. A cure was accomplished in this family with pharmacological doses of vitamin A (13).

Diagnosis

Plasma concentrations of vitamin A below 20 μg/dl (Table 3-6) are considered indicative of low stores. The Maternal and Child Health Survey (1971) showed that only 1% of children have values in the deficient range.

Treatment

Early manifestations of vitamin A deficiency are treated orally with a minimum of 2,500 to 4,000 IU daily for several weeks. In severe deficiency, body stores should be replenished quickly by giving 25,000 to 50,000 IU daily. Treatment must be continued until symptoms disappear, which may require weeks or months. Oral treatment with a water-miscible preparation is recommended in fat malabsorption syndromes; 1,500 μg daily is the preventive dose and 25,000 μg daily, the treatment dose. Intramuscular preparations are recommended in cases where intestinal mucosal damage prevents absorption of vitamin A. Water miscible preparations are better mobilized than oil-based vitamin A for intramuscular injections. The Ten-State Nutrition Survey reported vitamin A deficiencies in pregnant and lactating women. Low levels are seen in oral contraceptive users.

Vitamin D

Biochemistry

Vitamin D is the name for a pair of steroid alcohols—ergocalciferol from plant sources (D_2) and cholecalciferol from animal sources (D_3). They regulate calcium and phosphorus metabolism but require certain metabolic modifications before they can function as antirachitic factors. They are not true vitamins by definition, because adequate exposure to sunlight eliminates their dietary requirement. Moreover, their activation is under feedback control by the kidney in a manner reminiscent of the endocrine system. The physiologically active form may consequently be regarded as a hormone.

Activation of Vitamin D

Biosynthesis of D_3 occurs in the skin via photolysis of 7-dehydrocholesterol by UV light. D_3 accumulates in the liver where it undergoes the first hydroxylation reaction at the 25-position. The resultant 25-(OH)D_3 is the most abundant vitamin D in circulation (Fig. 10-4). Production is controlled to a limited extent by hepatic concentration of 25-(OH)D_3. This precursor of the active vitamin D may have some therapeutic value in human vitamin D-deficiency diseases. Bound to specific transport protein, 25-(OH)D_3 travels to the kidney where another hydroxylation reaction occurs at the 1 position. The resultant 1,25-$(OH)_2D_3$ is the active form of vitamin D (Fig. 10-5). It is at least five times as active as, and functions three times faster than, the immediate precursor, 25-(OH)D_3. In vitro bone resorption is approximately 100 times higher.

Biosynthesis

Regulation of biosynthesis occurs in part through modulation of 25-hydroxylase activity in the liver, where rising levels of 25-(OH)D_3 tend to shut off 25-hydroxylase. However, this mechanism is not tightly controlled,

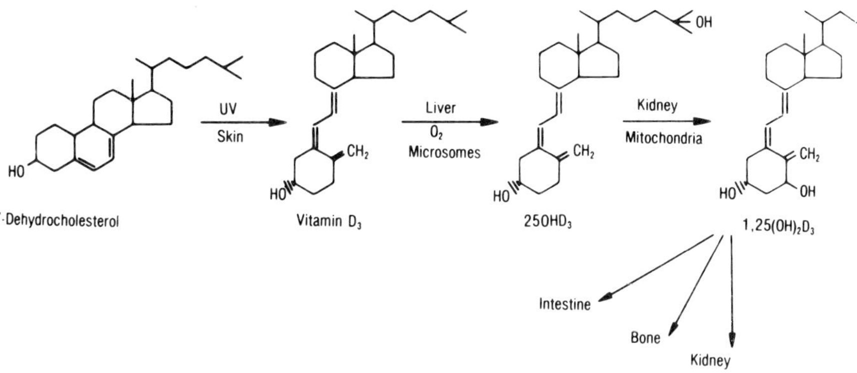

Figure 10-4. VITAMIN D METABOLISM: CONVERSION INTO THE ACTIVE FORM, 1,25$(OH)_2D_3$

nor does it seem to be influenced by the level of calcium or phosphorus in extracellular fluids. Circulating 25-$(OH)D_3$ is therefore largely a function of vitamin intake and exposure to sunlight.

Regulation of calcium and phosphorus metabolism through control of vitamin D biosynthesis is accomplished mainly by the kidney, which increases the output of 1,25-$(OH)_2D_3$ when serum calcium falls. This stimulation of 1-hydroxylase activity in the kidney is eliminated by the removal of the parathyroid gland, indicating that the parathyroid gland regulates 1,25-$(OH)_2D_3$ biosynthesis. Low serum phosphate levels also stimulate the conversion of 25-$(OH)D_3$ to 1,25-$(OH)_2D_3$, but this mechanism does not require parathyroid hormone (Fig. 10-5). Studies of egg-laying quails have shown that estradiol, in conjunction with either testosterone or progesterone, also stimulates 1-hydroxylase activity, an observation that may explain the occurrence of osteoporosis in postmenopausal women.

Function of Vitamin D

In the two vitamin D-deficiency diseases, rickets and osteomalacia, organic bone matrix fails to clacify because calcium and phosphorus are insufficient in the extracellular fluid. Vitamin D maintains adequate serum calcium levels and thus prevents rickets and contributes to the prevention of tetany and osteoporosis.

Major sites of vitamin action that have been identified with certainty are intestine, bone, and kidney. The cessation of muscle weakness after treatment of refractory rickets with vitamin D suggests that muscle may be another site where this vitamin has a direct effect.

In the intestine, vitamin D activates the calcium pump that actively transports calcium across the brush border of the intestinal villus cells through the cytoplasm and across the basal–lateral border into the extracellular space. The relationship between intake and absorption in

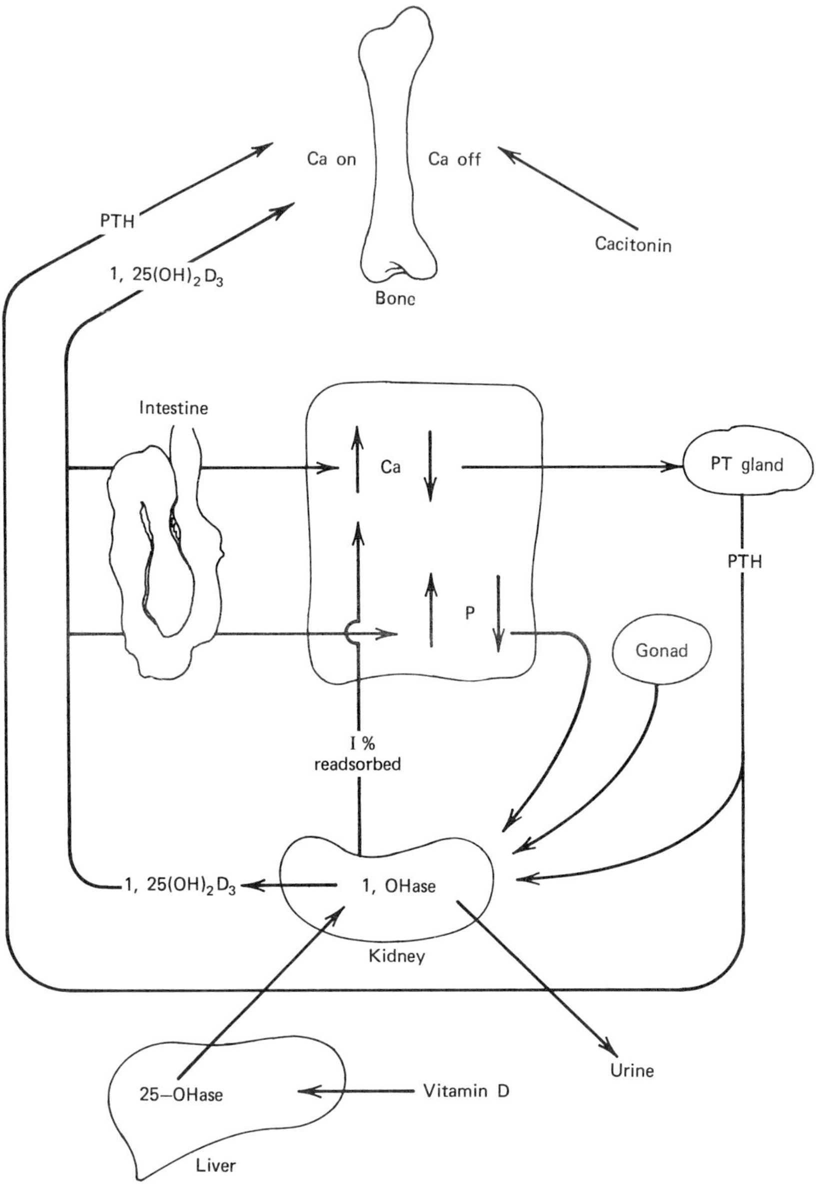

Figure 10-5. DIAGRAMMATIC REPRESENTATION OF CALCIUM–PHOSPHORUS HOMEOSTASIS AND BIOSYNTHESIS OF 1,25(OH)$_2$D$_3$
Hypocalcemia acts on the parathyroid (PT) gland, which releases parathyroid hormone (PTH). Hypophosphatemia and PTH activate 25-(OH)D$_3$-1-hydroxylase in the kidney. The resultant 1,25(OH)$_2$D$_3$ stimulates intestinal absorption of calcium and phosphorus, mobilizes calcium from bone, and contributes approximately 1% to renal tubular reabsorption of calcium. Calcitonin opposes the action of PTH. There is evidence that gondal function affects renal hydroxylase activity.

such a carrier-mediated transport process is nonlinear, so that an increased dietary intake of calcium does not cause a proportional increase in calcium uptake. There is now evidence (14) that vitamin D has, in addition to its effect on calcium, a direct function in the intestinal phosphate transport system. It should be noted that, in contrast to other sites of vitamin D activity, parathyroid hormone is not needed for the action of vitamin D at the intestinal site.

The skeleton is the major source of calcium for the prevention of hypocalcemia. Calcium mobilization by vitamin D requires the permissive action of parathyroid hormone (15), although evidence to the contrary has been presented (16). Rapid adjustments of plasma calcium levels may be possible because the parathyroid acts as an intermediary and is able to respond more quickly than vitamin D because of the short biological half-life of parathormone. Bone is not depleted of calcium by action of vitamin D because calcium mobilization also serves the formation of new bone. Moreover, the long-acting effect of vitamin D on calcium absorption replenishes the calcium extracted from bone.

The action of vitamin D in the kidney is of questionable importance, because the vitamin controls only a relatively small portion of total calcium reabsorption. The role of vitamin D in phosphorus reabsorption is still obscure.

Source and Requirements

Vitamin D occurs in appreciable amounts only in fish liver and in animals who feed on fish. Neither human milk nor cow's milk provides an adequate quantity of vitamin D. Of commercially available infant foods, only egg yolk supplies vitamin D in significant amounts (approximately 200 IU per 100 g or 20 IU per yolk). The daily requirement during infancy is 100 to 200 IU. The RDA, which does not vary with age, is liberally set at 400 IU or 10 μg/day. Since little storage of vitamin D occurs, and since exposure to sunlight cannot be relied upon in an industrialized society, regular supplementation is advised. This is accomplished in the United States through fortification of dairy milk and commercial infant formulas, which provide at least 400 IU per U.S. quart. A 4- to 6-month-old infant thus can be expected to receive its RDA in the daily milk consumption. Consequently, nutritional vitamin D deficiency is virtually nonexistent in infants fed vitamin D-fortified milk, with the possible exception of low birth weight infants, whose requirements have not yet been determined with certainty.

Manifestations of Deficiency

Rickets is a deficiency disease of growing bone, which is therefore seen only in young children. Adults with vitamin D deficiency develop osteomalcia, a rarefaction of preformed bone. Normally, growth proceeds at the epiphysis in orderly fashion, where proliferating cartilage cells form straight columns (Fig. 10-6). The surrounding matrix calcifies in the zone of preparatory calcification. As the stacked cartilage cells degenerate, capillaries grow straight into the tunnel spaces vacated by the cartilage cells. They carry with them osteoblasts and osteoclasts, which reabsorb the calcium of the surrounding matrix and deposit new bone along the intercolumnar matrix. In rickets, cartilaginous matrix does not calcify. Cartilage cells continue to proliferate, uncalcified osteoid tissue accumulates, and capillaries penetrate in a patchy manner. The result is a deep and widened metaphysis, made up of nonrigid, radiolucent osteoid tissue and cartilage. The border with the diaphysis of the long bones is cupped and frayed. On long bone x-rays these changes are reflected by a wide, radiolucent distance between the epiphyseal ossification center and the frayed, concave end of the diaphysis. Mineralization is also lacking in the subperiosteal area of membranous bones and the shafts of long bones where osteoid tissue accumulates. As the preexisting bone is reabsorbed through natural calcium mobilization, this shell of uncalcified osteoid tissue fails to provide support, causing deformities and fractures.

Clinical manifestations include metaphysical widening at the wrists, ankles, and the costochondral junction of the ribs. The thickening of the costochondral junction can be palpated at an early stage, and has been called "rachitic rosary." Craniotabes, a softening and thinning of the skull,

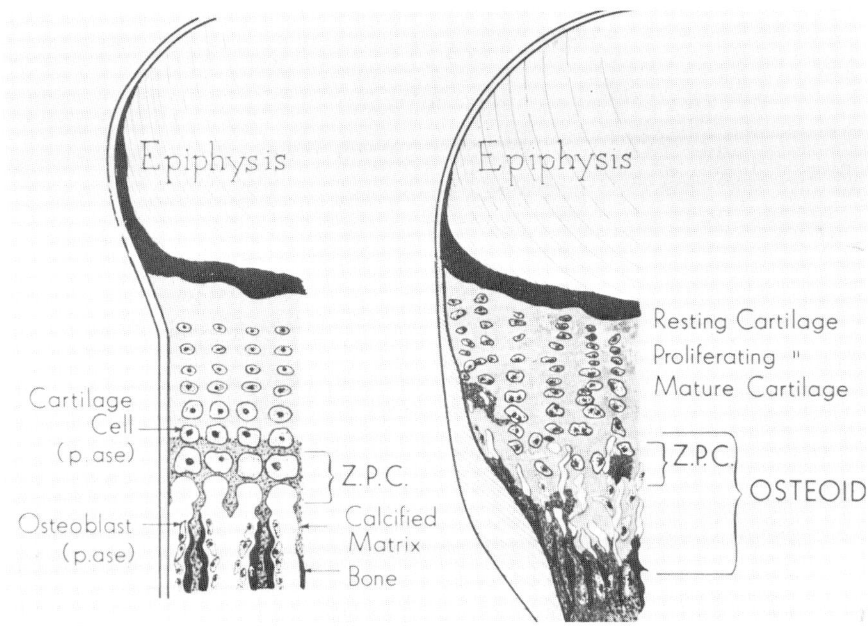

Figure 10-6. RICKETS: HISTOLOGIC CHANGES IN GROWING LONG BONES Shows epiphyseal widening due to cartilage proliferation (see text).

is an early sign of rickets in young infants. When pushing down on the skull tables with the fingertip, a Ping-Pong ball sensation can be felt, which is diagnostic of craniotabes. Due to the softness of bone, there may be a flattening of the thorax with projection of the sternum, curvature of the spine, bowing of the long bones, and projection of the promontory into the pelvic entrance. The central portion of membraneous skull bones is covered with osteoid tissue, causing a boxlike appearance referred to as "caput quadratum." Muscle weakness, a specific manifestation of vitamin D deficiency, is responsible for delayed standing and walking. A pot belly is frequently observed, which is also due to poor muscle tone in both abdominal muscles and intestinal walls.

Fraser, Kooh, and Scriver (17) described what they consider to be three typical stages in the development of rickets (Table 10-2). An early event is a slight degree of hypocalcemia, which stimulates the parathyroid gland and results ultimately in normalization of the plasma calcium level. Phosphorus values are usually normal at that point, and bone lesions are not evident. In the next phase of rachitogenesis, phosphorus values become low as a result of phosphate diuresis secondary to hyperparathyroidism. As long as calcium can be mobilized from bone, plasma levels will remain normal. However, continuing mobilization, unaccompanied by increased calcium absorption and new bone deposition, aggravates the rachitic process. In the third and final stage, calcium and phosphorus levels are low because the compensatory mechanisms fail. Amino aciduria is not uncommon in nutritional rickets. Its presence requires exclusion of rickets caused by acquired or genetic renal tubular diseases.

Causes of Rickets

Nutritional Vitamin D Deficiency

The rare cases of vitamin D deficiency seen in the United States today occur in infants who are exclusively fed either breast milk or nonfortified cow's milk. Black infants seem to be more susceptible, apparently due to several factors operating jointly. These factors include urban air pollution and heavy skin pigmentation, both of which filter out ultraviolet light and hinder vitamin D synthesis. Diets rich in unprocessed cereals cause formation of insoluble calcium complexes with phytates and oxalates that are not absorbed. Rickets may develop in a variety of conditions associated with steatorrhea, since this causes poor vitamin D absorption and the formation of calcium soaps contributes to the calcium deficiency. Biliary atresia, chronic pancreatitis, celiac disease, nontropical sprue and intestinal lymphangiectasia, are among such conditions.

Rickets due to deficient vitamin intake or poor absorption must be distinguished from genetic or acquired deficiencies of hydroxylase in

Table 10-2. Differential Diagnosis of Rickets and Osteomalacia

	Serum Calcium	*Serum Phosphorus*	*Urine Phosphorus*	*Urine Amino Acids*	*Alkaline Phosphatase*	*Plasma 1,25(OH)₂D₃*	*Treatment*
Vitamin D deficiency							2,000–4,000 IU vitamin D per/day until radiologic improvement.
Stage I	N/↓	N	N	N	↑	N/↓	
Stage II	N	↓	N/↑	↑	↑	N/↓	
Stage III	↓	↓	↑	↑	↑	↓	
Vitamin D dependency	↓↓	N	N/↑	↑	↑	↓	1 μg $1,25(OH)_2D_3$
X-linked (familial) hypophosphatemia	N	↓↓	↑↑	N	↑	N/↓	Phosphorus plus >1 μg $1,25(OH)_2D_3$
Renal osteodystrophy	N/↓	↑↑	↓		↑	↓	1 μg $1,25(OH)_2D_3$ Chelation of phosphorus
Renal tubular disease (Fancony syndrome)	N	↓	↑	↑↑	↑		Phosphorus supplements
Hypophosphatasia	N/↑	N	N	N	↓↓		
Hyperparathyroidism (primary)	↑↑	↓	↑		↑		Surgical

either the liver or kidney, causing insufficient production of the active form, 1,25-$(OH)_2D_3$. The disorders that follow should be considered.

Liver Disease

Parenchymal liver disease is known to be associated with decreased 25-hydroxylase activity. However, rickets is rarely seen in the pediatric age group unless cholestasis is an associated factor and causes decreased absorption of calcium and/or vitamin D. The rarity of clinical deficiency disease is probably due to the fact that 25-$(OH)D_3$, which can be stored, is abundant relative to the 1,25-hydroxylated compound. Deficiency of 25-hydroxylation has been observed in premature infants.

Drug-Induced Deficiency

Anticonvulsant drugs, such as phenobarbital and phenytoin, increase the need for viamin D by causing molecular changes that reduce the activity of vitamin D. Evidence of vitamin D deficiency has been observed by several investigators in institutionalized patients on chronic anticonvulsant therapy even though they received maintenance doses of vitamin D (18). Depressed plasma levels of 25-$(OH)D_3$ (19) and elevation of alkaline phosphatase have been reported. Symptomatic vitamin D deficiency is rare, because the deficiency of 25-hydroxylase must be severe and long-standing before body stores of 25$(OH)D_3$ are depleted.

Renal Glomerular Disease

Chronic renal disease that is associated with parenchymal involvement and glomerular dysfunction causes *renal osteodystrophy*. The term describes a combination of pathology consisting of varying degrees of osteitis fibrosa cystica and/or rickets. Osteitis fibrosa cystica is due to secondary hyper-parathyroidism in response to phosphate retention. Parathyroid hormone prevents reabsorption of phosphorus by the renal tubule. However, the compensatory attempt to reduce phosphorus levels also has the undesirable side effect of mobilizing calcium from bone, which results in bone erosion and cyst formation, typical of osteitis fibrosa. The degree of secondary hyperparathyroidism is variable. Undermineralization of bone or rickets, the second component of renal osteodystrophy, is consistently present and generally more pronounced than osteitis fibrosa. The responsible mech-anism is deficient biosynthesis of 1,25$(OH)_2D_3$, caused by loss of renal mass, uremia, and/or hyperphosphatemia. Decreased circulating levels of 1,25$(OH)_2D_3$ have been reported (20). Markedly decreased values are seen in end-stage renal disease. Successful renal transplantation corrects this abnormality. However, as a complication of renal transplantation, newly formed 1,25$(OH)_2D_3$, acting synergistically with an excess of parathyroid hormone (the product of preexisting hyperparathyroidism), often causes hypercalcemia. Laboratory findings of renal glomerular disease include normal or slightly decreased serum calcium levels, markedly elevated serum phosphorus, and decreased urinary phosphorus excretion.

Renal Tubular Disease

In contrast to the rickets of glomerular disease, which is marked by elevated serum phosphorus values, renal tubular disease causes phosphaturia and hypophosphatemia. Serum calcium is usually normal. Associated with phosphaturia are glucosuria, amino aciduria, hyposteuuria and renal tubular acidosis, a complex called *Fanconi's syndrome.* Tubular disease may be genetic or acquired. Genetic disorders of renal tubular reabsorption are cystinosis, hereditary tyrosinemia, hereditary fructose intolerance, and galactosemia.

Vitamin D refractory rickets also occurs as a result of an X-linked disorder of renal tubular phosphate uptake, called *familial hypophosphatemia.* Amino aciduria is not a feature of this disorder. The finding of low normal $1,25(OH)_2D_3$ serum levels suggests that insufficient stimulation of renal hydroxylase is an etiologic factor. Treatment requires oral phosphorus supplementation in conjunction with pharmacological doses of vitamin D, preferably $1,25(OH)_2D_3$, which acts by improving intestinal phosphorus absorption. Suppression of parathyroid hormone with improved renal phosphorus reabsorption at tubular sites unaffected by the mutation may also play a beneficial role. $1,25(OH)_2D_3$ has been used in place of dihydrotachysterol with some success and is therefore recommended.

The rickets of isolated renal tubular disease is generally not caused by deficiency of active vitamin D. Experimental maleic acid toxicity is an exception since it is manifested by acquired renal tubular disease as well as deficiency of renal hydroxylase activity (21).

Vitamin D-Dependency

This disease appears to be the result of an autosomal recessive deficiency of renal hydroxylase that is cured by physiologic doses of $1,25(OH)_2D_3$. Plasma calcium is markedly decreased, phosphorus is normal, and alkaline phosphatase is increased (22). Values promptly revert to normal with daily doses of 1.0 μg $1,25(OH)_2D_3$.

Diagnosis

Radiological bone changes and a characteristic combination of laboratory findings establish the diagnosis of rickets (Table 10-2). A typical diet history is usually sufficient for the diagnosis of nutritional vitamin D deficiency. If in doubt, renal rickets must be ruled out by appropriate tests. The family history and phosphaturia are diagnostic of x-linked hypophosphatemia. Determination of plasma $1,25(OH)_2D_3$ is rarely required.

Treatment
The Committee on Nutrition of the American Academy of Pediatrics recommended in 1963 that premature infants receive daily vitamin D supplements of 100 to 200 IU (2.5–5.0 μg) during the first 2 weeks of life. Treatment of rickets due to nutritional deficiency consists of oral administration of 2,000 to 4,000 IU vitamin D daily, until clinical improvement can be demonstrated radiologically. A single oral dose of 60,000 IU may be given when parents cannot be relied upon to give the medication regularly. This approach is also advantageous when the diagnosis of nutritional deficiency is in doubt, and when monitoring of the treatment response is crucial for diagnosis. An adequate response to treatment should be demonstrated in all cases by x-rays showing deposition of calcium in the zone of preparatory calcification. New calcium deposition is first detectable approximately 3 weeks after the onset of therapy. Patients with fat malabsorption should receive the vitamin in water-soluble preparation.

Vitamin D is ineffective when renal or liver hydroxylase activity is deficient due either to acquired or genetic abnormality. High doses (100 μg/day) of dihydrotachysterol, a reduction product of vitamin D, were used in the past with some success in vitamin D-resistant rickets. This drug is effective in renal rickets because it contains a hydroxyl group in the pseudo 1-position and therefore requires only the 25-hydroxylation step in the liver. Availability of synthetic 1,25-$(OH)_2D_3$ makes this compound the current drug of choice. Physiologic doses of 0.5 to 1.0 μg/day should suffice in most cases of renal osteodystrophy.

In disorders where phosphorus loss is the primary cause of clinical rickets, physiologic doses of 1,25-$(OH)_2D_3$ may be helpful, but must be supplemented with oral phosphate, 1 to 1.5 g/day, in five to six divided doses. It is available as sodium or potassium phosphate, in both tablet and powder form. By contrast, if renal rickets is caused by a reduction in the glomerular filtration rate, treatment should be aimed at decreasing the hyperphosphatemia by complexing phosphorus in the gut with aluminum carbonate or hydroxide gel. The use of calcium salts has been recommended, but it may be difficult to prevent excess calcium absorption when the patient is also receiving treatment with 1,25-$(OH)_2D_3$. To minimize the risk of hypercalcemia during treatment with vitamin D, frequent determinations of serum calcium levels should be made. Serum parathyroid hormone levels may be monitored in select patients.

Vitamin E

Biochemistry and Function
The E vitamins are naturally occurring forms of tocopherol, a methylated alcohol. They function primarily as antioxidants that prevent the peroxidation of polyunsaturated fatty acids (PUFA). The alpha, beta, gamma,

and delta substituted forms are all biologically active, although the delta form is the strongest antioxidant. Alpha-tocopherol is most important physiologically, because it makes up 90% of the vitamin E stored in body tissues.

Animal experiments and observations in humans suggest that the E vitamins have a protective effect in patients undergoing hyperbaric treatment and that they prevent hemolysis that occurs as a consequence of the peroxidation of lipid components in the red cell membrane. Studies are underway to test the potential value of vitamin E in the prevention of oxygen toxicity in premature infants. Vitamin E has been shown to enhance the absorption and use of vitamin A (23). While vitamin E is important for fertility of subprimates, claims of its usefulness in the treatment of recurrent abortion have not been sufficiently documented. A value in the prevention of cardiovascular disease has not been substantiated either.

Source and Requirements

The E vitamins are present in plants and, to a minor degree, in animal tissues. Requirements are a function of the intake of PUFA. A ratio for vitamin E/PUFA of >0.6 is recommended. Nature seems to have provided for this, because most foods with a high content of PUFA are also rich in vitamin E. The ratio of some commercial infant formulas remains low because of their high content of PUFA. The ratio is also too low in parenteral fluids if the customary vitamin concentrate (1 ml M.V.I.) is mixed with more than 20 ml intralipid and 130 ml fluid (24). RDA values are based on the average intake of a healthy population, because requirements have not been established. Daily intakes of 3 to 5 mg tocopherol equivalents are advised for infants and children under 3 years, and of 6 to 10 mg for older children and adults.

Manifestations of Deficiency

Typical manifestations are irritability, generalized edema, and decreased red cell survival, caused by the breakdown of phospholipids in red cell membranes. Signs of hemolysis include red cell fragmentation, bone marrow hyperplasia, and an increased reticulocyte count. Aniso- and poikilocytosis, spherocytes, and irregular and contracted erthyrocytes may be seen on the peripheral blood smear, while inclusion bodies often appear in the reticuloendothelial cells of the bone marrow. Infants with a birth weight of less than 1,500 g are at risk of developing between 4 and 6 weeks of age hemolytic anemia due to vitamin E deficiency (25,26).

Causes

Clinical manifestations of vitamin E deficiency are almost never seen in adults, because prolonged intake of a deficient diet is rare and it requires years to deplete the body. Vitamin E deficiency may develop in conditions accompanied by steatorrhea—mainly cystic fibrosis, celiac syndrome, and biliary obstruction. Vitamin E antagonists are found in alfalfa, kidney beans, peas, and legumes.

In premature infants, hemolytic anemia due to vitamin E deficiency is related to a lack of active transport in the placenta that leads to insufficient vitamin E stores. Their stores amount to approximately 3 mg as compared to 20 mg in the full term infant. Low intestinal absorption is a contributory factor. The PUFA content of vegetable oils, that are used in many commercial infant formulas, may have played a role in the past when the high PUFA content was not matched by vitamin E. Presumably, this causes damage to the cell membrane only if the lipids are not used for thermogenesis and are deposited in tissues. Iron contributes to the development of hemolytic anemia due to vitamin E deficiency. It has been suggested that peroxidation of lipids in the red cell membrane, which is initiated by the availability of unpaired electrons, causes the hemolysis. Iron is a potent generator of free electrons and thus enhances the disruption of red cell membranes if there is a lack of antioxidants, such as the E vitamins.

Diagnosis

A serum vitamin E level less than 0.5 mg/dl is considered indicative of deficiency. Neonates often have values as low as 0.2 mg/dl. However, blood levels are not reliable indicators of tissue stores or of dietary intake. A functional test has been proposed that measures the degree of hemolysis after exposure to hydrogen peroxide. Since factors other than vitamin E deficiency may contribute to the development of hemolysis, diagnostic usefulness of this test is also limited (Table 3-6).

Treatment

Routine administration of 5 to 10 IU/day is recommended for premature infants (1 IU = 1 mg tocopherol). Infants with vitamin E-deficient hemolytic anemia should be given 25 IU/day. Iron supplementation is contraindicated unless there is an associated iron-deficiency anemia. Water-soluble preparations of vitamin E in doses of 1 mg/kg correct vitamin E deficiency in cystic fibrosis. Lower doses are sufficient for chronic maintenance therapy in cystic fibrosis and other fat malabsorption syndromes. If the anemia is unresponsive to oral medication, 50 IU may be given IM, twice weekly. Alpha-tocopherol for oral administration is best absorbed as the polyethylene glycol succinate.

Vitamin K

Biochemistry and Function

The K vitamins comprise a group of methylnaphthoquinone derivatives. K_1 is the name of naturally occurring vitamin K, phytylmenaquinone. K_2 is the vitamin synthesized by bacteria, including those of the intestinal flora. The K vitamins are necessary for the hepatic synthesis of Factor VII (Proconvertin), which is measured by the Quick one-stage prothrombin time. This is the time taken for plasma to clot after the addition of calcium and thromboplastin. The Quick prothrombin time is abnormal in vitamin K deficiency. In the second stage of coagulation, Factor VII converts Factor X to Xa, which then forms a compound with Factor V and phospholipids. In the presence of calcium ion, this compound converts Factor II (prothrombin) into thrombin. The activities of Factors II, VII, IX, and X are vitamin K-dependent and can be assayed separately. Hemorrhagic manifestations do not generally occur until vitamin K activity is reduced to about 20%.

Source and Requirements

High concentrations of vitamin K are found in alfalfa and soy beans, and somewhat lower levels in spinach, tomatoes, and kale. Although an RDA has not been determined, an intake of about 30 μg/day has been considered adequate between 1 week and 3 years of age. The amount of vitamin K in 1l of human milk is 15 μg. Cow's milk contains roughly four times as much.

The normal infant is born relatively vitamin K-deficient. Approximately 1 in 400 infants develop "hemorrhagic disease of the newborn." The Committee on Nutrition (27) considered 200 μg/day of an oral preparation necessary for prophylaxis, based on the assumption that only 10% would be absorbed. This recommendation is especially important for breast-fed infants, since deficiency is prevalent in this group due to the lower vitamin K content of human milk and the fact that infants do not consume sufficient quantities of milk during the first few days of life, when they are at their highest risk.

Manifestations of Deficiency

The major symptoms are due to bleeding, which tends to be gastrointestinal, nasal, intracranial, or subgaleal. The bleeding tendency is due to a decrease of Factors II, VII, IX, and X. Laboratory evidence of vitamin K deficiency exists in almost all newborns between the second and tenth day of life, although only a few develop bleeding.

Causes

During the immediate neonatal period, vitamin K deficiency is common, especially in breast-fed infants. Later in life it usually occurs in disorders of fat absorption, such as cystic fibrosis, or is caused by factors that limit production of vitamin K by bacteria, including the prolonged use of antibiotics. Coumarin compounds are vitamin K antagonists that are used therapeutically to prevent clotting. Acetylsalicylic acid and sulfonamides also may act as vitamin K antagonists. Anticonvulsant therapy with either phenobarbital or diphenylhydantoin has been implicated as a cause of vitamin K deficiency. A mother receiving any one of these drugs thus may give birth to a child with an increased bleeding tendency.

Diagnosis

Vitamin K deficiency is established by measuring prothrombin time and observing the reversal of abnormality after treatment with vitamin K. Determination of the activity of Factors II, VII, IX, and X may be used to corroborate the diagnosis, but it is not necessary.

Treatment

Hypoprothrombinemia is treated with 1 mg vitamin K_1 either subcutaneously or intramuscularly. This dose will correct clinical bleeding within 1 hour and will promote the reversal of laboratory abnormality within several hours. If there is no response, larger doses are unlikely to be effective. Instead, other causes of hypoprothrombinemia must be excluded, mainly hepatic disease. The single parenteral doses of 1.0 mg, which may be used as prophylaxis for newborns, is not sufficient in infants whose mothers received drugs that cross the placenta and have antivitamin K activity, such as anticoagulants and diphenylhydantoin.

Infants with fat malabsorption may be given a water-miscible preparation of phytylmenaquinone (AquaMephyton by Merck, Sharp & Dohme or Konakion by Roche), 50 to 100 μg/day, or a parenteral dose of 1 mg of vitamin K_1 per month. Water-soluble analogues of menaquinone (Synkayvite by Roche or Hykinone by Abbott) should not be used before age 1 month, because they have been associated with hemolytic anemia, hyperbilirubinemia, kernicterus, and even death.

REFERENCES

1. Brunette MG, Delvin E, Hazel B, et al: Thiamine-responsive lactic acidosis in a patient with deficient low-KM pyruvate carboxylase activity in liver. *Pediatrics* 50:702, 1972.
2. Cooper JR, Itokawa Y, Pincus JH: Thiamine triphosphate deficiency in subacute-necrotizing encephalomyelopathy. *Science* 164:74, 1969.
3. Pincus JH, Itokawa Y, Cooper JR: Enzyme inhibiting factor in subacute necrotizing encephalomyelopathy. *Neurology* 19:841, 1969.
4. Scriver CR, Mackenzie S, Clow CL, et al: Thiamine-responsive maple-syrup urine disease. *Lancet* (i):310, 1971.
5. Bamji MS: Transketolase activity and urinary excretion of thiamine in the assessment of thiamine-nutrition status of Indians. *Am J Clin Nutr* 23:52, 1970.
6. Yoshida T, Tada K, Arakawa T: Vitamin B_6 dependence of glutamic acid decarboxylase in the kidney from a patient with vitamin B_6 dependent convulsions. *Tohoku J Exp Med* 104:195, 1971.
7. Linkswiler H: Biochemical and physiological changes in vitamin B_6 deficiency. *Am J Clin Nutr* 20:547, 1967.

8. Dillon MJ, England JM, Gompertz D, et al: Mental retardation, megaloblastic anaemia, methylmalonic aciduria and abnormal homocysteine metabolism due to an error in vitamin B_{12} metabolism. *Clin Sci Mol Med* 47:43, 1974.
9. Inoue S, Krieger I, Sarnaik A, et al: Pancytopenia in a patient with methylmalonic acidemia and inhibition of *in vitro* marrow cell growth by methylmalonic acid. *Pediatr Res* 15:95, 1981.
9a. Walter, TR: Congenital megaloblastic anemia responsive to N^5 formyltetrahydrofolic acid administration. *J Pediatr* 70:686, 1967.
10. Bartlett K, Ng H, Leonard JV: A combined defect of three mitochondrial carboxylases presenting as biotin responsive 3-methyl crotonyl glycinuria and 3-hydroxyisovaleric aciduria. *Clin Chim Acta* 100:183, 1980.
11. Elsas LJ, Miller RL, Pinnell SR: Inherited human collagen lysyl hydroxylase deficiency ascorbic acid response. *J Pediatr* 92:378, 1978.
12. Sobel AE, Strazzulla M, Sherman BS, et al: Vitamin A absorption and other blood composition studies in mongolism. *Am J Ment Defic* 62:642, 1958.
13. Getzler NA, Flint A: Keratosis follicularis: A study of one family. *Arch Dermatol* (Chicago) 93:545, 1966.
14. DeLuca HF, Schnoes HK: Metabolism and mechanism of action of vitamin D. *Annu Rev Biochem* 45:631, 1976.
15. Garabedian M, Tanaka Y, Holick MF, et al: Response of intestinal calcium transport and bone calcium mobilization to 1,25-dihydroxy vitamin D_3 in thyroparathyroidectomized rats. *Endocrinology* 94:1022, 1974.
16. Reynolds JJ, Pavlovitch H, Balsan S: 1,25-Dihydroxycholecalciferol increases bone resorption in hypoparathyroidectomised mice. *Calcif Tissue Res* 21:207, 1976.
17. Fraser D, Kooh SW, Scriver CR: Hyperparathyroidism as the cause of hyperaminoaciduria and phosphaturia in human vitamin D deficiency. *Pediatr Res* 1:425, 1967.
18. Lifshitz F, Maclaren NK: Vitamin D-dependent rickets in institutionalized, mentally retarded children receiving long-term anticonvulsant therapy: I. A survey of 288 patients. *J Pediatr* 83:612, 1973.
19. Hahn TJ, Hendin BA, Scharp CR, et al: Effect of chronic anticonvulsant therapy on serum 25-hydroxycalciferol levels in adults. *N Engl J Med* 287:900, 1972.
20. Brumbaugh PF, Haussler DH, Bressler R, et al: Radioreceptor assay for 1α,25-Dihydroxyvitamin D_3. *Science* 183:1089, 1974.
21. Brewer ED, Tsai HC, Szeto S, et al: Maleic acid-induced impairment of conversion of 25-hydroxyvitamin D_3 (25(OH)D_3) to 1,25-$(OH)_2D_3$ *in vivo* and *in vitro*: Implications for Fanconi's syndrome. *Clin Res* 24:395(A), 1976.
22. Fraser D, Kooh SW, Kind HP, et al: Pathogenesis of hereditary vitamin-D-dependent rickets: An inborn error of vitamin D metabolism involving defective conversion of 25-hydroxy vitamin D to 1,25-dihydroxy vitamin D. *N Engl J Med* 289:817, 1973.
23. Rodriguez MS, Irwin MT: A conspectus of research on vitamin A requirements of man. *J Nutr* 102:909, 1972.
24. Bell EF, Filer LJ: The role of vitamin E in the nutrition of premature infants. *Am J Clin Nutr* 34:414, 1981.
25. Melhorn DK, Gross S, Childers G: Vitamin E-dependent anemia in the premature infant: I. Effects of large doses of medicinal iron. *J Pediatr* 79:569, 1971.
26. Williams ML, Shott RJ, O'Neal PL, et al: Role of dietary iron and fat on vitamin E deficiency anemia of infancy. *N Engl J Med* 292:887, 1975.
27. Committee on Nutrition, American Academy of Pediatrics: Vitamin K supplementation for infants receiving milk substitute formulas and for those with low malabsorption. *Pediatrics* 48:483, 1971.

11
Mineral Deficiencies

TRACE METALS

Although the trace metals make up only a minute fraction of the body weight, each contributing less than 0.01% to the total, they are nevertheless vital to many metabolic processes. Trace metals which serve vital functions in human metabolism are iron, zinc, copper, iodine, fluoride, chromium, selenium, manganese, molybdenum, and cobalt. Only the first five are of practical importance to the health care professional. Nutritional requirements for these micronutrients are highest early in life, and the consequences of deficiency are more severe in infants than in adults. If one considers also that most genetic disorders of trace metal metabolism show up in the pediatric age group, it becomes apparent that trace metals are of particular concern to the pediatrician.

Iron

Function

Iron functions in the transport and use of oxygen and is the most abundant trace metal in the human body. The largest compartment is contained in the heme moiety of the hemoglobin molecule, and the second largest is the storage iron in liver and bone marrow. About 5% is in myoglobin and 1% in transferrin and other iron-containing compounds.

Metabolism

Transferrin, a β_1-globulin, is the transport protein for iron. It binds iron in the ferric form at two sites, but usually only 30 to 40% of the binding sites are saturated. Ferritin and hemosiderin, which contain about 20% of their weight as iron, are the compounds used for iron storage in liver and bone marrow. Ferritin makes up the greater percentage of the total when iron stores are low, while hemosiderin rises with increasing iron stores. Serum ferritin reflects the amount stored except in newborns, who have disproportionately high values of up to 200 ng/ml. At 3 months of age, when iron stores are mobilized, serum ferritin begins to decline and reaches a physiologic low of about 20 ng/ml at 6 months; the range in childhood is between 10 and 150 ng/ml.

The adult body contains 4 to 5 g and the newborn, about 300 mg iron. At birth, over two-thirds of the iron is contained in the red cell mass and less than 7% in stores, which is considerably less than the 30% stored by the adult. As the red cell mass decreases during the first 2 to 3 months of life, iron is released from hemoglobin, and iron stores increase. This is reflected by an increase in the concentration of iron in liver, which rises from 30 mg at birth to 100 mg at 3 months. The premature infant, who has a lower red cell mass, consequently cannot build up sufficient iron stores. Significant blood loss during delivery and in the neonatal period also decreases iron stores and will lead to iron deficiency after 3 months of age.

Iron is absorbed in the ferrous form, mainly in the duodenum. Absorption ranges from 1% to more than 20% of intake. The rate of absorption depends on a variety of factors, including age, iron stores, rate of erythropoeisis, and the vehicle. Thus, food iron is less well absorbed than iron salts. There is also variability among iron salts; sodium iron pyrophosphate, which is used in the fortification of some cereals, is less well absorbed than the ferrous sulfate contained in commercial infant formulas. Iron absorption from vegetable sources ranges from 2 to 7%, but is considerably higher from animal sources, with the lowest rate from cow's milk and the highest from meats. Absorption from soy formulas is similar to that from cow's milk, roughly 10%. By contrast, absorption from human milk may approach 59% (1). Given the same absolute amount of iron intake and the same vehicle, more iron is absorbed when body iron stores are low. However, if the absolute amount of iron intake is high, a lower percentage is absorbed. Tea inhibits iron absorption by up to 95%.

Providing iron stores are adequate and there is no blood loss, the adult absorbs about 1 mg/day and loses a comparable amount, mostly through cell extrusion. The infant loses only about 20 μg/kg. The intestinal mucosa serves as a temporary reservoir, responsive to regulatory mechanisms, where the rate of transfer from intestine to blood depends on demand and nonmobilized iron in intestinal cells is shed during mucosal turnover.

Source

Cow's milk and most commercially prepared infant foods are poor sources of iron. The use of iron-fortified formulas has become increasingly popular in the United States since the original recommendation of the Committee on Nutrition. Iron in the reduced form and small particle size, which is fairly well absorbed, is used in the United States to fortify infant cereals, which have become very popular. They are, unfortunately, not used as frequently after 6 months of age as before that time, although this is when their use should be encouraged, because formulas are usually replaced by cow's milk at this time of life. Meat and egg are rich iron sources. By comparison, the absolute amount of iron that could be absorbed from iron-rich vegetables is insignificant.

Requirements

The RDA for iron is relatively high because absorption is not constant under ordinary living conditions. The recommended value for adolescents is 18 mg/day. It is 10 mg/day for infants 0 to 6 months and for children 3 to 10 years old. After 6 months of age, iron stores have been depleted. Because of this and the rapid rate of growth, requirements are higher between 6 months and 3 years of age, 15 mg/day. If animal food sources account for more than 25% of total calories, lower iron intakes are sufficient because of better rates of absorption (2). These RDA values are equivalent to double the actual requirements as calculated from iron stores at birth, dermal losses, the need for growth, and an absorption rate of 10%. RDA values are similar to those recommended by the Committee on Nutrition (3), 1 mg/kg/day for term infants and 2 mg/kg/day for preterm infants.

Human milk and cow's milk contain 0.07 to 0.15 mg/100 kcal and consequently supply about 0.1 mg/kg body weight to the average infant taking 100 kcal/kg. This amount is thus only one-tenth the dose recommended by the Committee on Nutrition in 1976. Supplementation is obviously necessary, but the optimal amount is still under debate, mainly because of evidence suggesting that excess quantities reduce the amount of free transferrin and lactoferrin, which have anti-infectious properties.

In order to meet the requirements, it appears necessary to supplement full term infants by about 4 months of age, at the latest, and preterm infants after 2 months of age. Breast feeding by a healthy, iron-sufficient mother protects the full term infant against iron deficiency up to about 6 months of age. Currently, most iron-supplemented formulas on the market exceed requirements substantially, since they generally contain about 1.75 mg/100 kcal.

Normal Values
Commonly used indices of iron nutriture are hemoglobin (Hgb) in conjunction with erythrocyte morphologic characteristics, serum ferritin, free erythrocyte protoporphyrin (FEP), and serum iron (Table 3-6 and Chapter 8). Hemosiderin is low in normal infants less than 6 months of age and therefore not useful in the evaluation of iron status. A serum transferrin saturation >10% is considered normal. However, this parameter is of limited usefulness in the evaluation of iron status in infants, because active hemoglobin synthesis is possible even when the saturation is less than 10%. Both the WHO Scientific Group (2) and the Committee on Nutrition (3) have stated that a hemoglobin >11 g/dl is normal. The lower limit of normal for the hematocrit (Hct) increases during childhood from 33 to 37% and the mean corpuscular volume (MCV), from 70 to 78 μ^3. Serum ferritin is normally >10 ng/ml, and free erythrocyte protoporphyrin (FEP) <3 μg/g Hgb.

Microcytic, Hypochromic Anemia
Clinical manifestations of iron deficiency anemia are not unlike those seen in anemias of other etiologies and include pallor, fatigue, irritability, poor attention span, anorexia, and decreased exercise tolerance. They usually do not become apparent until the anemia is severe and imposes an increased load on the cardiorespiratory system. The level at which symptoms appear has not been determined for different age groups.

The laboratory manifestations of iron-deficiency anemia develop in three stages: The first is a decrease in iron stores, evidenced by a fall in serum ferritin. The second stage is characterized by a decrease in serum iron and an elevation in total iron-binding capacity. Finally, hemoglobin production decreases, FEP increases, and peripheral red cells become typical of iron deficiency, with hypochromasia, microcytosis, poikilocytosis, and a decrease in mean corpuscular volume. In infants serum ferritin may be normal in iron-responsive anemia.

Causes of Iron Deficiency
The major cause of iron deficiency in infancy is a diet consisting mainly of milk. This suspicion should arise whenever an infant in the age group at risk is reported to take significantly more than a quart of milk per day without iron supplements, because the caloric value of this amount is adequate, and it is unlikely that such an infant is hungry enough to take sufficient quantities of other iron-containing foods. The second major or contributory cause of iron deficiency is poor iron stores since birth because of prematurity or perinatal blood loss due to fetal–maternal hemorrhage, twin–twin transfusion, placenta previa, and other placental tears. Chronic postnatal blood loss must be considered when these two major causes of iron deficiency in infancy can be ruled out, or when the anemia occurs after the period of greatest risk, in preschool and preadolescent children.

Anatomic lesions (Meckel's diverticulum, ulcerative colitis etc.) should be considered. Hookworm infestation is a common cause of chronic blood loss in other parts of the world. In infants, chronic occult blood loss from the intestines has been associated with sensitivity to the protein in unheated milk, but the etiologic relationships are not certain. It is possible that the anemia itself causes intestinal epithelial damage, excess desquamation, and iron loss, because treatment of the anemia not infrequently results in the disappearance of microscopic blood losses.

Diagnosis

The definition of anemia is to some extent arbitrary, because the level of Hgb that is incompatible with good health has not been defined. A level of 11 g has been accepted as the cutoff point. Anemia may be diagnosed at higher hemoglobin levels when there is associated microcytosis and hypochromasia and when iron therapy causes a rise in the hemoglobin level.

Several diagnostic steps should be taken when a routine Hgb or hematocrit determination is abnormal and iron deficiency is being considered. Peripheral red cell morphology should be examined or the MCV determined in conjunction with FEP and serum transferrin saturation. A value below 7% for transferrin saturation suggests iron deficiency; the range between 7 and 15% represents the zone of overlap with normal values. Determination of serum ferritin is optional. The value is less than 10 ng/ml in iron-deficiency anemia. However, since this test is abnormal early during development of anemia patients may show transient abnormality without ever developing anemia. A low Hgb due to other causes is thus easily misinterpreted as iron deficiency. Serum iron determinations are popular, but the test suffers from poor reproducibility, in part because of diurnal fluctuations or other biological variations. A value less than 50 μg/dl suggests iron deficiency. Determination of FEP has become popular because the test can be done with a technically simple and rapid fluorometric procedure that is also inexpensive. The value rises when there is interference in the last step in heme synthesis, the combination of iron and protoporphyrin. A rise to levels above 80 μg/dl is apparent before Hgb depression becomes noticeable and leads to an increase in the FEP/Hgb ratio. The test loses diagnostic usefulness, because it is abnormal during infection and in lead intoxication. FEP values are higher in plumbism than iron deficiency anemia. Differential diagnosis is complicated by the fact that the anemia of plumbism is also microcytic and hypochromic. Moreover, pica, which should suggest lead ingestion, is also not uncommon in iron-deficiency anemia. Differential diagnosis requires determination of serum lead levels.

Aside from plumbism, differential diagnosis must consider thalassemia, idiopathic pulmonary hemosiderosis (IPH), congenital atransferrinemia, and some rare sideroblastic anemias, including the pyridoxine-responsive variety. The reticulocyte count is helpful because it is elevated in thalassemia and IPH. It is low in iron deficiency, but the rise during spontaneous recovery following introduction of iron-containing foods may be misleading. In the presence of elevated levels of reticulocytes and serum iron, Hgb electrophoresis and determination of fetal Hgb and Hgb A_2 are necessary to rule out thalassemia. An elevated reticulocyte count due to IPH can be ruled out by a normal sputum examination for sideroblasts and a chest x-ray. It is important, as part of the diagnostic process, to monitor the response to iron treatment because these other rare hypochromic, microcytic anemias might otherwise be missed. Chronic blood loss is often not recognized until there is recurrence of anemia after cessation of therapy.

Treatment

Simple ferrous salts, such as ferrous sulfate, gluconate, or fumarate, are well tolerated, readily absorbed, and inexpensive. The dose is 6 mg/kg/day for children and 3 mg/kg/day for adults, given in two to three doses, preferably between meals to achieve better absorption. Gastrointestinal upset is extremely rare in children. Staining of the teeth may occur, but it is reversible and can be prevented by administering the drug as a concentrated solution with a dropper on the back of the tongue. Parenteral administration of iron-dextran does not accomplish faster recovery but is occasionally advisable when questions concerning compliance arise. One dose of 2.5 mg/kg iron for each gram per deciliter of desired Hgb rise should be given before a therapeutic response can be considered negative. Dietary instruction is an essential part of therapy. To enforce better dietary habits, it is advisable to limit the milk intake to a pint or less per day. The infant who has become accustomed to satisfying its sucking needs throughout the day by using the milk bottle thus will get hungry enough and take iron-containing pureed foods that should be part of the diet after 6 months or, certainly, after 12 months of age.

The bone marrow responds within about 4 days, as evidenced by an increased peripheral reticulocyte count. The reticulocyte response, which is proportionate to the degree of anemia, may be missed, especially when the anemia is mild. It is therefore better to monitor the therapeutic effect by monitoring the rise in Hgb. The maximum recovery rate is 0.4 g/dl/day.

Blood transfusions may be necessary when the anemia is severe and a threat of heart failure exists. To avoid cardiac overload, patients should receive packed red cells, 5 ml/kg, at a slow rate, and the infusion should be repeated at daily intervals until a safe Hgb range of about 6 g/dl has been reached. Venipuncture coupled with red cell transfusion may be necessary when heart failure is manifest.

Zinc

Function

Zinc functions as a component of numerous metalloenzymes and an activator of enzyme complexes. Some of the better known zinc-requiring enzymes are alkaline phosphatase, carbonic anhydrase, carboxypeptidase, alcohol lactic dehydrogenase, and glutaric dehydrogenase. Zinc plays a central role in nucleic acid metabolism because it is a component of DNA and RNA polymerase and an activator of thymidine kinase; it also appears to be necessary to prevent excessive ribonuclease activity. It is therefore not surprising that zinc is important for many vital processes, including protein synthesis, CNS function, growth, and organogenesis. Zinc also plays a role in host defense, wound healing, osteogenesis and keratogenesis.

Metabolism

Approximately 20 to 30% of dietary zinc is absorbed. Observations in acrodermatitis enteropathica suggest that zinc absorption can be improved by zinc-binding ligands that are present in human milk. Recently, picolinic acid was identified as a zinc-binding ligand in human milk (4). A function in absorption is suggested by its presence in pancreatic secretions (5). Other components of food which complex with zinc and promote absorption are cystine and histidine. Zinc absorption is impaired by iron and apparently by copper, as well as by substances that form insoluble complexes with zinc, including polyphosphates, laundry starch, fiber, and phytates that are present in unleavened bread. Dietary zinc determines the uptake by intestinal mucosa apparently through regulation of de novo synthesis of metallothioneines, which act as a temporary reservoir and prevent excessive release into the blood stream. Zinc is carried in blood, bound largely to albumin and some to α_2-macroglobulin and transferrin. The highest concentration of zinc is found in the choroid of the eyes and in spermatozoa. Concentrations in excess of 100 ppm occur in plasma, hair, nails, prostate, semen, and bone. Concentrations in liver, kidney, and muscle are approximately half that amount. The major excretory route is the feces. Endogenous zinc is excreted in pancreatic secretions and reabsorbed together with dietary zinc.

Source

Only a few classes of food supply significant quantities of zinc. Dietary zinc intake is therefore variable from day to day. Foods that are rich in zinc are beef, chicken, shellfish, and whole-kernel breads. Commercial infant formulas have been supplemented with zinc since 1975. They were zinc deficient because zinc bound to protein is removed when the protein content of formulas based on cow's milk is artificially decreased. Although both cow's milk and human milk are good sources of zinc, the bioavailability of zinc from human milk is superior because of the presence of zinc-binding substances. The bioavailability of zinc is very poor in formulas containing soy protein because soy contains phytic acid. Zinc concentration in colostrum may be as high as 20 mg/l. With progressive lactation, zinc content drops below the average of 3 mg/l and may fall as low as 1 mg/l or less, presumably because of deficient zinc nutrition of the mother.

Requirements

No satisfactory method for estimating zinc requirements exists. According to calculations based on zinc concentrations in increments of fat-free body mass after birth, the young infant requires a retention of 0.3 mg/day or an intake of at least 1.2 mg/day. The actual intake ranges from 2 to 5 mg/day in infants under 3 years of age, and from 5 to 7 mg/day in 3- to 5-year-old children (6). The recommended daily allowance (RDA) is liberally set at 3 mg/day for infants under 7 months and at 5 mg/day for infants 7 to 12 months. Cow's milk and human milk, which contain from 3 to 5 mg/l, thus provide adequate amounts of zinc. FT infants on intravenous alimentation should receive 100 μg/kg/day and LBW infants 300 μg/kg/day.

Normal Values

The accuracy of quantitative zinc measurements in biological materials has been greatly improved since the advent of atomic absorption spectrophotometry. Normal plasma values from various laboratories nevertheless still vary by as much as 20%, necessitating caution in the interpretation of random determinations. Nail clippings and hair from the nape of the neck, which must be cut close to the root, are accessible tissues and fairly accurate in the assessment of zinc status. Urinary zinc is not a useful indicator. Red blood cell zinc drops only after prolonged deficiency. Plasma has limitations because zinc concentration during infection or tissue breakdown does not reflect zinc status. Moreover, tissue concentrations may be normal if the deficiency has caused growth arrest. There are indications that leukocytes will prove to be the best indicator of zinc nutriture.

Normal plasma and hair zinc values of asymptomatic adults from a variety of studies range between 100 and 200 ppm (i.e., μg/g). Plasma and hair zinc levels are highest in newborn infants (7). In a survey of 338 healthy people from birth to adulthood, the lowest hair zinc values were observed in infants and preschoolers, age 3 months to 4 years (mean 88 μg/g). Plasma zinc values of breast-fed infants are higher than those of artificially fed infants. Premature infants on pasteurized milk tend to be in negative zinc balance for the first 2 months of life, and even FT infants rarely retain significant amounts of zinc in the first 4 months, a factor that contributes to the apparent "physiologically" low hair zinc concentration in infancy.

Nutritional Zinc Deficiency

This entity was first recognized in Middle Eastern countries (8), where the syndrome affects up to 3% of adolescents living in rural areas. The cardinal features were dwarfism and lack of sexual maturation, including impaired testosterone synthesis. Hepatomegaly and anemia, which were also observed, are probably due to unrecognized deficiencies of other nutrients. Dermatitis is a major manifestation of genetic zinc deficiency, acrodermatitis enteropathica, and of deficiency following prolonged use of parenteral alimentation with zinc-free solutions. It is apparently not a feature of the middle eastern form. Skin lesions include roughening, keratosis, and alopecia. Lesions subject to irritation tend to become erythematous and infected. Fungal infections are particularily common, presumably because of deficient cell-mediated immunity (10). Zinc deficiency appears to be a major cause of immunodeficiency, described in infants with protein-calorie malnutrition from underdeveloped countries. Effects of zinc deficiency on the central nervous system are evident in acrodermatitis enteropathica, where irritability, emotional instability, and even ataxia have been described. Marginal zinc deficiency has been shown to cause decreased taste acuity, anorexia, and mild growth failure in infants and children from the United States (7).

Prenatal Zinc Deficiency

The teratogenic effects of zinc deficiency are evidenced by the high incidence of abortion, anencephaly, and skeletal anomalies in offspring of adult women suffering from acrodermatitis enteropathica (11). Epidemiological data suggest that maternal zinc deficiency could be a cause of the high incidence of anencephaly observed in certain geographic areas. The teratogenic potential of zinc deficiency has also been demonstrated in rat studies.

Causes of Zinc Deficiency

Marginal deficiency in the United States occurs in low-income families and appears to be the result of insufficient intake relative to individual need. Requirements are higher during periods of rapid growth, which explains the greater vulnerability of young, especially prematurely born, infants. Low intake is the cause in occasional surgical patients on institutional diets with low zinc content, especially when oral feedings are frequently withheld without addition of zinc to parenteral solutions. Development of deficiency is accelerated in these cases when requirements are increased because of wound healing or excessive zinc losses. Thus, zinc may be lost in urine, tissues, feces, and other secretions, especially those from burns. In chronic enteritis, zinc deficiency may develop through the loss of blood and zinc-containing protein complexes into the intestine. Hyperzincuria occurs in hepatic cirrhosis, conditions associated with chronic albuminuria and tissue breakdown (e.g., multiple injuries), starvation, and severe protein deprivation. In the severe cases of deficiency that occur in Middle Eastern countries, factors other than low intake play an important contributory role. The high content of phytates in unleaved bread was shown to be a factor. Iatrogenic zinc deficiency occurs in patients on chelating agents, such as penicillamine or ethambutal. Diseases that are not infrequently associated with subclinical zinc deficiency are sickle cell anemia (12) and cystic fibrosis.

Genetic Zinc Deficiency: Acrodermatitis Enteropathica (AE)

AE is a genetic disorder associated with severe zinc deficiency (9) due to poor absorption. Next to dermatitis and emotional instability, diarrhea is a major manifestation and is partly responsible for the failure to thrive. Onset is after birth or—in breast-fed infants—after weaning from the breast. Failure to thrive is progressive, and death results if the condition remains untreated. The earliest signs are maceration and fissuring at the angles of the mouth, followed by symmetrical extension of well-demarcated erythematous lesions to the face. Involvement of the distal ends of the extremities has given the disorder its name. The dermatitis also affects genitalia and areas subject to irritation.

Zinc values in plasma, hair, and intestinal mucosa are very low. The cause is believed to be the lack of a factor that is necessary for zinc absorption. This factor is present in breast milk, whereas cow's milk contains insufficient quantities. Before hypozincemia was recognized, these patients were treated successfully with breast milk. Diiodohydroxyquin, a versatile chelating agent, had also been used with some success prior to the use of oral zinc. Absorption must be reevaluated because endogenous zinc was not considered in earlier studies. Genetic heterogeneity is suggested by the description of AE without hypozincemia (5,13).

Diagnosis

Recognition of sporadic cases of marginal deficiency may be difficult, because the zinc concentration of commonly used tissues and body fluids is influenced by factors other than zinc nutriture. For instance, hypozincemia occurs in the absence of zinc depletion as a result of infection, surgery, or burns and when serum proteins are low or circulating levels of estrogen are high. In view of these diagnostic difficulties, suspected cases of marginal zinc deficiency may warrant treatment with zinc for a limited period of time, providing objective parameters are monitored. Lower limits of normal for zinc are 75 μg/dl in plasma, 75 μg/g in hair and 25 μg/g Hgb. However, normal controls should be established by each laboratory.

The diagnosis of AE rests on the demonstration of hypozincemia in the presence of characteristic clinical manifestations and a dramatic response to treatment with zinc. Repeated testing of the response to zinc treatment and withdrawal of therapy is advised. This is especially important in cases of AE without hypozincemia (5,13). The triad of diarrhea, dermatitis, and neuropsychiatric symptoms is seen in pellagra, but the disorder is rare in the United States. The dermatitis of essential fatty acid deficiency enters the differential diagnosis and should be ruled out by a careful diet history.

Treatment

The provision of elemental zinc in amounts corresponding to the normal daily dietary intake of this metal is adequate for the long-term treatment of zinc deficiency. This amounts to 2 to 5 mg for infants, 5 to 7 mg for preschoolers, 10 mg for older children, and 15 mg for adults. The starting dose for patients with acrodermatitis is 20 to 40 mg/day, but some patients require substantially higher doses. Zinc infusions aimed at correcting low plasma values should be avoided during severe infections. Treatment causes disappearance of clinical symptoms within days. Since the mechanism of the absorption defect in AE is not yet understood, care should be taken not to overdose because in normal individuals, large doses of one trace metal affect absorption of others. Zinc may be given in tablet form as the sulfate or as a solution of zinc acetate, which contains 30 mg per teaspoon and supplies 8.8 mg elemental zinc. Plasma zinc should be monitored.

Copper

Function

Correlations between biochemical function and clinical features of deficiency are more apparent with regard to copper than most other trace metals. Approximately 90% of the copper in plasma is bound to ceruloplasmin, which is both a transport protein and has ferroxidase activity. In addition to its importance as a component of ferroxidase I, copper is an essential part of cytochrome oxidase, ascorbic acid oxidase, tyrosine hydroxylase, lysyl oxidase, amine oxidase, superoxide dismutase, and dopamine-β-hydroxylase. Ferroxidase catalyzes the oxidation of ferrous to ferric iron, thus making it available for binding to transferrin and transport to the bone marrow. Lack of copper ferroxidase contributes to the anemia of copper deficiency, which resembles iron deficiency. As part of cytochrome oxidase, copper functions in the electron transport chain and is necessary for many energy-requiring processes and synthetic functions. It is thus not surprising that deficiency causes hypothermia, loss of cortical neurons, and neutropenia. Dysfunction of tyrosine hydroxylase causes hypopigmentation. Deficiency of ascorbic acid, lysyl andamine oxidases is probably responsible for scorbutic changes, fragmentation of the internal elastic lamina, and for instability of collagen in connective tissue.

Metabolism

About 40% of ingested copper is absorbed from the stomach and upper small intestines by an active, energy-requiring process, possibly involving ligands. There is evidence that copper competes with other trace metals for a ligand or transport site. This mechanism would explain the observation that excess ingestion of one trace metal, like zinc, may be associated with hypocupremia. About 40% of ingested copper is absorbed, and of this amount 80% is excreted in bile, amounting to 1.6 mg/day in the adult. The remainder is excreted with the desquamating intestinal mucosa. The liver, cortical gray matter, heart, and kidneys contain the highest concentrations of copper, although the bulk of it is in muscle and bone. The liver of the full term infant contains a relatively large amount of total body copper–approximately 50% compared to 10% in the adult. These copper stores accumulate during the latter part of gestation and represent a considerable margin of safety against the development of deficiency of which the premature infant is deprived (14).

Source

The diet generally consumed by people of all ages provides about 2 to 5 mg/day, which is more than the required amount of copper. An adequate intake is more difficult to ensure in infants who remain, after 6 months of age, primarily on a diet of cow's milk with a copper content of 0.1 to 0.3 mg/l. Breast milk is only slightly superior, with 0.2 to 0.4 mg/l. Most commercial infant formulas are now supplemented to provide an adequate copper supply. Basic foodstuffs, such as fresh vegetables, meats, and refined cereals, provide two to four times the concentration in milk. The richest sources are liver, kidney, shellfish, and unrefined cereals.

Requirements

During the first 6 months, requirements are low because of large hepatic copper stores. Requirements during the latter part of infancy have been calculated to be 0.05 mg/kg body weight. This amount is readily supplied by mixed infant feeding. The RDA has been liberally set at 0.08 mg/kg body weight. Premature infants may require more. A high protein intake seems to increase requirements.

Normal Values

Serum copper concentrations at birth average 30 μg/dl. Subsequently, there is a gradual rise, so that after 8 months of age values range from 125 to 240 μg/dl. The fact that newborns have low serum values but large liver stores shows that hypocupremia is not always diagnostic of copper depletion. Corticosteroids also reduce serum copper levels. Hypercupremia is induced by infections, neoplasia, and rheumatoid arthritis. Estrogen elevation raises serum copper levels through stimulation of ceruloplasmin synthesis. The average copper concentration in the liver after birth is about 20 μg/g dry weight. Other indices, such as RBC and urinary copper, are rarely used in the evaluation of copper nutriture. Hair copper seems to reflect total body copper, but may be unreliable unless increasing concentrations in the shaft with distance from the scalp are taken in account (15).

Nutritional Copper Deficiency

The earliest signs are iron-deficiency anemia, neutropenia, and osteoporosis. Iron accumulates in the liver and intestinal mucosal cells because ferroxidase deficiency prevents mobilization and transport. Regulatory mechanisms then cause a further decrease in iron absorption. Erythrocyte morphologic characteristics resemble those of iron-deficiency anemia, but the response to iron is poor. The bone marrow may show vacuolization and megaloblastic changes in erythroid precursors. Other physical findings include depigmentation of skin and hair, seborrhea, and hepatomegaly. Deficiency of amine oxidase and lysyl oxidase is thought to be responsible for lack of cross-linkage in collagen and elastic tissue thus causing bladder diverticula, pulmonary emphysema, vascular tortuosity, aneurisms, and the rupture of major vessels. Radiologic changes resemble scurvy because of subperiosteal densities, osteoporosis, metaphyseal spurs, and submetaphyseal fractures. Since multiple fractures of the ribs are not uncommon, the battered child syndrome may be suspected. Osteoporosis, cupping, and flaring of the metaphyses of the long bones may be confused with rickets (Table 11-1).

Causes of Copper Deficiency

Copper deficiency has been reported in malnutrition that is complicated by prolonged diarrhea. Most cases occurred in infants over 6 months of age and young children recovering from malnutrition while on a diet based on cow's milk, which has a relatively low copper content (18). Prematurity predisposes to the development of deficiency under these circumstances (19). Protein malnutrition may lead to hypocupremia because there is insufficient production of apoceruloplasmin. Excessive loss of ceruloplasmin is responsible for hypocupremia in protein-losing enteropathy and nephrosis. Patients who were maintained for extended periods of time on parenteral nutrition without copper supplementation also have developed deficiency symptoms (20). Iatrogenic deficiency may occur after the prolonged use of chelating agents. Liver dysfunction increases intestinal losses of copper.

Genetic Copper Deficiency: Menkes' Syndrome

Severe manifestations of copper deficiency occur in Menkes' kinky-hair syndrome (16), a genetic disorder characterized by pili torti and profound depression of copper levels in serum, liver, and brain. The disease starts

Table 11-1. Manifestations of Copper Deficiency

Pathology	*Nutritional*	*Genetic (Menkes' Syndrome)*
Anemia	+	0
Liver enlargement	+	0
Neutropenia	+	0
Seborrheic dermatitis	+	+
Hair depigmentation	+	+
Pili torti	?	+
Mental retardation	?	+
Convulsions	?	+
Hypothermia	0	+
Optic nerve atrophy	?	+
Scorbutic changes	+	+
Failure to thrive	+	+
Vascular tortuosity	+	+
Hemorrhages, (incl. CNS)	+	+
Bladder diverticula	?	+
Pulmonary emphysema	?	+
Lab:		
Serum copper	low	low
Serum ceruloplasmin	low	low
Red blood count	low	normal
Urinary copper	low	increased
Hepatic copper	low	low

early in infancy, causes progressive CNS degeneration, and is usually fatal in late infancy or early childhood. A genetic absorption defect has been suspected. However, the fact that urine copper may be elevated, that the anemia of nutritional deficiency is absent, and that copper is not deficient in kidney, intestines, or erythrocytes suggests that the pathogenic mechanism is more complex. The genetic abnormality of copper metabolism was first recognized by Danks et al. (17) who noted the similarity with nutritional copper deficiency in "sway-back" sheep (Table 11-1).

Diagnosis

Copper deficiency should be considered in cases with iron-deficiency anemia that do not respond to iron, and in infants with osteoporosis that cannot otherwise be explained. The association of osteoporosis and neutropenia is typical of copper deficiency, but is also seen in several ketotic hyperglycinemias (i.e., methylmalonic, isovaleric, and propionic acidemias). Decreased ceruloplasmin, low serum copper, and low urinary copper excretion confirm the diagnosis. However, hypocupremias that are not due to nutritional deficiency exist and must be ruled out, including the physiologic hypocupremia of early infancy. Tentative lower limits of normal are a serum copper of 45 μg/dl for infants over 3 months of age, 80 μg/dl for children, and 70 μg/dl for adults. The values in ceruloplasmin deficiency due to hypoproteinemia are low long before the body becomes depleted. On the other hand, since ceruloplasmin behaves like an acute phase reactant, ceruloplasmin values may be normal or even high in copper deficiency if there is a coexistent infection, neoplasia, or rheumatoid arthritis.

Wilson's disease must be considered in the differential diagnosis of nutritional copper deficiency, especially in the pediatric age group, when clinical manifestations of Wilson's disease may be too mild to be recognizable. Serum copper and ceruloplasmin are low in both diseases. However, urinary copper is increased in Wilson's disease (up to 1.5 mg/day) but low in nutritional deficiency. A liver biopsy confirms the diagnosis of Wilson's disease, because copper concentration is increased—usually in excess of 100 μg/g dry weight. The hypocupremia of Menkes' kinky-hair syndrome is invariably associated with severe mental retardation and characteristic hair abnormalities. Moreover, the onset is soon after birth, while nutritional deficiency is rare before 6 months of age.

Treatment

Nutritional copper deficiency in infants may be treated orally with a 1% solution of copper sulfate, containing 0.2 mg elemental copper per 0.1 ml. The recommended dose is 0.1 mg/kg/day. Infants on parenteral therapy may be given copper in the infusate in doses of about 0.02 mg/kg/day. There is no satisfactory treatment for Menkes' kinky-hair syndrome. Parenteral copper treatment has been tried without success. It was given subcutaneously for 427 days to one patient, who showed a persistently negative copper balance due to large fecal losses (21).

Iodine

Function

The only known function of iodine is as an essential part of thyroid hormones, thyroxine and triiodothyronine. Of the 10 to 20 mg contained in the adult human body, more than two-thirds is concentrated in the thyroid gland. The remainder is distributed throughout the body in tissues where thyroid acts, with somewhat greater concentrations in the salivary and gastric glands.

Source

Sea water, fish, and seafood are rich sources of iodine. Concentrations in soil and fertilizer are variable, depending on the geographic area. The iodine content of plants reflects that of soil, and the content of milk reflects that of the diet, which includes plants. Seasonal variations affect cow's milk, which has concentrations ranging from 10 to 200 μg/l. The waters of the Pacific West, the Great Lakes, and high mountain regions of the Alps, Himalayas, and Andes are deficient in iodine. Commercially made bread is a significant source of iodine in modern society because of the addition of iodine to the bread mix as a conditioner. In the United States potassium iodide is added to table salt in concentrations of 0.01%.

Requirements

Determination of requirements has been difficult. It is known that infants have done well on breast milk and formulas with an iodine content of 40 to 80 μg/l. One may therefore assume that an intake in this range is sufficient during periods of rapid growth. Data for nongoitrous children and adolescents from a geographic area of low iodine content (22) caused some observers to arrive at a similar figure for the daily requirement of older individuals, approximately 60 μg/l.

Normal Values

Since the iodine in the human body is linked to thyroxine, assessment of iodine nutriture is not as simple as the measurement of other trace metals in tissues or body fluids. In the absence of thyroid enlargement and when the values for thyroxine and thyroid stimulating hormone (TSH) are normal, one may assume that iodine status is normal.

Nutritional Iodine Deficiency

Iodine deficiency, which is prevalent in certain geographic areas and which causes goiter, has been recognized for more than 50 years. *Endemic goiter*—as the condition is called—develops because the body compensates for the deficiency by recycling iodine liberated in the tissues and resynthesizes thyroid hormone at an increased rate. Enlargement is due to hypertrophy and hyperplasia in response to stimulation by the pituitary gland, which releases thyroid stimulating hormone (TSH). Goiter may decrease or even subside during periods of decreased demand for thyroid hormone. Characteristically, the serum thyroxine level is normal or low, and TSH shows varying degrees of elevation.

There are two types of "cretinism" that are endemic in the same areas where iodine-deficiency goiter is prevalent. One is the "nervous" variety, which is prevalent in New Guinea and is due to CNS damage that was evidently sustained during the first trimester before development of the thyroid gland. The syndrome consists of ataxia, spasticity, deafmutism, and mental retardation. Signs of hypothyroidism are minimal or absent. The other is myxedematous cretimism, which delays growth, bone maturation, and sexual development and causes mental retardation. Only about one-quarter of the cases in a given area have thyroid enlargement, which is usually not severe. The serum thyroxin level is low, and TSH is elevated.

Endemic goiter and both types of endemic cretinism are caused by nutritional iodine deficiency. This has been documented by the disappearance of these conditions in populations at risk following iodine prophylaxis, which is usually carried out through the use of iodine supplementation of table salt.

Genetic Disorders of Iodine Utilization

Pendred's syndrome of congenital deafness and goiter is due to an inherited defect of iodine organification, transmitted as an autosomal recessive gene. Administration of perchlorate causes discharge of iodide from the thyroid gland. The disorder may be confused with the "nervous" type of endemic cretinism, because signs of hypothyroidism are mild or even absent in both. Congenital goitrous hypothyroidism is the hallmark of two other genetic disorders that have effects comparable to those of iodine deficiency, although dietary iodine is available and absorbed. One is a deficiency of iodide trapping, characterized by low radioiodine uptake. The other is an isolated organification defect due to the absence of thyroid peroxidase, which prevents oxidation and thus incorporation into tyrosine and conversion to thyroid hormone.

Diagnosis

Determination of TSH and iodine as either thyroxine or protein-bound iodine is not sufficient for the diagnosis of nutritional deficiency. Clinical and epidemiological features must be taken into consideration. The differential diagnosis includes genetic and acquired disorders of iodine utilization and other, non-iodine-related causes of congenital and acquired goiter.

The differential diagnosis of congenital goiter includes (*1*) genetic defects in the synthesis of thyroid hormone, (*2*) neonatal goiter due to maternal ingestion of iodides and antithyroid drugs that cross the placenta and interfere with thyroid synthesis, (*3*) goiter due to congenital hyperthyroidism (which poses no diagnostic problem because of the symptoms of hyperthyroidism), and finally (*4*) thyroid tumors, such as teratomas.

The differential diagnosis of endemic goiter includes (*1*) iodine goiter, (*2*) lymphocytic thyroiditis, (*3*) simple goiter of unknown etiology (which is usually euthyroid and prevalent in girls), and (*4*) adenomatous goiter (which also poses no diagnostic problem because of its firm consistency and lobulated or nodular surface).

Fluoride

Function

Fluoride has not been clearly established as essential, although certain benefits have been demonstrated. Tooth enamel and calcified tissues of bone are made up of hydroxyapatite and fluorapatite in varying composition, depending on the amount of fluoride available at the time and site of formation. Small amounts of fluoride enhance mineralization of tooth enamel. Resistance to caries is decreased if the amount of fluoride in the outer layer of the tooth is inadequate. Consumption of 0.5 to 1.0 mg fluoride per day during infancy and childhood thus can be expected to decrease the caries attack rate in permanent teeth by up to 60%. The mechanism of action is not understood, although most observers believe that the low acid solubility of fluorapatite is responsible for the resistance to caries. Fluoride has a beneficial effect on osteoporosis by improving calcium balance and bone density. Animal studies indicate that it may be necessary for maintenance of a normal hematocrit, fertility, and growth.

Source

Almost all foodstuffs contain trace amounts of fluoride, but with the exception of seafood, they do not supply significant amounts. Drinking water is therefore the only major source of fluoride for the prevention of caries. Both human and cow's milk are better sources than most other foodstuffs, supplying 0.05 to 0.2 mg/l, but this is not sufficient to provide the recommended dose of 0.5 to 1.0 mg/day. Formulas made up of powdered or concentrated milk products have varying amounts, depending on the amount and fluoride content of the water used for dilution. Currently, most formulas provide fluoride in amounts comparable to that in cow's milk.

Requirements

The optimal fluoride intake during the first 3 years of life is 0.5 mg/day, according to the 1972 recommendations by the Committee on Nutrition (23). The prescribed dosage should be individualized, depending on the fluoride content of the local water supply (24). In areas where the water contains 0.3 to 0.7 ppm, infants may be expected to consume the recommended amount, and no supplements are necessary. In areas where the water contains less than 0.3 ppm, supplementation is recommended in amounts of 0.25 mg/day. Prophylaxis should begin at or soon after 2 weeks of age, because the period of mineralization of unerupted deciduous teeth includes early infancy. The recommended fluoride intake after 3 years of age is 1 mg/day. The supplemental dosage schedule (Table 11-2) is based on the assumption that about 1 l of water is consumed. The margin of safety appears to be sufficiently wide to guard against fluorosis. However, in warm climates or in the case of medical conditions such as diabetes, where water consumption is excessive, adjustments should be made. Commercially available preparations come in dosages that supply the recommended supplements in one dose per day: 0.25, 0.5, and 1.0 mg per tablet, either as such or in combination with vitamins. Fluoride solutions that can be dispensed by dropper are available for infants. They contain a predictable amount of fluoride per drop and thus allow indivi-

Table 11-2. Supplemental Fluoride Dosage (in mg/day)

	Fluoride Concentration in Drinking Water (ppm)		
Age	*0.3*	*0.3 to 0.7*	*0.7*
2 weeks to 2 years	0.25	0	0
2 to 3 years	0.50	0.25	0
3 to 16 years	1.00	0.50	0

dualization of the dose. The recommended dosage schedule is in accord with the Council on Dental Therapeutics (25).

It has been suggested that infants receive the total recommended dose as a supplement because their water intake is negligible. This applies particularly to many breast-fed infants. The Committee on Nutrition (23) does not support this view because available evidence does not indicate a different rate of caries in breast-fed infants compared to infants on formulas made with fluoridated water.

Other Trace Metals

Chromium is a cofactor to insulin that potentiates its peripheral activity. In the naturally occurring form, it is called *glucose factor*. Low concentrations of chromium in hair have been observed in children with juvenile diabetes (26). Since insulin activity is associated with urinary chromium excretion, this observation may have been the result of prolonged insulin therapy in these children. It is possible that the known insulin resistance of obese subjects is related to chromium deficiency, which could develop as a result of chronic insulin overactivity. Chromium deficit appears to be associated with a decrease of high-density lipoproteins (HDL) (27) and an increase in blood lipids, an intriguing observation in view of the vascular complications of obesity that are enhanced by low HDL levels. Improvement of impaired glucose tolerance by chromium has been observed in malnourished infants and was interpreted as a sign of prior deficiency (28).

Selenium is an essential part of glutathione peroxidase. This function may explain the sparing effect of selenium on vitamin E requirements, since this enzyme, like vitamin E, protects the erythrocyte from oxidative damage. Premature infants are most prone to lipid peroxidation in red cell membranes due to a variety of factors, including vitamin E deficiency. A recognized selenium-deficiency disease is the so-called Keshan's disease (29). Sodium selenite, containing 50 μg selenium, is used in its treatment.

Manganese plays a role as activator of several enzymes, including superoxide dysmutase, arginase, succinic dehydrogenase, and two enzymes that are required for mucopolysaccharide synthesis: polymerase and galactotransferase. Deficiency of these two enzymes may explain symptoms of disequilibrium that are seen in experimental deficiency and that appear to be due to abnormalities of the matrix of otoliths, bone, and cartilage. Spontaneous nutritional deficiency or genetic enzyme deficiencies involving manganese binding have not been recognized to date in children. An adult male has been described who had hypocholesterolemia, some weight loss, reddening of facial hair, and a poor response to vitamin K (30).

Molybdenum is an essential part of xanthine oxidase and may be necessary for the conversion of ferric to ferrous ferritin, which must precede the release of iron from ferritin.

Cobalt is part of vitamin B_{12}. It is not known whether this is the only vital function of cobalt in human metabolism.

MAJOR MINERALS

Sodium

Source and Requirements

The organism can tolerate wide variations in sodium intake, so that problems in meeting dietary requirements are virtually nonexistent. Hyponatremia occurs therefore mainly in disorders that are associated with sodium loss in excess of water retention. Sodium retention is very efficient, especially when intakes are low. Retention from breast milk, which has a low sodium content, is in the order of 95%. Assuming normal losses from skin, urine, and feces and 95% retention, requirements of infants under 3 years do not exceed 3 mEq/day. However, the advisable sodium intake is in the order of 6 to 8 mEq/day (31). Infants on breast milk obtain on the average 1 mEq/kg/day. By 4 months, when solid foods supply usually 20% of the caloric needs, average sodium intake amounts to about 5 mEq/kg/day. Prior to the restriction of sodium in commercial baby foods, infants in the United States received anywhere from 9 to 60 mEq/day (32).

Regulatory Mechanisms

The major regulatory mechanism of sodium balance is through renal tubular absorption. The major objective is the maintenance of an effective arterial volume (EAV). Thus, when cardiac output drops during heart failure, the patient retains sodium. A reduction in EAV leads to an increase in renin release and hence to an increase in aldosterone, which acts on the distal tubule and causes sodium retention. Other regulatory mechanisms are listed in Table 11-3.

The renin-angiotensin-aldosterone system, which is the major regulator of sodium balance, is influenced by a number of factors. The three most important stimuli for the release of renin are salt concentration, renal

Table 11-3. Mechanisms* Causing Excessive Renal Sodium Loss

↓ Renin output
↓ Angiotensin production
↓ Aldosterone secretion
↑ Effective arterial volume
↑ Serum sodium
↑ Glomerular filtration rate
↓ Serum potassium
↓ Oncotic pressure

* Reverse mechanism causes sodium retention.

perfusion pressure, and nerve activity. The mechanism may be summarized as follows: (*1*) A decreased salt concentration of the fluid that passes special salt-sensing cells in the distal renal tubule stimulates renin release. This proteolytic enzyme is produced and stored in the juxtaglomerular cells of the afferent renal arterioles and converts angiotensinogen to angiotensin I, which in turn is converted by another enzyme into angiotensin II. In addition to being a potent vasoconstrictor, this peptide stimulates the adrenal gland to produce aldosterone (salt retaining hormone). (*2*) A decreased perfusion pressure in the kidney somehow also triggers the release of renin. Thus, stenosis of the aorta or renal artery, hemorrhage, upright position, extracellular fluid loss, and a decrease in cardiac output all serve to trigger renin release. (*3*) Catecholamines and adrenergic nerve activity are the third major stimulus of the renin-angiotensin system.

Causes of Sodium Imbalance

Tolerance of variable intakes is possible because of regulatory mechanisms that match excretion to intake. A deficient intake is thus rarely the cause of hyponatremia. Sodium imbalances are usually due to disorders that affect the regulatory mechanism—mainly, kidney diseases, oliguria due to dehydration, adrenal diseases, or disorders in which either sodium or water is lost in excess. Causes of hyponatremia due to excessive sodium loss are listed in Table 11-4.

Manifestations of Hyponatremia

In contrast to reductions of potassium, calcium, or magnesium, hyponatremia per se has no physiological consequences. The manifestations of hyponatremia are due to intracellular hypoosmolarity, of which it is a sign. They consist of weakness, fatigue, muscle cramps, disorientation, loss of consciousness, and—in rare cases—convulsion and death. Rapid changes in osmolarity carry the greatest risk. (Further discussion of hyponatremia and the correction of the fluid imbalance is beyond the scope of this book.)

Potassium

Source and Requirements

Potassium requirements are similar to those for sodium. They consist of the amount needed for the formation of new tissues and the replacement of losses. Advisable intakes for infants under 3 years of age are in the area of 6–8 mEq/day (31). Based on the concentration in human milk, the Committee on Nutrition recommended twice this amount. The parallel between potassium and sodium also applies to the diet, which is rarely deficient in these two minerals, and to the efficiency of absorption (95%). Potassium content is remarkably constant in all animal and vegetable tissues. Potassium and sodium also share the same renal regulatory mechanisms, although the direction of movement is opposite.

Metabolism and Function

Most of the body's potassium is contained in muscle. It is the major intracellular cation, with a concentration of about 160 mEq/l, compared to less than 5 mEq/l in extracellular fluid. The most important physiological function of potassium is its role as a determinant of intracellular ionic strength and transmembrane potential. The charge across the cell is determined by the ratio between intra- and extracellular potassium, which is about 30 to 1. This ratio is affected most by changes in the smaller extracellular portion, which occur first in most clinical situations of potassium imbalance. Even minor changes in extracellular potassium concentration consequently may have serious effects.

External potassium balance is determined by intake and, to a variable extent, by fecal excretion and losses in sweat, which are minor. Urinary excretion varies greatly, depending on the adequacy and the need for

Table 11-4. Causes of Excessive Sodium Loss

Renal	Salt-losing renal disease
	Bartter's syndrome
	Diuresis, osmotic or drug induced (incl. diabetes mellitus)
	Diuretic phase of acute tubular necrosis
	Relief of acute urinary obstruction
	Metabolic acidosis (incl. diabetic ketoacidosis)
Hormonal	Adrenal insufficiency
Gastrointestinal	Diarrhea
	Vomiting
	Suction
Skin	Excessive sweating (mainly in cystic fibrosis)
	Burns
	Wound drainage

regulatory adjustments. The potassium is filtered through the renal glomerulus and is reabsorbed in the proximal tubule and the loop of Henle. The amount that is finally excreted in the urine is that which is secreted by the distal tubule and the collecting duct.

Causes of Hypopotassemia

Renal disease and conditions associated with increased renin and aldosterone secretion, as well as a variety of other disorders of homeostatic control, can cause excess potassium loss (Table 11-5). In the absence of potassium depletion, hypopotassemia occurs due to shifts from the extra- to the intracellular space. The two major mechanisms that lead to renal potassium loss are (*1*) increased sodium concentration in the distal nephron in the presence of normal aldosterone secretion and (*2*) an increased concentration of poorly reabsorbable anions in the distal nephron.

Manifestations of Hypopotassemia

Intracellular potassium is depleted in most clinical conditions that are associated with hypopotassemia. However, since the decrease is always proportionally greater outside than inside the cell, the 30 to 1 ratio, which determines membrane potential, increases. This increase in membrane

Table 11-5. Causes of Hypopotassemia

Poor potassium intake	
Increased potassium loss	
Gastrointestinal	Vomiting
	Diarrhea, purgative abuse
	Ureterosigmoidoscopy, intestinal fistulas
Renal	Increased renin release
	Hyperaldosteronism, primary or secondary
	Bartter's syndrome
	Diuretis (thiazide, furosemide, ethycrinic acid)
	Magnesium deficiency
	Direct tubular damage
	Increased sodium in distal nephron
	Poorly absorbable anions in distal nephron
	Bicarbonate administration
	Metabolic or respiratory alkalosis
	Diabetic ketoacidosis
	Penicillin, carbenicillin, nafcillin therapy
Skin	Excess sweating
Shift into cells	Acute alkalosis
	Glucose administration
	Bicarbonate administration
	Insulin administration
	Familial periodic paralysis

potential blocks impulse transmission and causes general muscle weakness—usually when serum potassium is in the range of 2.5 mEq/l. More profound hypopotassemia causes paralysis, which may include respiratory muscles. Intracellular acidosis is due to replacement of potassium with hydrogen, which causes paresthesia, pain, cramps, tenderness, and muscle swelling. Muscle necrosis and associated myoglobinuria also occur. The effects on heart muscle are most severe when hypopotassemia develops rapidly. Abnormalities in rhythm develop, which are due to supraventricular or ventricular ectopic beats, tachycardia, and atrioventricular conduction disturbances. The ECG shows depression of the ST segment, flattening and inversion of the T wave, and appearance of a U wave. Death due to ventricular fibrillation may result.

Chronic potassium depletion causes cardiomegaly and congestive heart failure. Involvement of intestinal smooth muscle is responsible for abdominal distention, cramps, and finally paralytic ileus. Patients complain of anorexia, nausea, and vomiting. In the kidney, potassium deficiency leads to vascular changes of the tubular epithelium, and to inability to concentrate, amino aciduria, phosphaturia, and mild proteinuria.

Calcium

Source and Requirements

The RDA for calcium is 360 mg/day in the first half-year of life, which is the amount contained in 1 l of human milk. For the second half-year of life, 540 mg/day is recommended, and 800 mg/day thereafter, except during the pubertal growth period, when it is 1,200 mg/day. RDA values provide a ratio of 1.5 for calcium to phosphorus during the first year of life. The recommendation thus stands in contrast to the belief that the ratio of calcium to phosphorus in human milk (>2.0) is particularly effective. The recommendation is supported by data of Widdowson et al. (33), who showed that the addition of phosphorus to the diet of breast-fed infants enhances absorption of calcium and magnesium. Recommended values for calcium intake by young infants are based on (*1*) the increment of total body calcium during growth, (*2*) a value of about 45% for absorption, and (*3*) an extra 20% to cover circumstances when calcium is less well absorbed. Major sources of calcium in the American diet, aside from milk, are vegetables, fish, and certain fruits. The following items are especially high in calcium content: salmon; shellfish; beans; cabbage; celery; sweet potatoes; spinach; beets; broccoli; chard; collard, dandelion, mustard, and turnip greens; kale; artichokes; figs; dates; and raisins.

Metabolism and Function

About 99% of the body's calcium is contained in the skeleton. The 1% that is contained in intra- and extracellular fluid and plasma is readily exchangable with bone calcium, which serves as a reservoir for the maintenance of calcium homeostasis. The need for a sensitive and efficient control mechanism is reflected by the many vital functions of calcium, which include the release of neurochemical transmitters at synaptic junctions, synthesis and action of hormone and enzymes, muscle contractility, blood coagulation, and the integrity of intercellular cement substances. Total intracellular calcium amounts to about 4 mg/dl, of which 10% is ionized. Calcium in extracellular fluid is 10 mg/dl, and 47% is ionized, while the remainder is complexed—mainly to protein and some to phosphates and citrate. The ratio between total and ionized calcium is influenced by pH and the protein concentration of plasma. Alkalosis decreases the ionization of calcium and its release from bone. In the presence of hypoproteinemia, total calcium may be low although ionized calcium is adequate. Only the ionized fraction is physiologically active, and its concentration is tightly controlled by the complex interrelated action of vitamin D (Chapter 10), parathyroid hormone (PTH), and calcitonin.

PTH acts to raise serum calcium by increasing bone resorption and, to a minor degree, renal tubular reabsorption. Hypocalcemia is the primary stimulus for the secretion of PTH. The hormone functions principally by stimulating renal hydroxylase to activate vitamin D. In the kidney, PTH increases the renal clearance of inorganic phosphorus, sodium, potassium, and bicarbonate, and it decreases the clearance of magnesium in addition to that of calcium. The clinical role of calcitonin is poorly understood because measurement has been difficult to date. This hormone is produced mainly by the parafollicular cells of the thyroid gland. Secretion is stimulated by hypercalcemia and inhibited by hypocalcemia. Excluding its action in the kidney, calcitonin opposes PTH and vitamin D. It decreases bone resorption and intestinal absorption of calcium, phosphorus, and magnesium (34).

Renal excretion of calcium is influenced by serum levels. It amounts to no more than about 200 mg/day. Total loss in bile and pancreatic juices is slightly less, and dermal losses average 20 mg/day. High-protein diets increase urinary calcium excretion (35). Excess renal losses do not cause hypocalcemia, and vice versa: renal failure does not lead to hypercalcemia. By contrast, intestinal calcium loss in the presence of dietary deprivation is a major cause of negative calcium balance. Adjustments following a sudden reduction in intake are slow and cause temporarily a negative balance. Intestinal calcium absorption is inhibited by calcitonin and glucocorticoids. Dietary factors that cause fecal calcium losses are unabsorbed fats; the fiber, oxalate, and phytate content of certain foods; and—most of all—vitamin D deficiency. Calcium may be lost in feces due to intestinal calcium secretion even when there is no calcium intake.

Causes of Calcium Imbalance

The only significant nutritional causes of imbalance are vitamin D deficiency (Chapter 10) or excess (Chapter 12) and phosphorus excess. Deficient calcium intake during pregnancy may be a factor in neonatal rickets. The rarity of nutritional calcium deficiency is attributable to the large calcium pool in the skeleton and the ability of calcium homeostatic mechanisms to adapt to and compensate for low intakes. Consequently, disorders of these homeostatic mechanisms are the major causes of hypocalcemia (Table 11-6). Levels below 7.0 mg/dl are diagnostic of hypocalcemia.

Neonatal Hypocalcemia

Special circumstances exist during the newborn period that predispose to hypocalcemia. Early neonatal hypocalcemia develops in premature and

Table 11-6. Causes of Hypocalcemia

- *Neonatal*
  - *Early*
    - Prematurity
    - Respiratory distress
    - Complicated delivery
    - Toxemia of pregnancy
    - Diabetic mother
    - Cerebral birth injury
    - Neonatal jaundice
  - *Late*
    - Phosphorus excess (cow's milk)
    - Maternal hyperparathyroidism
    - Maternal vitamin D excess
    - Congenital absence of parathyroid with (Di George syndrome) or without thymus aplasia
    - Congenital Hypocalcemia with cortical thickening of tubular bones (McKusick 12700)
- *Any time*
  - Vitamin D deficiency (Chapter 11)
  - Vitamin D dependency (autosomal dominant)
  - Hyperphosphatemia
    - Increased intake
    - Renal failure
    - Hypoparathyroidism
  - Hypoparathyroidism, primary
  - Autoimmune (polyglandular) disease
  - Pseudohypoparathyroidism
  - Magnesium deficiency
  - Acute pancreatitis
  - Massive transfusion of citrated blood
  - Calcitonin excess
    - Post-thyroidectomy
    - Thyroid cancer
    - Glucagon excess
  - Surgical parathyroidectomy

stressed infants, including infants with respiratory distress syndrome, infants born after a complicated delivery or to diabetic or toxemic mothers, and infants with cerebral birth injury or neonatal jaundice. Late neonatal hypocalcemia develops toward the end of the first or during the second week of life. The high phosphorus content of cow's milk and transient hypoparathyroidism seem to be responsible, but other factors may play an etiologic role. Dietary phosphorus excess rarely causes hypocalcemia in adults, excluding extreme cases of phosphorus ingestion due to laxative abuse. Newborns, on the other hand, are unable to meet the increased need for phosphorus excretion imposed by undiluted cow's milk. A diminished renal response to PTH during the first 48 hours compared to the third day has been reported (36,37). However, an increase in serum phosphorus following hormone administration indicated that phosphorus could be mobilized. Since these earlier studies, PTH has been measured in normal, in sick, and in hypocalcemic newborns (38), and it has been shown that PTH is low to undetectable during the first 48 hours when serum calcium shows a progressive fall. After 48 hours there was a parallel increase in serum calcium and PTH. In hypocalcemic infants with levels below 7.5 and 4 mg/dl for total and ionized calcium, no rise in PTH was observed. Transient hypoparathyroidism thus may explain the low phosphorus clearance during the first 48 hours, but since calcium values were not consistently correlated with PTH levels, other factors appear to play an additional role, especially in sick neonates. Whether excess calcitonin is a factor in some cases remains to be determined.

Manifestations

Clinical symptoms of neonatal hypocalcemia are those of tetany: irritability, tremors, twitching, convulsions, laryngospasm, and carpopedal spasm. Convulsions may be generalized or unilateral. They develop when ionized calcium falls below 4 mg/dl, which usually corresponds to a total calcium level below 7 mg/dl. To distinguish the disorder from benign tremors signs of latent tetany should be checked: (*1*) production of carpopedal spasms by causing ischemia of motor nerves with a tourniquet, (*2*) contraction of the eye and/or upper lip through tapping of the facial nerve anterior to the external ear canal, and (*3*) ECG changes that consist of a prolonged Q-T interval.

Treatment

The specific diagnosis determines the treatment. In neonatal hypocalcemia prompt correction is required, using 10% calcium gluconate (2ml/kg) given slowly by intravenous route, while the pulse is monitored for bradycardia. Oral calcium, which precipitates phosphate in the gut, should be added. Hypomagnesemia, which occasionally accompanies neonatal hypocalcemia, requires no treatment unless it is severe, in which case 25% magnesium sulfate may be given, 0.2 ml/kg. Persistence of hypocalcemia beyond the third week should suggest other causes (Table 11-6). Until a firm diagnosis is established in such cases, oral calcium in combination with vitamin D in doses of 10,000 IU/day or more may be used, followed by specific treatment, as indicated by the diagnosis.

Phosphorus

Source and Requirements

Phosphorus is widely present in the diet, and—in the absence of starvation—nutritional deficiency is almost never a cause of body depletion. The RDA for children over 1 year of age is equal to that for calcium, i.e., 800 mg/day, and 1,200 mg during puberty. RDA values for infants under 1 year of age add up to a calcium/phosphorus ratio of 1.5, which is similar to that of cow's milk but substantially less than that of human milk. Requirements for the two minerals are interdependent, but the ideal proportion in the diet for efficient absorption and utilization remains uncertain.

Metabolism and Function

Phosphorus functions as a structural element of bone and cell walls, as part of ATP in oxygen delivery, and as an anion in carbohydrate, lipid, and nucleic acid metabolism. About 85% of total body phosphorus is found in bone. As one of the major intracellular anions, it is part of organic compounds. Serum concentrations in adults are usually less than 4 mg/dl, while the values of infants on cow's milk are between 7.0 and 7.5 mg/dl and of breast-fed infants, between 6 and 7 mg/dl. The concentration is not as tightly controlled as that of calcium and often varies in the course of a day by up to 2 mg/dl. About 12% of serum phosphorus is protein bound, and the remainder is ionized or complexed to diffusable cations, such as sodium, calcium, and magnesium. Acute changes occur as a result of shifts between the intra- and extracellular space and during glycolysis, which causes a decrease of extracellular phosphorus. Exchange between extracellular space and bone occurs as part of calcium homeostasis, phosphorus and calcium moving in parallel to and from bone.

Phosphorus absorption, which is stimulated by vitamin D (39), varies between 50 and 90%, depending on intake. Low dietary phosphorus concentrations are associated with a higher value for percentage absorption. Phosphate binding in the intestines by calcium and antacids decreases absorption.

Urinary excretion of phosphorus is mainly determined by PTH. High serum concentrations of phosphorus cause PTH release, indirectly, by lowering serum calcium concentration through the deposition of calcium in bone as hydroxyapatite. Hypocalcemia is the principle stimulus for PTH release. PTH and calcitonin inhibit, and vitamin D and growth hormone enhance, tubular phosphorus reabsorption. Phosphorus reabsorption in the proximal tubule is linked with sodium reabsorption. Inhibition of sodium reabsorption consequently also leads to phosphaturia. Factors that inhibit sodium reabsorption and thus cause phosphaturia are metabolic acidosis, potassium depletion, and use of diuretics, such as thiazide, acetazolamide, and furosemide (40).

Magnesium

Source and Requirements

Magnesium is derived in the American diet mainly from foods with a relatively low magnesium content (i.e., dairy products, meats, and vegetables). Foods with a high magnesium content are corn, whole-grain wheat and barley, nuts, dry beans, peas, and spinach.

Metabolism and Function

Magnesium is a structural element of bone, which contains about 60% of total body magnesium. It affects neuromuscular function and is a cofactor of many enzymes. Total body content is roughly 0.05% or 35 g in the average adult. Next to potassium, it is the second most abundant intracellular cation, with a concentration of 30 to 40 mEq/l. Normal plasma concentration ranges between 1.4 and 2.0 mEq/l. Normally, 55% of the total is ionized, and the remainder is bound to protein. Changes in plasma proteins consequently have a corresponding effect on renal magnesium values.

Plasma concentration is affected by intestinal absorption, renal excretion, and exchange with bone, but there is no regulatory mechanism with physiologic significance. Yet many of the movements of magnesium are similar to those of calcium, except for muscle magnesium, which follows the movement of potassium. Thus, PTH decreases urinary magnesium excretion. Acute hypomagnesemia is associated with increased PTH activity, but PTH secretion is low in chronic magnesium deficiency (41,42). Low serum magnesium values are usually paralleled by low calcium values, even in cases of primary hypocalcemia. The presence of a regulatory mechanism aimed at the protection of body stores is indicated by observations in malnourished infants who had a reduced muscle content of magnesium. Although their blood levels were normal, urinary excretion was extremely low (43), and after a parenteral loading dose, these infants retained significantly larger amounts than normal infants (44).

Absorption occurs mainly in the ileum, but magnesium can be absorbed from the colon, as evidenced by the effectiveness of magnesium sulfate given by enema. The efficiency of absorption, which usually ranges between 30 and 40% of intake, varies inversely with the amount ingested. Absorption is enhanced by acidity and dietary lactose and decreased by oxalic and phytic acid. Vitamin D or high calcium intakes also reduce absorption, apparently by competing with magnesium at their common transport site. Renal excretion is a function of blood concentration and may vary from one to several hundred milliequivalents per day during magnesium loading. PTH decreases urinary magnesium concentration, while calcitonin and diuretics increase it.

Causes of Hypomagnesemia

On the American diet, hypomagnesemia could occur through a combination of factors: a diet consisting mainly of certain vegetables, highly milled grains, and milk products, which all have a low magnesium content; and coexistent factors that impede absorption, such as alcohol consumption or a high vitamin D or calcium intake. In neonates, hypomagnesemia occurs in the absence of any identifiable cause. Maternal hyperparathyroidism or hypophosphatemia is responsible in some cases, presumably because it leads to transient hypoparathyroidism in the infant and increased urinary losses, decreased intestinal absorption, and decreased release of magnesium from bone. Low plasma magnesium levels are also seen in familial hypoparathyroidism. Neonatal hypomagnesemia has been linked with other diseases in the mother, including diabetes mellitus, malabsorption, and disorders causing intrauterine growth failure. Older infants and children may develop hypomagnesemia as a consequence of malabsorption or after extensive intestinal surgery.

Manifestations

Body depletion of magnesium is accompanied by hypocalcemia and hypopotassemia. Clinical manifestations simulate those of hypocalcemia. Neuromuscular signs may, in fact, be due to the accompanying hypocalcemia. Anorexia, nausea, lethargy, and psychological changes, on the other hand, may be a direct result of magnesium deficiency.

Newborns frequently have a transient depression of magnesium levels that accompanies both the early and late forms of neonatal hypocalcemia, with levels ranging between 0.8 and 1.4 mEq/l. Magnesium levels rise in most neonates with hypomagnesemia spontaneously after calcium therapy (45). In primary hypomagnesemia, plasma levels are lower, 0.2 to 0.8 mEq/l, and response to calcium therapy is poor. Treatment with magnesium corrects any coexistent hypocalcemia (46). Primary hypomagnesemia is probably due to a genetic defect of intestinal magnesium transport. Patients have severe manifestations—twitching, eye rolling, convulsions, cardiac arrhythmias, and bony abnormalities.

Treatment

In neonatal hypomagnesemia with hypocalcemia, treatment with calcium should be tried first. If there is no response, intramuscular injections of 25% magnesium sulfate, 0.2 mEq/kg (0.1 ml/kg), are given every 6 hours for three to four doses.

REFERENCES

1. Schulz J, Smith NJ: A quantitative study of the absorption of food iron in infants and children. *Am J Dis Child* 95:109, 1958.
2. FAO/WHO: *Requirements of Ascorbic Acid, Vitamin D, Vitamin B_{12}, Folate and Iron,* Technical Report Series, No 452. Geneva: WHO, 1970.
3. Committee on Nutrition: Iron supplementation for infants. *Pediatrics* 58:765, 1976.
4. Evans GW, Johnson PE: Characterization and quantitation of a zinc-binding ligand in human milk. *Pediatr Res* 14:876, 1980.
5. Krieger I, Evans GW: Acrodermatitis-enteropathica without hypozincemia: Therapeutic effect of a pancreatic-enzyme preparation due to a zinc-binding ligand. *J Pediatr* 96:32, 1980.
6. Schlage C, Wortberg B: Zinc in the diet of healthy pre-school and school children. *Acta Paediatr Scand* 61:421, 1972.
7. Hambidge KM, Hambidge C, Jacobs M, et al: Low levels of zinc in hair, anorexia, poor growth and hypogeusia in children. *Pediatr Res* 6:868, 1972.
8. Prasad AS, Holsted JA, Nadimi M: Syndrome of iron deficiency, hepatosplenomegaly, hypogonadism, dwarfism and geophagia. *Am J Med* 31:532, 1961.
9. Moynahan EY: A lethal inherited human zinc deficiency disorder. *Lancet* 2:399, 1970.
10. Golden MHN, Golden BE, Harland PSEG, et al: Zinc and immunocompetence in protein energy malnutrition. *Lancet* 1:1226, 1972.
11. Hambidge KM, Neldner KH, Walravens PA: Zinc, acrodermatitis enteropathica, and congenital malformation. *Lancet* 1:577, 1975.
12. Brewer JH, Brewer LF, Prasad AS: Suppression of irreversibly sickled erythrocytes by zinc therapy in sickle cell anemia. *J Lab Clin Med* 90:549, 1977.
13. Garrets M, Molakhia M: Acrodermatitis without hypozincemia. *Pediatrics* 91:492, 1977.
14. Widdowson EM, Dauncey J, Shaw JCL: Trace elements in fetal and early postnatal development. *Proc Nutr Soc* 33:275, 1974.
15. Hambidge KM: Increase in hair copper concentration with increasing distance from scalp. *Am J Clin Nutr* 26:1212, 1973.
16. Menkes JH, Alter M, Steigleger GK, et al: A sex-linked recessive disorder with retardation of growth, peculiar hair and local cerebral and cerebellar degeneration. *Pediatrics* 29:764, 1962.
17. Danks DM, Stevens BJ, Campbell PE, et al: Menkes' kinky hair syndrome. *Lancet* 1:1100, 1972.
18. Graham GG, Cordano A: Copper depletion and deficiency in the malnourished infant. *Johns Hopkins Med J* 124:139, 1969.
19. Al-Rashid RA, Spongler J: Neonatal copper deficiency. *N Engl J Med* 285:841, 1971.
20. Karpel JT, Peden VH: Copper deficiency in long-term parenteral nutrition. *J Pediatr* 80:32, 1972.
21. Williams DM, Atkins CL, Frens DB, et al: Menkes' kinky hair syndrome: Studies of copper metabolism and long-term copper therapy. *Pediatr Res* 11:823, 1977.
22. Malvaux P, Beckers C, Devisscher M: Iodine balance studies in non-goitrous children and in adolescents on low iodine intake. *J Clin Endocrinol Metab* 29:79, 1969.
23. Committee on Nutrition American Academy of Pediatrics: Fluoride as nutrient. *Pediatrics* 49:456, 1972.
24. Dean HT: Endemic fluorosis and its relation to dental caries. *Int Dent J* 4:311, 1954.
25. Council on Dental Therapeutics: Prescribing fluoride supplements, in *Accepted Dental Therapeutics.* Chicago, Amer Dental Assoc, 1977, p 293.

26. Hambidge KM, Rodgerson DO, O'Brien D: Concentration of chromium in hair of normal children and children with juvenile diabetes mellitus. *Diabetes* 17:517, 1968.
27. Offenbacher EG, Pi-Sunyer F: Beneficial effect of chromium-rich yeast on glucose tolerance and blood lipids in elderly subjects. *Diabetes* 29:919, 1980.
28. Hopkins LL, Jr, Ransome-Kuti O, Majaj AS: Improvement of impaired carbohydrate metabolism by chromium in malnourished infants. *Am J Clin Nutr* 21:203, 1968.
29. Keshan's Disease Research Group of the Chinese Academy of Medical Sciences, Beijing: Observations on the effect of sodium selenite in prevention of Keshan's disease. *Chin Med J* 92:471, 1979.
30. Doisy A: Micronutrient control of biosynthesis of clotting proteins and cholesterol, in Hemphill DD (ed): *Trace Substances in Environmental Health, VI.* Columbus, Mo, Univ Press, p 193.
31. Ziegler EE, Fomon SJ: Major minerals, in Fomon SJ (ed): *Infant Nutrition.* Philadelphia, WB Saunders Co, 1974, p 268.
32. Filer L: Salt in infant foods. *Nutr Rev* 29:27, 1971.
33. Widdowson EM, McCance RA, Harrison GE, et al: Effect of giving phosphate supplements to breast-fed babies on absorption and excretion of calcium, strontium, magnesium and phosphorus. *Lancet* 2:1250, 1963.
34. Haas HG, Bambacher MA, Guncaga J, et al: Renal effects of calcitonin and parathyroid extract in man: Studies in hypoparathyroidism. *J Clin Invest* 50:2689, 1971.
35. Margen S, Kaufman NA, Costa F, et al: Studies in the mechanism of calciuria induced by protein feeding. *Fed Proc* 29:566, 1976.
36. Tsang RC, Light IJ, Sutherland JM, et al: Possible pathogenetic factors in neonatal hypocalcemia of prematurity. *J Pediatr* 82:423, 1973.
37. Linarelli LG, John B, Caroline B: Newborn urinary cyclic AMP and developmental renal responsiveness to parathyroid hormone. *Pediatrics* 50:14, 1972.
38. David L, Anast CS: Calcium metabolism in newborn infants: The interrelationship of parathyroid function and calcium, magnesium and phosphorus metabolism in normal, "sick", and hypocalcemic newborns. *J Clin Invest* 54:287, 1974.
39. Ahmed KY, Varghese Z, Wills MR, et al: Persistent hypophosphatemia and osteomalacia in dialysis patients not on oral phosphate-binders: Response to dihydrotachysterol therapy. *Lancet* 2:439, 1976.
40. Barzel US: Parathyroid hormone, blood phosphorus and acid base metabolism. *Lancet* 1:1329, 1971.
41. Anast CS, Mohs JM, Kaplan SL, et al: Evidence for parathyroid failure in magnesium deficiency. *Science* 177:606, 1972.
42. Suh SM, Tashjian AH Jr, Matsuo N, et al: Pathogenesis of hypocalcemia in primary hypomagnesemia: Normal end-organ responsiveness to parathyroid hormone, impaired parathyroid gland function. *J Clin Invest* 52:153, 1973.
43. Garrow JS, Smith R, Ward EE: *Electrolyte Metabolism in Severe Infantile Malnutrition.* Oxford, Pergamon Press, 1968.
44. Caddell JL, Suskind R, Sillup H, et al: II. Parenteral magnesium load evaluation of malnourished Thai children. *J Pediatr* 83:129, 1973.
45. Friedman M, Hatcher G, Watson L: Primary hypomagnesemia with secondary hypocalcemia in an infant. *Lancet* 1:703, 1967.
46. Zimmet P, Breidahl HD, Nayler WG: Plasma ionized calcium in hypomagnesemia. *Br Med J* 1:622, 1968.

12 Disorders of Nutrient Excess

OBESITY
Etiology
Diet, Eating Patterns, and Energy Balance
Activity
Psychological and Cultural Factors
Diagnosis and Differential Diagnosis
Endocrine and Metabolic Consequences
Adverse Effects on Health and Longevity
Treatment
Dietary Management
Exercise
Behavior Modification
Surgical Therapy
Drug Therapy

SPECIFIC NUTRIENT EXCESS
Vitamins
Vitamin B Group
Hypervitaminosis A
Hypervitaminosis D
Vitamin C
Vitamin K
Trace metals
Iron (incl. hemochromatosis)
Zinc
Copper (incl. Wilson's disease)
Iodine (incl. iodide goitre and iodinism)
Fluoride (incl. fluorosis)
Other Select Trace Minerals
Major minerals
Sodium (incl. Relation of chronic high salt intake to disease)
Potassium
Calcium
Phosphorus
Magnesium

OBESITY

Obesity is defined as an excessive accumulation of adipose tissue that contains fat in the form of triglycerides. During this century it has become a chronic health problem in the United States and other industrialized societies, with a rapidly increasing incidence among children and adults (1). Onset is often before puberty, and estimates show that as many as 80% of obese children may remain obese (2). Whether the degree of weight gain during infancy is predictive of adult weight remains controversial, but there is no question that extreme infantile obesity tends to persist. Surveys of obese adults show that 20 to 40% were obese adolescents.

Etiology

Obesity is always due to an imbalance between food intake and energy expenditure, although the food requirements may be abnormally low in persons with a tendency to obesity. Whether such a "tendency" exists and whether it is genetic or acquired in early infancy, rather than psychological, remains controversial. Exogenous obesity, which is the most common form, is attributable to a combination of hyperphagia and hypomotility that are frequently conditioned by cultural or psychological factors. Endocrine and genetic causes are rare. Most of the hormone and metabolic abnormalities observed in obese patients appear to be a consequence rather than a cause of obesity.

Diet, Eating Patterns, and Energy Balance
Most studies, whether psychologically or physiologically oriented, indicate that the eating habits of obese individuals are not normal. Even observations suggestive of a prenatal onset of obesity can be explained by overeating rather than genetic factors. In these cases, mothers overeat during pregnancy and probably overfeed the infant, because a correlation between infant weight and weight gain during pregnancy exists. Reactive overeating explains the obesity that commonly follows feeding problems or deprivation in infancy, although secondary physiologic changes, conditioned by starvation, are a possibility in these cases. An exogenous cause of infantile obesity is suggested by the observation that breast feeding rarely leads to obesity, because it is physically difficult to overfeed an infant on the breast.

Irregular patterns of eating, which are characteristic of many obese individuals, promote fat accumulation both because an excess of total calories is usually consumed and because eating after a fast augments lipogenesis and enhances the ability to assimilate food efficiently. Evidence in support of this mechanism has been reported in several studies of humans (3) and experimental animals. Thus, rats trained to eat their entire daily ration in one meal convert ingested carbohydrates into fat, as evidenced by a respiratory quotient above 1. Adult men gain more weight on equal amounts of calories and have higher plasma cholesterol levels when they eat two meals rather than multiple small meals evenly spaced throughout the day. The habit of professionals and schoolchildren to eat only one meal at the end of the day, followed by snacking throughout the evening, therefore presents a disadvantage. Another undesirable eating habit is a preference for sweets, characteristic of many obese people who eat for oral gratification rather than to satisfy hunger. This choice promotes obesity because carbohydrates stimulate appetite more than fat or protein-rich foods, presumably because of reactive hypoglycemia.

Several studies have shown that the eating behavior of obese individuals tends to be stimulus-bound. Thus, they are more influenced by the taste, smell, and sight of food than normal individuals (5). The effect of taste was tested in one study through the use of quinine added to milkshakes. Obese individuals drank less than normal-weight persons when the drinks tasted bitter (6). A variety of other studies have shown that normal-weight individuals have a relatively steady intake, presumably determined by need, whereas obese persons respond to such cues as food availability (7), time of day for eating, and the example of others' eating. It is not known whether the lack of adequate hunger control is psychological or due to metabolic or neurological abnormality. In either case, many obese people apparently do not have the mechanism that operates like an automatic "hunger-stat" and prevents obesity in the fortunate ones who thus do not need to be "weight watchers."

Psychological conflict does not explain all forms of obesity. An example are very young infants with morbid obesity who allow themselves to be overfed, while most infants resist forced feeding. Calculation of what it takes to become obese also suggests that in some cases, especially children, other factors may be involved. If a toddler were to take 4 saltine crackers, or 50 kcal in excess of requirements throughout childhood, and if the excess were converted into fat, he would be extremely obese after only 10 years, weighing 50 lbs more than normal. Similar calculations have led to the concept of a "hunger-stat," which would explain the ability of most healthy people to maintain such a delicate energy balance. Many studies from earlier decades have attempted to explain the tolerance of "luxus consumption" by measuring energy balance. Some observations indeed suggest differences between individuals that allow some to eat more than others without getting fat because they seem able to adjust by increasing oxygen consumption (8). The explanation is not likely to be found in measurement of the basal metabolic rate (BMR) because of difficulties in interpretation. Absolute BMR values are increased, but the BMR per unit of body weight is lower in obese than in normal individuals because tissues with a low metabolic rate make a comparatively greater contribution to total weight. One approach to the question has been the measurement of postprandial heat production, which indeed was found to be lower in obese than in nonobese women (9). This observation may be attributable to differences in the use of meal calories, because the investigators found high plasma triglycerides, a faster and more sustained elevation of plasma amino acids, an increased BUN, and higher insulin levels in the obese women who had a low "specific dynamic action" following a test meal.

Observations in infants recovering from malnutrition indicate that postprandial heat production is, to a large extent, due to the assimilation of amino acids for growth, probably less for transamination than for protein synthesis (10). Assuming that this mechanism is operative in normal and obese individuals, which is likely, one may anticipate postprandial heat production to be different in obese individuals because lipogenesis predominates. The low "specific dynamic action" is therefore most likely a secondary event rather than the cause of obesity. However, the finding of a lower postprandial heat production and explanation of its mechanism have therapeutic implications, because high-protein foods are often advised for weight reduction in hopes that protein calories are inefficiently used, thus allowing a greater total calorie intake. Actual observation of postprandial heat production in obese subjects argues against the usefulness of this approach (9). Deamination of ingested amino acids for use as fuel and the associated increase of nitrogen excretion are not positively correlated with a corresponding increase in postprandial excess heat (10).

Failure to demonstrate convincingly in many cases a psychological cause for overeating has resulted in numerous other studies and theories that attempt to explain why some individuals have difficulty maintaining the delicate balance between energy intake and output. These investigations led to the recognition of a satiety center in the ventromedial hypothalamus and a hunger center in the lateral hypothalamus. It has been postulated that stimulation occurs directly by way of the blood stream when the concentration of sugar or some hypothetical metabolite changes. Peripheral sensors in the intestines, which signal gastric distention or other changes, also may play a role. However, there is little evidence to date that either mechanism plays a role in exogenous obesity. Other theories, which attempt to explain the regulation of body weight and offer reasons for abnormality, are the "pull and push theory" of Van Itallie (11), the glucostatic theory of Mayer (12), the thermostatic theory of Brobeck (13), and the lipostatic theory of Kennedy (14).

Recently, the fat cell theory has attracted considerable attention (15). The original studies in rats seemed to show that excess food intake before weaning increases the number of adipocytes in the body, whereas the fat deposition that follows overfeeding at a later stage causes an increase in the size of adipocytes. This led to a classification of obesity into a hyperplastic type and a hypertrophic type. An intriguing aspect of this theory was the proposal that early overfeeding would program the individual for life because the number of fat cells developed during the hyperplastic phase remains constant thereafter. If the degree of fat cell filling with triglycerides were the sensor that signals hunger or satiety, it would explain the difficulty certain individuals have in maintaining normal weight, because a larger number of cells have to be kept at a critical degree of "filling." In view of technical difficulties in counting fat cell number, this theory has been questioned. The most convincing data (16) came from the study of human fetuses by a method that allows recognition of much smaller cells than were hitherto detectable. Very small cells that did not contain fat were found in tissues before birth and in the first months of life. They appear to be the precursors of the mature fat-containing adipocytes that were recognized by earlier workers.

Activity

The calorie intake of most obese persons is excessive relative to the individual's energy output. Obesity in the physically handicapped is a typical example of energy imbalance due to inactivity. The importance of this factor as a cause of obesity has been measured by a variety of techniques, including the use of pedometers and film recordings. Thus, it could be shown that obese individuals walk only about half as much as normal-weight persons (17) and that obese children in a summer camp spent more time floating than actively swimming (18). Hypoactivity may contribute originally to the development of obesity, which in turn is a factor that further decreases activity, thus adding to the positive energy balance. Since obesity itself decreases mobility and causes inactivity through social isolation, a vicious cycle develops.

Psychological and Cultural Factors

The importance of relative hyperphagia as a cause of obesity has never been questioned. However, the causes and mechanisms responsible for hyperphagia are not clear. Only this knowledge can provide a rational basis for treatment.

Psychological problems may be the reason that obese individuals follow cues other than hunger. The term *situational obesity* has been coined to describe obesity that develops as a reaction to specific situational stress, such as when a person stops smoking or faces other types of frustration. Eating binges are stress related. Neurotics may eat to punish themselves or people close to them. Boredom or feelings of isolation also cause overeating, especially at night, on weekends, and holidays. Juvenile obesity is commonly due to difficulties with interpersonal relationships, school adjustment, or frustrated career goals. Lack of motivation to reduce and maintain a good figure may be related to the fact that the adolescent does not feel good about himself or herself. Thus, the obese adolescent is often dressed sloppily and pays little attention to grooming. An impaired self-image probably antedates the obesity in most cases, but feelings of inferiority do increase with increasing fatness because society discriminates against the obese and pushes them into social isolation. Psychological factors should be explored early in the development of obesity by the pediatrician who may be dealing with a youngster who was pushed into abnormal eating habits by parental attitudes that can be corrected by early intervention.

Significant obesity in infants probably originates very early after birth, at a time when the infant is unable to reject feeding due to immaturity. Why infants fail to recognize satiety and do not react appropriately after neuromuscular function has matured sufficiently to allow food rejection is difficult to explain. Whereas acceptance of excess food by infant is not likely psychogenic, the parental behavior that leads to overfeeding is usually psychological in origin. The misconception that a chubby baby is healthy probably plays a minor role. Inability to interpret the infant's cry correctly is also an insufficient explanation. The problem thus appears to be more complex. Parents may use feeding as an affirmation of their love. Thus, obesity not infrequently follows a life-threatening illness during infancy. Parents may feel guilty for wanting to hit a crying infant or for not feeling the romanticized emotions toward their newborn that they anticipated. Guilt also may be related to a failure to breast feed successfully. Unable to communicate their feelings, parents who do not realize that these are common emotions tend to overcompensate and may use food as an expression of their desire to do well by the infant.

The psychodynamics of adult onset obesity in many instances are different because cultural and socioeconomic factors play an increasingly greater role. Situational obesity is also common, such as after the loss of a spouse or the departure of grown children or as a reaction to growing older. What appears to be a racial difference may, on closer examination, turn out to be psychosocial or cultural. For instance, black boys and men are not as heavy as their white counterparts (19), but a reversal of this seemingly racial difference takes place after puberty in females. In modern Western culture, success is identified with bigness, and a portly figure is no handicap for men, whereas riches and glamour are associated with slender women's figures. By contrast, in certain ethnic groups, fatness in the mature woman fits the image of motherhood and propriety. Obesity also develops throughout life because of shared attitudes toward food and exercise among family members; husbands are as fat as their wives, and parents are like their adoptive children; even the family dog may look like its master. These are important considerations for the pediatrician, who should not look at the child without considering the family unit.

Diagnosis and Differential

Various criteria have been suggested for the diagnosis of obesity. According to the Ten-State Nutrition Survey (20), "skinfold measurements appear to be the best single, simple and practical determination of adiposity."

They are of proven value because they reflect the amount of subcutaneous fat, which in turn is correlated with the fat in body cavities (21). Normal standards are available for all age groups (Chapter 3). Any one scoring at the 90th percentile or above should be considered obese. Out of convenience, when such tables are not at hand, physicians frequently use body weight, although this measure does not discriminate between fat and muscle weight. A body weight 20% or more in excess of the normal weight for height and sex or above the 90th percentile for height-age and sex is probably equivalent to obesity. However, visual appraisal by an experienced observer is more reliable than weight standards, which do not distinguish between the muscularity of a college athlete and an obese person.

The diagnosis of exogenous obesity requires exclusion of endocrine and genetic causes. Complications of obesity (Table 12-1) also should be sought. Thus the determination of plasma triglycerides and cholesterol is indicated. A glucose tolerance test should be done if there is a family history of diabetes mellitus or findings suggestive of Prader–Willie syndrome. Height and bone age are normal or increased in exogenous obesity and distinguish this entity from obesity due to hypothyroidism. The diagnosis of hypothyroidism should pose no problem, because the clinical manifestations are characteristic of hypometabolism. Serum thyroxine determinations are often done to dispel the patient's belief that the problem is "glandular" and to motivate him or her to dietary control. Serum thyroxine is normal in exogenous obesity.

The generalized nature of exogenous obesity is similar to that in Cushing's syndrome, but the flushed moon facies and characteristic buffalo hump distinguish that syndrome. Moreover, hypercortisolism causes gradual deceleration of linear growth. Plasma cortisol and urinary corticosteroid determinations and a dexamethasone suppression test may be necessary to rule out Cushing's syndrome. In exogenous obesity, the plasma cortisol level is normal, the urinary corticosteroid level tends to be elevated, and the hypothalamic–pituitary axis suppresses appropriately with dexamethasone.

A number of genetic disorders that are associated with obesity should be ruled out. They are recognized by a characteristic combination of structural and/or endocrine abnormalities (Table 12-2). Only one of these, Prader-Willie syndrome, is associated with obesity due to hyperphagia and may present a diagnostic problem early in the development of obesity because of the absence of characteristic dysmorphic stigmata.

The syndrome consists of hypotonia, hypomentia, hypogonadism, and obesity (HHHO). The majority of cases are sporadic, but a genetic component seems to be present. A hypothalamic dysfunction has been assumed. The clinical course can be divided into two phases. The first is characterized by severe hypotonia, which is in some cases manifested in utero by decreased fetal movements. A flat face and triangular mouth may be evidence of facial diplegia. Young infants are almost motionless,

Table 12-1. Disorders Caused or Exacerbated by Obesity

Cardiovascular System
Angina pectoris
Early coronary heart disease
Sudden death
Left ventricular hypertrophy
Hypertension
Stroke
Venous stasis and thromboembolic disease
Respiratory System
Alveolar hypoventilation (Pickwickian syndrome)
Obstructive sleep apnea
Hepatobiliary System
Cholelithiasis
Fatty liver
Metabolic and Endocrine System
Hyperlipidemia
Gout
Diabetes
Irregular menstruation and reduced fertility
Increased obstetrical risk
Musculoskeletal System
Osteoarthritis of spine and knees
Bone spurs of the heel
Decreased mobility
Skin
Intertrigo and papillomata
Benign acanthosis nigricans
Striae
Psychosocial Function
Social isolation
Professional discrimination
Feelings of inferiority

and primitive reflexes are decreased or absent. Because of a poorly developed sucking and swallowing reflex, feeding is difficult and may necessitate gavage feeding during the early months after birth. The manifestations of hypogonadism are not very impressive at this stage. With time, the infants become more lively and responsive, and feeding difficulties subside. This marks the second phase, when there is a complete reversal of feeding behavior. Hyperphagia becomes so pronounced that patients steal food, pilfer garbage cans, and consequently become obese. Gross obesity characteristically involves the trunk and proximal part of the limbs more than the lower legs and forearms. The hands and feet always remain disproportionately small (acromicria). In contrast to exo-

Table 12-2. Obesity Syndromes: Differential Diagnosis

Major Manifestations	*Type of Obesity*	*Growth Characteristics*
Prader–Willie Syndrome		
Hypotonia Hypogonadism (LHRH defect) Mental retardation Microcephaly	Onset between 1 and 4 years; trunk, buttocks, and proximal limbs involved; small hands and feet hyperphagia, severe	Feeding problems and failure to thrive in early infancy; diabetic glucose tolerance, adult type diabetes, with onset in adolescence
Klinefelter's Syndrome or Seminiferous Tubular Dysgenesis		
One or more extra X chromosomes Small, firm testes Azoospermia (increased FSH) Gynecomastia, eunuchoidal habitus Mental retardation, mild Personality disorders common	Onset in adolescence, BMR may be decreased	Underweight for height in childhood; tall stature
Laurence–Moon–Biedl Syndrome (autosomal recessive)		
Retinitis pigmentosa Hypogenitalism, hypogonadotrophic Mental retardation Polydactyly, syndactyly	Partial expression may include obesity and only one other manifestation in affected siblings	Occasionally, short stature

Carpenter's Syndrome		
Acrocephaly Hypogenitalism Mental retardation Polydactyly, syndactyly	Obesity mild, often present in infancy, progressive; inactivity plays a major role	
Pseudohypoparathyroidism, or Albright's Hereditary Osteodystrophy (X-linked dominant)		
Hypocalcemia despite high PTH Mental retardation Brachydactylia Calcium deposits in tissues	Round facies	Short stature, stocky build; osteitis fibrosa may develop
Pickwickian Syndrome		
Narcolepsy Hypoventilation	Obesity severe	
Fröhlich's Syndrome (hypothalamic lesions)		
Visual field defects Signs of intracranial pressure	No obesity in early childhood; onset of obesity is sudden	Growth retardation; failure of pubertal development
Cushing's Syndrome (hypercortisolism)		
Characteristic obesity	Trunkal obesity, buffalo hump, purple striae, mild hyperphagia	Short stature, retarded bone age, osteoporosis

genous obesity, longitudinal growth is impaired so that height is always below the 50th percentile. Because of a decreased or absent pubertal growth spurt, short stature becomes more pronounced in the teens. Hypotonia decreases with age, but impairment of psychomotor and intellectual development becomes more pronounced. Psychometric tests yield IQs between 20 and 90. Speech development is particularly retarded. These children are no serious management problem, because they tend to be, on the whole, friendly, content, and phlegmatic. However, tempers and seemingly uncontrollable phases of negativism and destructiveness occur. Minor dysmorphic stigmata may be present, including a high arched palate, simian creases, poorly modeled ears, narrow external ear canals, scoliosis, and mesobrachyphalangia. Hypogonadism may already be evident during the first phase in boys, who have a small penis and scrotum. The testes are undescended in most cases, and the gubernaculum may be too short to permit orchidopexy. Testes may be small or absent. Seminiferous tubules are immature, with decreased or absent spermatogenesis. Thus, male patients are infertile. Female patients have primary amenorrhea or delayed menarche and irregular anovulatory cycles. Development of secondary sex characteristics is delayed and incomplete in both sexes. Endocrine abnormalities of the hypothalamic–pituitary–gonadal axis have been reported but are not consistent. Urinary gonadotropins may be normal or increased, but are rarely decreased. Plasma testosterone levels are decreased and remain so after clomiphene administration. Diabetes mellitus of the adult type tends to develop during the second decade. Treatment of the obesity is rarely successful, and it is unlikely that weight reductions can be maintained, because hyperphagia is severe and seems to be of central origin. These patients tend to have paradoxic reactions to amphetamines and vehemently resist caloric restrictions. Gastric bypass procedures should be considered (22).

Endocrine and Metabolic Consequences

A wealth of data on endocrine dysfunctions and metabolic abnormalities have appeared over the years in the literature. To date, no single finding can be considered the cause of obesity. Rather, most of the observed changes appear to be consequences of obesity, as they revert to normal after weight reduction.

Basal insulin levels are increased a fewfold, and insulin response to stimulation with oral glucose, intravenous arginine, and a glucose-protein meal is excessively high (23). A deficient glucose uptake by adipocytes is evidence of tissue resistance to insulin, apparently because the number of membrane receptors decreases with increasing degrees of obesity. Clinical tests thus show a modestly impaired response to exogenous insulin, but glucose tolerance tests are normal as long as an excess of insulin can be produced by pancreatic β-cells. High circulating levels of essential amino acids are apparently another sign of tissue resistance, because they suggest that insulin fails to inhibit the release of amino acids from tissue.

The glucagon response to starvation and alanine infusion is diminished (24). Fasting blood sugar is within the normal range, although the mean may be significantly lower than normal control values (25). Cortisol metabolism seems to be accelerated, because urinary corticosteroid excretion is increased although plasma cortisol is normal. This is indicative of increased cortisol secretion by the adrenal glands.

Thyroid studies of obese patients do not reveal a primary etiologic role nor any significant secondary changes. Plasma levels of T_4, T_3 and thyroxine-binding globulin (TBG) are slightly elevated when compared to those of healthy normal-weight control subjects, whereas the T_4/TBG ratio, the T_3/TBG ratio, and thyroid stimulative hormone are normal (26).

Growth hormone responses to insulin-induced hypoglycemia, arginine infusion, exercise, and a glucose-protein meal are diminished (25). In view of the fact that obese children have normal or even increased growth rates, this may seem to be a paradoxical or unexpected finding. "Growth without growth hormone" is a reversal of the endocrine adjustment to protein-calorie malnutrition. These phenomena can be explained by the activity of somatomedin, which is normal in obesity but low in malnutrition (27). The fact that insulin levels in obese subjects are also opposite the levels in malnutrition suggests that these endocrine adjustments are determined by the state of nutrition. Since growth hormone raises free fatty acids because of its stimulating effect on triglyceride lipase, decreased levels of growth hormone should lower plasma fatty acids, which are instead elevated in obese subjects (25). Other observed hormone changes, such as the insulin increase, also seem to be aimed at decreasing the activity of lipase (Fig. 12-1). Thus, by inhibiting hydrolysis of fat, these hormone changes further promote lipogenesis.

Pubertal maturation, along with gonadal size and gonadotropin releasing hormone, is normal, although in cases of gradual and long-standing obesity, onset of puberty may be advanced by 1 year. In these cases skeletal maturation and height age are also advanced, and lean body mass is increased by at least 10% of the predicted value (28).

Adverse Effects on Health and Longevity

Obesity has been linked with a variety of conditions that pose a major public health hazard in developed countries. The list of disorders that are either caused or exacerbated by obesity include heart and vascular diseases, diabetes mellitus, hyperlipidemia and gout, gallbladder disorders, hepatic steatosis, ventilatory defects, disorders of weight-bearing joints and structures, and psychosocial disability. Obese persons are also believed to be at greater risk from anesthesia, surgery, and accidents, possibly because of venous stasis and a greater risk of developing thromboembolisms. The

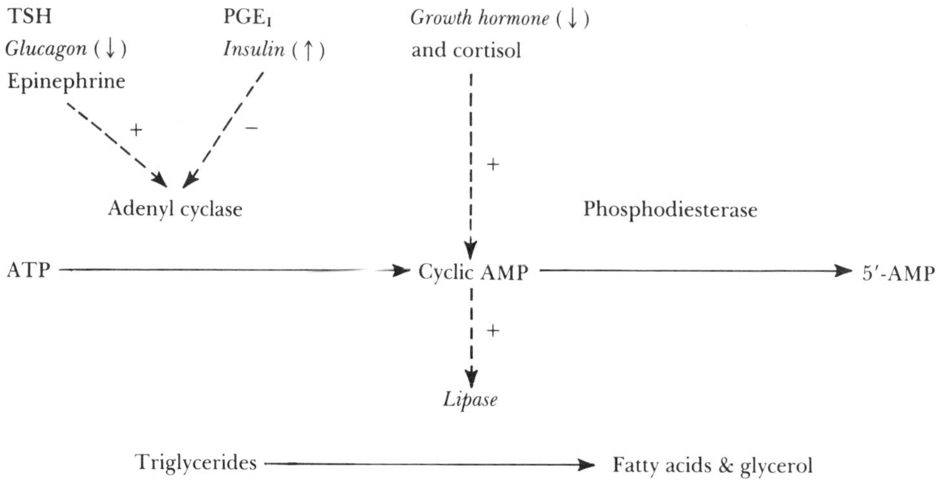

Figure 12-1. ABNORMAL HORMONE EFFECTS ON LIPASE ACTIVITY IN EXOGENOUS OBESITY

higher incidence of these disorders is responsible for decreased longevity (29). The relationship between overweight and mortality is not linear, because the risk increases more rapidly as the degree of obesity increases.

There is little understanding of the role that obesity plays in the development of coronary heart disease (CorHD). It is well known that obesity presents a hemodynamic burden and causes left ventricular hypertrophy. It is also recognized that it elevates blood pressure, causes hyperlipidemia, and predisposes to diabetes. However, the mechanisms that cause these changes are not known. Moreover, evidence from longitudinal studies suggests, at best, a weak positive relationship between obesity and CorHD and no correlation with myocardial infarcts (30,31). One reason relates to the fact that the American population samples included relatively few lean individuals, and the effect of obesity may have been obscured by other risk factors, mainly smoking. It is also very likely that many people are either protected or at risk because of genetic factors. A case in point is the protective effect of high-density lipoproteins or the genetic predisposition for diabetes. Characteristics peculiar to women also confer a certain protection. Thus, in the Framingham study angina and sudden death were related to antecedent weight gain in men but not in women (30,32).

The relationship between various indices of hyperlipidemia and obesity or CorHD has been the subject of intense study for many years. The data show that the correlation between fatness and triglyceride concentration is weak. Plasma cholesterol is related to weight changes, but the correlation with actual body weight is poor. It is becoming increasingly evident that the relationship is much stronger between certain lipoprotein carriers and either obesity or CorHD. The three main carriers are low-, very-low-, and high-density lipoproteins (LDL, VLDL, and HDL). A strong positive correlation between LDL and the degree of overweight exists in both sexes and all age groups. A positive correlation with VLDL was observed only in men. HDL is a protective factor against CorHD and is negatively related to the degree of overweight (33). One of the best predictors of CorHD appears to be the ratio between total cholesterol and HDL (32). A recent study of young adults, including 16- to 19-year-olds, suggests that in men this ratio is strongly related to the degree of obesity at all age levels. By contrast, a positive correlation for women was evident only in the 40- to 49-year-old group.

Equally fascinating though less well understood is the relation between obesity and diabetes. Obese subjects develop diabetes three times more often than normal-weight individuals. The diabetes is the so-called adult variety and is associated with increased insulin levels that do not compensate for a decrease in insulin receptors. It was possible to show in the Framingham study that for every 10% increment in relative weight, there was a 12 mg/dl rise in plasma cholesterol, a 6.5-mm rise in systolic blood pressure, and a 2 mg/dl rise in blood sugar. Obesity, carbohydrate intolerance and hyperlipidemia are major atherogenic traits. A majority of obese subjects who lost weight also achieved a normal blood pressure (34).

Obese infants seem prone to respiratory problems; croup is especially more common in chubby infants and young children. Obstructive sleep apnea is another respiratory complication of obesity. Aveolar hyperventilation is one manifestation of the Pickwickian syndrome that also occurs in other types of morbid obesity. It causes polycythemia and, occasionally, right ventricular hypertrophy or even right heart failure. An increased incidence of cholelithiasis has been described and was attributed to high cholesterol saturation of bile.

Treatment

The many different diets for obesity control that have been popularized over the years attest to the fact that treatment is difficult and lasting effects are rarely obtained. Dietary treatment modalities include starvation regimens, modified starvation, one-emphasis diets, and combination diets that restrict calories to varying degrees. Although the rationale for some of these diets is dubious and without scientific foundation, each may work in an individual case. This is usually attributable to the fact that fewer calories are consumed, even in diets that advertise unlimited intake. The reason for spontaneous restriction is the inability to make up for imposed deficits by using the allowed foods. This happens, for example, when fats, which are repulsive and cause ketosis, are the only alternate choice (35).

Calorie restriction and induction of increased losses or use of calories are the objective of other treatment modalities, including drugs, surgery, jaw wiring, exercise, psychotherapy, and hypnosis. With the exception of extreme approaches, such as surgery and jaw wiring, the success rate of each form of therapy alone in limited. Even if one treatment or combination of treatments is successful, the relapse rate is very high. Because of these experiences, a program consisting of calorie restriction, regular exercises, and modification of eating habits through behavior therapy has been advised in recent years. Moreover, weight maintenance after reduction can be expected only if the induced behavior modification is lasting. This may require follow-up, at long intervals, for many years and the establishment of a strong relationship with the patient. The components of this three-pronged treatment are discussed separately.

Dietary Management

No matter which approach is used, total calorie intake must be restricted sufficiently to exceed expenditures if weight loss is to occur. Even if future research should prove that certain obese people are genetically or metabolically different, the basic thermodynamic rules on the conversion of energy apply. Consequently, an obese individual must restrict food until weight loss occurs.

The caloric restriction needed for weight reduction varies from person to person and the deficit required for each pound of loss is not the same at each stage of a weight reduction regimen. Since it is necessary to set a specific goal at the outset of the program, this limitation of knowledge makes it difficult to predict the necessary restriction. To avoid disappointment over achieving less than the expected weight loss, the problem must be explained to patients, who should expect that calorie intake will be "titrated" against weight changes.

The goal varies depending on the degree of obesity. Adolescents with morbid obesity can lose 50 lb in 8 to 12 months, which is a pound per week. The same time frame should be used for lesser degrees of obesity, which are often harder to lose. Consequently, the goal for a child who is 25 lb overweight should only be about half a pound per week. Gradual reduction is preferred in children and adolescents, because it reduces the stress and allows time for behavior modification. The first three-fourths of the desired loss should be lost within the first half of the allotted time. The calculated amount per month may be doubled for the first month. These goals should be discussed with the patient and the family.

Patients should personally monitor their progress by weighing daily every morning before breakfast. Use of a graph is preferred because it shows the trend of weight change better than a list of figures, which are misleading when normally occurring daily fluctuations in weight are large.

In severely obese adults and adolescents who have completed the pubertal growth spurt, a modified fast may be advisable at the start. Genuth et al. (36) recommended a supplementation of 300 to 600 kcal maximum, and Bistrian et al. (37) devised a protein-sparing modified fast.

The high protein–low carbohydrate supplementation appears superior, because hunger is less severe when carbohydrates are restricted; however, some carbohydrates are necessary to avoid ketosis. Fasting regimens have two advantages: the initial weight loss is fairly rapid, and after the first 2 days patients have relatively little hunger. Eventually, however, hunger returns. This is the time when retraining must begin in order to develop eating habits that can be maintained. A prolonged period of severe restriction carries the risk of anemia, postural hypotension, electrolyte imbalance, and hyperuricemia. Fatty liver enlargement also occurs, and elevated serum bilirubin levels have been reported. Recently, the so-called last chance diet (38), which provides supplements in the form of protein hydrolysates of low nutrient value, led to a number of deaths and complications, such as thrombophlebitis. The deaths occurred (39) even though high-quality protein supplements were given. They were attributed to cardiac arrhythmias and cerebral ischemia.

A calorie-restricted diet for severely obese children that presents no hazard to their health while they are still growing consists of half the recommended lower limit for age (Table 1-2) or 100 kcal for every year, starting with 400 kcal/day for a 4-year-old, up to 1,000 kcal/day for children 10 and over. Children less than 4 years old should be allowed to "grow into" their size and therefore should be only modestly restricted. The diet should be balanced, relatively low in carbohydrates, low in cholesterol, and high in unsaturated fatty acids. Infants may be placed on 2% milk. Skim milk is not advised because this may lead to a deficient intake of essential fatty acids. If 20% of the restricted calorie allowance is protein, the child will get the RDA of protein based on ideal weight for height. As long as sugars are avoided, the remaining calories may be divided about equally between starches and fat. Roughage and foods of low caloric density should be encouraged. They suppress hunger intensity and are superior to medicinal bulk fillers because they supply minerals and vitamins. Low-calorie vegetables are lettuce, cucumbers, celery, squash, tomatoes, cauliflower, cabbage, green beans, and brussels sprouts. Use of diet drinks, diet salad dressings, diet jams, and so forth frees calories for foods that the person has difficulty giving up. Idiosyncrasies should be respected. Although the effect of meal frequency on calorie efficiency has not been conclusively demonstrated, it is advisable to offer at least three small meals per day, if only because longer intervals between meals increase hunger and may lead to a once-daily eating binge. Reducing diets usually do not supply adequate amounts of B vitamins and iron. To guard against that and other unpredictable deficits, daily supplementation with a multiple vitamin tablet with iron is recommended.

Exercise

Lack of physical exercise encourages the deposition of fat. Exercise is especially important for usually active individuals whose lifestyle changes, because the mechanism responsible for the regulation of appetite and satiety does not adjust readily to a lower level of activity (40). Although regular exercises help to prevent the development of obesity, exercise alone is of limited success in weight reduction.

Regular exercises are an important component of the three-pronged regimen. Calorie restriction alone causes muscle wasting, whereas the weight loss consists mainly of fat if exercise is coupled with a reducing diet. Activity should be increased gradually. It is absolutely necessary to make the prescription for exercise specific. For the patient unable to afford attendance at organized programs, a schedule of indoor exercises, bicycling, walking, or jogging must be devised.

Behavior Modification

This form of therapy has been used for obesity control for some 20 years, but only recently has it been applied to children (41–44). It seems to have its limitations in adults, although overall results are better than for other forms of treatment. Its use in children is to be encouraged, since it is easier to modify behavior and achieve lasting results in children because they are less set in their ways than adults.

Behavior modification, in general, is based on the premise that abnormal habits are not symptomatic or specific of the underlying psychological problem but are a learned response that helps the person cope with the problem. Consequently, pathologic habits can be unlearned. Its application to obesity requires careful analysis of the patient's eating behavior, of the stimuli that start overeating, and of the rewards that serve to maintain it.

Self-monitoring is an important aspect of behavior modification. During the initial phase of the program, the patient is asked to keep a record of body weight, food intake, its caloric value, and the circumstances surrounding the eating, including time of day, people present, feelings, degree of hunger, and preceding events that may have disturbed the patient. The amount of exercise also may be recorded. The purpose is twofold. It provides information for structuring an individualized treatment program, and it brings to the patient an awareness of those abnormal eating behaviors that went unnoticed or were denied before. Snacking is often automatic, or it is done rapidly and forgotten, as though calories did not count when the time used for eating is short. Patients should record the behavior right after it has taken place. Some observers advise "premonitoring" (45), because this may help the patient during the treatment phase of the program to stop the behavior before it takes place. Thus, self-monitoring becomes a treatment tool that forces self-awareness. Moreover, it is a log for recording the patient's success.

After an initial self-monitoring period of about 2 weeks' duration, when certain provocative stimuli have been recognized, treatment begins. Stimulus control is a major part of the program. It includes the kind of cue elimination that has been fairly routine in traditional weight reduction—namely, the elimination of sweets and other high-calorie snack foods from the shopping list to avoid temptation and replacement with low-calorie finger foods, such as celery and carrots. Meal plans should consist of foods that require preparation and cannot be eaten on impulse. Specific stimulus control must be individualized. Patients are urged to "recondition" themselves. By always eating at the same time, by taking each meal at the same place and table, and even by using the same napkin and place setting, it is hoped that new cues will take over so that the patient will not want to eat in other settings. Family participation can be helpful in cue elimination, although it has been shown that parental involvement is not essential for the success of behavior modification (42). However, if family eating is a major cue, then it becomes important for other members to change and become models. Consequently, in certain cases, the whole family should participate in the modification program.

Slowing the rate of eating has also been advised, and various means to achieve this have been advocated. Thus, the patient is asked to put down the eating utensil after each bite or sip and to use very small portions at a time, even if it means refilling the plate or glass several times in the course of the meal. The patient is taught to enjoy consciously the act of eating and to make mealtimes an experience of relaxation. Distractions, such as reading a paper, are not allowed. These methods discourage automatic eating. Slow eating has the additional benefit of postponing a large portion of the meal to a time when food absorption has already begun and when satiety may be signaled before too much is eaten.

Finally, reinforcement is an important part of behavior modification. Ideally, a picture of a slim model, pinned on the refrigerator door, reflecting the child's goal, should be sufficient positive reinforcement. However, this is obviously not the case, as evidenced by the poor success rate of most treatment regimens. Parents can help to provide reinforcement through internal rewards, by developing pride in the child through praise. To this end, attractive clothes or a new hairdo can help, as can being taught other grooming routines. Nevertheless, this type of reinforcement may not help, because the reward does not materialize until after a considerable delay, while eating provides immediate pleasure. The use of more tangible rewards therefore has been tried. Such reinforcement programs for children have to be worked out jointly with the patient and parents. They may consist of toys, an increase in the weekly allowance, attendance at special events, trips, and so on. The agreement is best written out like a contract and signed by both parties, with the health care professional as the witness.

Some unusual reinforcement schemes have been devised that involve the deposition of money that is refunded for certain desired behavior. They have been tried successfully in children (43). A percentage of the deposit may be refunded for attending therapy sessions or completing self-monitoring records. It also may be useful to distinguish between weight loss and a desired change in eating behavior and to award each separately. The two published studies that used some type of monetary reward scheme were successful, if compared with controls on the basis of weight loss; but follow-up proved very disappointing in that all subjects regained most of their weight (42,43). This result probably comes as no surprise to those who consider behavior therapy too superficial an approach to make a lasting impact, especially if the cause of abnormal behavior is a deep-seated psychological problem that remains untouched. If success is permanent with behavior modification, it may occur only at the cost of another coping device—for example, the patient replaces overeating with compulsive behavior.

The positive aspects of behavior therapy are—to this observer—(*1*) self-monitoring to increase self-awareness and to counteract denial, (*2*) stimulus control, and (*3*) positive reinforcement, providing it is done through the development of meaningful internal rewards, such as an appreciation of increased physical well-being and mobility, of prospects for long-term health, and—most importantly—of social acceptance. If personal fulfillment develops hand in hand with the improvement of external appearance, the patient will attribute one to the other and is more likely to maintain the desired eating behavior. To accomplish this, it will be necessary to conduct an analysis that probes beyond the circumstances that started the overeating. This will usually require the services of a psychiatrist or a similarly oriented professional. In children prolonged analysis is rarely required.

Surgical Therapy

Nonsurgical therapy of morbid obesity has met with limited success, especially in disorders like the Prader–Willie syndrome. The most commonly performed surgical procedure in adults is the jejunoileal bypass, which is intended to exclude ingested calories from absorption. The degree of resulting malabsorption depends on the length of small bowel that is preserved. In the pediatric age group, this operation is still in the investigational stage. Aside from the mortality attached to any surgical procedure, which is increased in the obese, postoperative complications have been reported in adults, including liver failure, pancreatitis, bypass enteritis, pulmonary embolism, hemorrhage, and cardiac failure. Postsurgical diarrhea is a hazard that may become a chronic problem. Ensuing metabolic problems, like nitrogen wasting, potassium and calcium deficit, and so forth are especially dangerous to growing children. Unfortunately, if more bowel is retained in order to avoid these complications, weight loss will be less.

The gastric bypass procedure was introduced for the treatment of obesity in 1969 (46). Postoperative complications are less than for the jejunoileal bypass. They consist mainly of postprandial vomiting, but this disappears as the patient develops better eating habits with respect to mastication and quantity consumed. The patient learns through a Pavlovian type of reeducation to limit intake in order to avoid abdominal discomfort. Since intestinal digestion and absorption are retained, metabolic complications are avoided. The child with Prader–Willie syndrome, who is such an aggressive eater, seems especially well suited for this surgical approach. However, if obesity is already extreme, it is difficult to attain a normal weight in genetic obesity with this procedure alone (47). In genetically normal children, behavior modification should always be tried first, reserving gastric bypass to certain, select cases.

Drug Therapy

Of the many drugs marketed for obesity control, only a few have been proven more effective than placebos. Thyroid hormone increases the basal metabolic rate and appears to promote lipolysis by potentiating the effect of epinephrine. However, in time, endocrine adjustments seem to occur that compensate for the medication, probably by decreasing endogenous thyroid hormone production. Moreover, thyroid hormone increases the loss of lean body tissue and is therefore contraindicated in growing children.

Amphetamines are known appetite depressants, but the weight loss produced by their use alone has been modest unless conscious restrictions are also imposed. Anorexiants are helpful adjuncts to the treatment of morbid obesity with diet and behavior modification. However, the potential for abuse restricts their therapeutic value. If anorexiants are used at all in the pediatric age group, they should be prescribed only for a limited period (no longer than 2 months) until pathologic eating habits are broken and behavior modification is showing positive effects.

Bulk fillers have been prescribed with some success in adults to suppress hunger intensity. They should be a temporary "crutch" until the hunger feeling caused by a nondistended stomach is no longer felt.

The use of chorionic gonadotropins was recommended by Simeons (48) and supported by several articles that appeared in reputable journals (49,50). The Food and Drug Administration later found upon review of the literature, that there was no convincing scientific evidence of their effectiveness (51).

SPECIFIC NUTRIENT EXCESS

Vitamins

Vitamins are frequently not viewed by the laiety as drugs, and there is a tendency to believe that "more is better than less." Thus, vitamins are taken with impunity, especially in the United States. Adults take them for a variety of reasons, ranging from the improvement of sexual potency to the prevention of aging or the counteraction of side effects of chronic alcohol ingestion. Yet, a number of diseases due to vitamin excess are recognized. The two major disorders, hypervitaminosis A and D, are better known to pediatricians than to internists. It was believed that only these two fat-soluble vitamins are toxic if taken in excess over a period of time because they can be stored by the body. However, there are now more and more case reports appearing that suggest that other vitamins can be toxic as well. These reports are likely to increase, because abuse is spreading due to a trend set by food faddists and believers in orthomolecular theorics. Justified trials of pharmacological doses of vitamins in cases of proven or suspected genetic vitamin dependency can also lead to abuse.

Vitamin B Group

Niacin has been used in schizophrenia by people who consider it a form of "cerebral pellagra." There are reports of adult schizophrenics who received as much as 3 g/day and developed skin changes resembling acanthosis nigricans (52). Transient side effects, which may occur after doses of about 20 mg, consist of flushing, tingling sensations, headache, dizziness, and a drop in blood pressure. Of the B-group vitamins, pyridoxine is also potentially harmful. Offspring of mothers who receive large doses during pregnancy may develop transient dependency, with symptoms like those seen in genetic pyridoxine dependency, including irritability, hyperacusis, and convulsions (see Chapter 10).

Hypervitaminosis A

The acute form, which is more common in infants under 1 year, is manifested by a sudden intracranial pressure increase, as evidenced by bulging fontanels or papilledema, vomiting, headache, blurred vision, and drowsiness. The condition has been called "pseudo-tumor cerebri." Following chronic vitamin A ingestion, there may be fatigue, abdominal discomfort, anorexia, and failure to gain weight. Other symptoms include a seborrheic skin rash, itching and desquamation of the palms and soles, patchy hair loss and hepatomegaly. Infants develop a picture resembling that of Caffey's disease, a cortical hyperostosis of the long bones which involves mainly the ulna and one or more metatarsals. The disease is manifested by tender swelling over the affected areas, limitation of motion, and irritability. Hypercalcemia occurs occasionally and is due to stimulation of parathyroid hormone by vitamin A. In contrast to Caffey's disease, flat bones and the mandible are not affected. The disorder has occurred after chronic ingestion of daily doses of 300,000 IU or more, as soon as 2 months after onset. Toxicity may result from the cumulative effect of doses as low as 30,000 IU/day, taken over months and years. Aqueous solutions are more toxic, apparently because they are more readily absorbed. Diagnosis and differentiation from Caffey's disease rests on the demonstration of increased vitamin A levels, about 300 μg/dl.

Hypervitaminosis D

Toxicity develops although the enzymatic conversion of dietary vitamin D into the active form by renal 1,25-hydroxylase is well controlled. Thus, anephric patients can develop hypervitaminosis D (53). This is possible because liver 25-hydroxylase is poorly controlled and excess amounts of 25-(OH)D_3 enhance intestinal calcium absorption. Circulating levels of 1,25-$(OH)_2$ D_3 are normal in hypervitaminosis D, but 25-(OH)D_3 may be elevated as much as 30 times (54). Metastatic calcifications occur in the kidneys, blood vessels, heart, lung, and skin. Long bones show osteoporosis as well as metastatic calcifications. Early manifestations are mainly gastrointestinal and neurological. Symptoms include hypotonia, hyporeflexia, and intestinal hypomotility. Muscle weakness may resemble a proximal limb girdle myopathy. Many of the late manifestations are a consequence of kidney damage, including elevated BUN and albuminuria (Table 12-3). Confusion and coma develop when serum calcium reaches levels in excess of 16 mg/dl. Irreversible brain damage has been observed. The disorder used to be common in Great Britain in the 1950s because food fortification was excessive. When it was reduced to a degree where few infants could receive more than 1500 IU/day, incidence of hypervitaminosis D gradually decreased.

Hypervitaminosis D should be distinguished from idiopathic hypercal-

Table 12-3. Signs and Symptoms in Hypervitaminosis D

Early	Fatigue	Hypotonia
	Headache	Hyporeflexia
	Anorexia	Intestinal hypomotility
	Nausea	Constipation
	Vomiting	Muscle and bone pain
	Diarrhea	Metallic taste
Late	Polyuria	Photophobia
	Polydipsia	Conjunctivitis
	Nocturia	Rhinorrhea
	Hypertension	Pruritus
	Weight Loss	Reduced cognitive function
	Pancreatitis	Confusion and coma
	Hyperthermia	
Laboratory findings		
	Hypercalcemia, normal phosphorus	
	Elevated BUN	
	Albuminemia	
	Hypercholesterolemia	
	X-ray evidence of metastatic calcifications	
	Osteoporosis	

cemia, which has been attributed to vitamin D hypersensitivity. However, the pathogenetic mechanism is uncertain. Thus, hypersensitivity cannot always be demonstrated, and elevated serum calcium levels are not a consistent feature of patients with the physical stigma of idiopathic hypercalcemia. Prenatal vitamin D excess should be ruled out. Infants with the disorder have a characteristic facies, described as "elfin" face, and other abnormalities that suggest a dysmorphic syndrome of prenatal onset. Characteristics include a pug nose, epicanthal folds, and a flat nasal bridge with anteverted nostrils and full lips. Failure to thrive and constitutional symptoms, which usually develop after the first month of life, are similar to the manifestations of hypervitaminosis D. The finding of radiologic bone densities with normal serum phosphorus values is also similar to hypervitaminosis D and distinguish these two types of hypercalcemia from hyperparathyroidism, in which phosphorus is low and x-rays show characteristic rarefactions. Supravalvular aortic stenosis, mental deficiency, and short stature are common. These dysmorphic features suggest that a prenatal insult is the cause of this syndrome.

Therapy. Discontinuation of vitamin D is usually sufficient. A low-calcium diet is a helpful adjunct since vitamin D activity and its effect on intestinal absorption cannot be entirely eliminated. Foods to be avoided are milk and wheat products, enriched cereals, fruits and fruit juices (except apple, peach, and cranberry), fish, potatoes, nuts, chocolate, maple syrup, and artificial sweeteners containing calcium cyclamate. Hospitalization is advised if serum calcium elevation is severe. Cortisone has been used in severe cases because of its inhibitory effect on calcium absorption. However, the efficacy of such use in hypervitaminosis D is questionable, since cortisone causes PTH release and augments formation of $1,25\text{-}(OH)_2D_3$. Inorganic phosphorus may be given, either orally as sodium or potassium phosphate or IV as buffered 0.1 molar solution of disodium plus monopotassium phosphate. Mithramycin is the drug of choice in treating hypercalcemia due to metastatic malignancies. Other treatment methods that have been advised include EDTA, indomethacin, peritoneal dialysis, and hemodialysis.

Vitamin C

Megadoses of vitamin C are usually taken in an effort to prevent frequent upper respiratory infections. Its use should be discouraged, except at the onset of a cold, when high doses of over 1 g/day may decrease the severity of the symptoms and shorten the duration of the illness (55). Whereas brief exposure to high doses does not seem to be harmful, long-term use may have adverse effects, including vitamin B_{12} deficiency (56), renal stones, and acute hemolysis in patients with glucose-6-phosphate dehydrogenase deficiency. Long-term use is contraindicated during pregnancy.

Vitamin K

Toxicity to vitamin K appears to be a function of the form of the vitamin K administered, the amount given, and the patient's age. Newborn infants may develop hemolytic anemia with hyperbilirubinemia, kernicterus, and death if given large doses of water-soluble analogues of vitamin K (57).

Trace Metals

Iron

Of the trace metals known to cause toxicity, iron is one that is not infrequently ingested by children in excess amounts. Parents tend to handle iron tablets carelessly, since they do not consider it a drug. Acute iron poisoning occurs when soluble iron salts in amounts of 2 to 4 g or more are ingested. The mechanism that normally regulates absorption is overwhelmed at these doses, and binding sites in plasma and tissues become saturated. Excess free iron produces shock and central nervous system depression, which may lead to death. Fatality rates of 50% have been reported. Recovery is more likely in cases that are treated before appearance of coma and shock. Early manifestations are gastrointestinal irritation and hemorrhagic necrosis of the mucosa, causing vomiting and bloody diarrhea. Direct hepatic damage is possible. The disease may progress rapidly to coma, shock, and death, or there may be a latent period of several hours followed by shock, which is due to the action of vasopressor substances. Patients therefore must be watched closely for at least 24 to 48 hours. Even with the best of therapeutic attention, death is often unpreventable. Metabolic acidosis, which is common in severe cases, is probably a result of deficient tissue perfusion during shock and accumulation of lactic and citric acid.

Immediate treatment consists of lavage with sodium bicarbonate. This medication has several useful actions: it forms insoluble ferrous carbonate; it counteracts the metabolic acidosis that develops in severe cases; and it improves the chelating action of deferoxamine, which is the major drug used in treatment. Deferoxamine is a chelating agent with a stronger affinity for iron than either transferrin, hemosiderin, or ferritin. It may combine with iron in the intestinal tract or bind with iron in the tissues and form a complex that is readily excreted by the kidney. Theoretically, 100 mg of deferoxamine combines with 9.3 mg of trivalent iron. Whereas the complex is considered nontoxic, both iron and deferoxamine itself have hypotensive action, probably mediated through the release of vasopressors. This limits the usefulness of the drug in cases where massive amounts of iron have been ingested and a safe dosage of deferoxamine is insufficient for detoxification.

Chronic iron excess leads first to iron accumulation in tissues, unassociated with secondary damage. This condition is generally referred to as *hemosiderosis*. Ultimately, iron accumulation causes tissue damage and dysfunction in certain organs, such as the heart, lung, and pancreas. *Hemochromatosis* is the term that describes this association. Hemochromatosis may be primary, as in the familial disorder, which is presumably caused by a genetic defect of iron absorption; or it may develop secondary to repeated blood transfusions or long-term oral iron therapy in hemolytic disease for which iron treatment is required. It is questionable whether excessive oral ingestion alone, without increased hemolysis and erythropoiesis or a genctic abnormality, can lead to hemochromatosis. A disorder seen among the Bantu tribe, which presumably results from the use of iron pots for cooking and fermentation of alcoholic beverages, also may be the result of several factors, excessive intake and uncontrolled absorption due to a single or double dose of the hemodromatosis gene.

Isolated hemosiderosis occurs occasionally in organs that are affected by chronic bleeding into the tissues in amounts that exceed the capacity for iron removal. This happens in the lung when bleeding is due to congestion from left ventricular heart failure or allergy. Primary bleeding and localized hemosiderosis occur in idiopathic pulmonary hemosiderosis and Goodpasture's syndrome.

Accumulation of hemosiderin is generalized in *primary hemochromatosis*. The nature of the metabolic defect that causes excessive absorption in this familial disorder is not understood. Because of the long time required until iron accumulation reaches toxic levels, children are never symptomatic and rarely have increased serum iron levels. Except for the history, the disorder cannot be distinguished on clinical grounds from iatrogenic (transfusion) hemochromatosis. The disease presents as a tetrad: (*1*) bronze pigmentation of the skin, (*2*) liver disease, (*3*) diabetes mellitus due to hemosiderosis of the pancreas, and (*4*) myocardial hemosiderosis that can cause heart failure. *Secondary hemochromatosis* develops invariably in patients with thalassemia major. It may develop during the teens in patients who require blood transfusions every 2 to 3 months. Chronic treatment with intramuscular deferoxamine is now considered appropriate prophylactic therapy for these children, but it should not be started until there is evidence of iron overload and more than 1 mg iron can be mobilized per day.

Zinc

The margin between physiologic requirements and toxic quantities is wide. Toxicity is consequently rare, but it has been observed—for instance, following prolonged ingestion of lemonade that was stored in galvanized cans. The type of liquid stored may have been a factor, because citric acid appears to be a zinc-binding ligand, and its presence in lemonade may have promoted zinc uptake. Sustained administration of zinc also occurred in a few cases where dialysis fluid from galvanized tanks was used. This led to fever, gastrointestinal symptoms, and anemia. Since saturation of metal-binding sites in the intestinal mucosa by one metal may interfere with the absorption of another, copper or iron deficiency may have been the cause of the anemia. Symptoms after acute ingestion of elemental zinc in doses as high as 12 g are minor. However, in experimental animals receiving an excess of elemental zinc, survival after exposure to pathogenic bacteria was decreased. Immunodeficiency may have been responsible, since leukocytes appear to require a specific zinc concentration for optimal function. Possible implications for humans relate to the speed of zinc infusion during parenteral alimentation.

Copper

Wilson's disease is an example of chronic trace metal excess due to a genetic defect. The disease has provided insights into the potential toxicity of copper, although accumulation in tissues is rarely caused by dietary excess. The pathogenesis of the disease is related to ceruloplasmin deficiency and an abnormality of copper transport and/or mobilization. However, the level of ceruloplasmin in patients with Wilson's disease is poorly correlated with either tissue copper or the severity of the disease. Although serum copper and ceruloplasmin are low, copper can be transported to the kidney and is excreted in excess. Occasional cases with a compensatory increase in albumin-bound copper have normal serum copper. Inheritance appears to be autosomal recessive. Similarly to hemochromatosis, the accumulation of the trace metal to levels where it is toxic to the tissue takes years. Thus, the disorder is rarely symptomatic before 6 years of age, and onset may be delayed until the fifth decade. Pathologically, the disease is characterized by liver cirrhosis, renal tubular disease, and degenerative changes in the brain, mainly the basal ganglia. Corneal copper deposits (Kayser-Fleischer ring) are pathognomonic. Toxic accumulations in brain and kidney account for the neurological manifestations and signs of Fanconi's syndrome: amino aciduria, phosphaturia, and glucosuria (Table 12-4). Hepatic disease is most severe in some patients, while in others neurological symptoms are more prominent. Both types may be present in the same family, but the hepatic form is common in patients with onset during childhood. Diagnosis requires demonstration of excess copper in the liver.

Treatment has become possible following introduction of penicillamine in 1956. Since this chelating agent removes copper as well as cystine, patients may become methionine-deficient. The drug also increases the requirements for pyridoxine and possibly other vitamins. Because of this and a variety of potentially serious other side effects, use of the drug requires careful monitoring. It is of considerable interest that some of the side effects of chronic penicillamine therapy are those of zinc deficiency, including depression of T-cell activity, hypogeusia, cheilosis, and stomatitis.

Table 12-4. Signs and Symptoms of Chronic Copper Excess in Wilson's Disease

Corneal copper deposits (Kayser–Fleischer ring)
Liver cirrhosis
CNS involvement (basal ganglia)
Choreoathetosis, tremors
Dystonia ("wing beating" of the shoulders)
Dysarthria
Hypertonicity
Emotional lability
Renal disease, mainly tubular dysfunction
Bone changes
Laboratory findings
Normal to decreased serum copper
Decreased ceruloplasmin
Increased urine copper
Markedly increased tissue copper (liver biopsy)
Low serum phosphorus
Low serum uric acid
Increased renal clearance for phosphorus and uric acid
Aminoaciduria
Glucosuria, occasionally
Increases of select plasma amino acids (in liver disease)
Anemia, may be hemolytic
Pancytopenia (in advanced liver disease)

Treatment should be supplemented by a low-copper diet, which excludes the following foods: chocolate, shellfish, nuts, mushrooms, liver, enriched cereals, onions, broccoli, molasses, and curry.

The manifestations of chronic copper excess differ from those caused by acute toxicity, which has been observed following exposure to copper salts in fumes and vineyard spray and after accidental ingestion of over 1 g. A metallic taste appears to be a characteristic early sign. Combinations of the following signs and symptoms have been reported: nausea, vomiting, epigastric pain, diarrhea, and melena. Acute hemolytic anemia may develop and cause jaundice, hemoglobinuria, and anuria.

A few cases of chronic copper poisoning due to excess intake have been reported. They were attributed to the use of copper for hot water tanks and pipes. In one case, manifestations were reminiscent of mercury sensitivity—pink disease (58). Another patient showed severe micronodular liver cirrhosis at 14 months of age (59). Diagnosis must rely on a history of exposure rather than copper levels, because infection and stress also raise circulating plasma copper and estrogen increases the synthesis of ceruloplasmin.

Iodine

The occurrence of chronic iodine excess due to its ingestion with food is unlikely. It usually develops from the use of iodide-containing cough medicines and antiasthmatic drugs. The two known manifestations are iodide goiter and iodinism. Both seem to require a certain "sensitivity" on the part of the individual. Thus, an autoregulatory mechanism which limits the amount of iodine trapping in normal individuals appears to be ineffective in patients with iodide-induced goiter. Their failure to inhibit the organification of iodine may be genetic or acquired, possibly as a result of lymphocytic thyroiditis or treatment with radioactive iodine. Hypersensitivity is also a contributing factor in iodinism. Symptoms consist of acneiform or erythematous rashes, rhinitis, conjunctivitis, and excessive salivation.

Acute toxic actions of iodine are due to its corrosive action on the gastrointestinal tract. Ingestion may be followed by a burning sensation, abdominal pain, vomiting, bloody diarrhea, and even shock. Diagnosis is facilitated by the brown staining of mucous membranes and the blue color of the vomitus. Anaphylactoid shock has followed the use of iodinated substances in diagnostic radiography.

Fluoride

Although a considerable margin of safety seems to exist with regard to fluoride ingestion during infancy, long-term exposure to fluoride-containing drinking water has led to fluorosis, which consists of mottling of the teeth and pitting of the enamel. Bone manifestations include osteosclerosis and exostosis of the long bones. Growth may be impaired. Available data indicate that it is desirable to restrict fluoride intake during infancy to 0.5 mg/day. Analysis from several studies on the relationship between fluoride content of drinking water and the incidence of tooth decay or fluorosis suggests that the optimal fluoride concentration is close to 1 ppm (60). Above that level, incidence of fluorosis increases rapidly. Thus, 189 children, ages 9 to 12 years, were studied in a community in Texas where the fluoride content of drinking water was 4.4 ppm; 46% were found to have severe dental fluorosis (61).

Other Select Trace Minerals

Acute or chronic excess of the remaining trace minerals does not play an important role in pediatrics. Only a few observations appear to be relevant. Thus, it has been noted that increased *selenium* intake during tooth development was associated with an increased incidence of dental caries (62). *Manganese* excess has been observed only in adults. These were miners who inhaled manganese-containing dust over a period of time and developed an encephalitis-like condition with extrapyramidal signs. Acute toxicity may follow ingestion of potassium permanganate. Manganese sulfate or chloride in amounts of 4 to 5 mg is contained in several adult multivitamin preparations that could fall into the hands of children or be given on a long-term basis to children out of ignorance. Symptoms are irritation of gastric mucosa, hemolytic jaundice, and capillary damage. Chronic *molybdenum* ingestion may cause copper deficiency, because it forms a strong copper–molybdenum–sulfate complex that is not absorbed.

Major Minerals

Sodium

Acute dietary sodium excess severe enough to cause hypernatremia is rare. It may develop after excessive use of salt tablets, especially when water loss due to sweating is also excessive. Hypernatremia in diarrhea is usually due to multiple factors. Diet may play a role because of the common use of electrolyte solutions or boiled skim milk in the treatment of diarrhea. Since most watery stools are hypotonic, water replacement is insufficient when these high osmolar solutions are used in an undiluted form. Acute sodium excess occurred in a tragic accident involving infants who were fed formula containing salt in place of sugar (63). It may be a manifestation of child abuse. Iatrogenic hypernatremia follows administration of parenteral solutions with high sodium content or when excess sodium is absorbed from hypertonic solutions given for the induction of abortion. Hypernatremia is more common as a result of a decrease in body water relative to sodium, for example in diarrhea, diabetes insipidus and in patients receiving urea or mannitol for osmotic diuresis.

Clinical manifestations reflect the hyperosmolarity of the extracellular fluid. The skin has a doughy or rubbery feel, and the loss of skin turgor is not impressive, even in cases with significant dehydration. Symptoms include high fever, convulsions, stupor, and paralysis. Whether sodium is taken in excess or deficient intake and retention of water are the cause of hypernatremia, an acute elevation of osmolarity results in cell shrinkage due to dehydration which may cause tearing of bridging vessels in the brain and hemorrhage.

Treatment of hypernatremia requires an estimation of the free water deficit from serum sodium concentration. Each 1 mEq/l above a serum sodium of 145 mEq/l reflects a deficit of about 4 ml/kg. This amount of water is necessary in addition to maintenance requirements of water and electrolytes in order to dilute the serum to 145 mEq/l. However, correction must proceed slowly to prevent cerebral edema. This can be achieved by planning the complete correction to be finished no sooner than after 48 hours or longer if the serum sodium concentration is in excess of 175 mEq/l. Thus, additional water should never exceed 60 ml/kg/day, and it should be given slowly over the entire 24 hours.

Because of the serious consequences of hypernatremia, prevention is of paramount importance. Thus infants requiring feedings of high-caloric density should be given low-solute formulas which may be concentrated without increasing sodium content excessively (Chapter 2). Particular attention to sodium intake is required in the following conditions: fever, high environmental temperature, hyperventilation, diarrhea, renal disease, and conditions associated with a low fluid intake.

Relationship of Chronic High Salt Intake to Disease. The effects of chronic sodium excess are not well understood. Early in the 1920s Allen (64) demonstrated the effectiveness of salt restriction in hypertension and suggested that "the morbidity and mortality from renal and vascular disease would be reduced by general abstinence from salt." Investigators subsequently showed that reduction in sodium intake lowers blood pressure in patients with essential hypertension. This disorder is also effectively treated with diuretic agents that facilitate the renal excretion of sodium. Moreover, population studies have shown that in areas where adults eat less than 30 mEq of sodium per day, hypertension is virtually nonexistent and the "normal" rise in blood pressure with advancing age does not occur. However, sodium intakes that raise blood pressure acutely in normotensive adults are much higher, over 600 mEq/day. Chronic intakes in excess of 300 mEq/day increase the incidence of hypertension and the death rate from stroke (65). The effects of chronic intakes in the intermediate range are not known. The possibility has been raised that mild to moderate abuse, starting in early childhood, can have long-range consequences.

The debate on the need for salt restriction in childhood intensified when it was shown in the late 1960s that processed baby foods contain a disproportionately large amount of salt (66), leading to sodium intakes of 9 to 60 mEq/day in infants on supplementary baby foods, who require at most only 6 to 8 mEq/day. Kagan had shown earlier (67), in studies of premature infants, that total body water was influenced by the protein and electrolyte concentration of their formula. The normal decrease of total body water and of the percentage of extracellular fluid during maturation did not occur in infants fed milk with a high sodium content. Salt (average 0.4 to 0.6%) had been added to baby foods by manufacturers to please the palate of parents who taste the food and tend to add excessive amounts themselves to home-prepared pureed infant foods. As a result of publicity, manufacturers now limit salt concentration to 0.25%. In view of the low minimum sodium requirements (Chapter 11), this appears to be a prudent approach to an unsettled question.

Since a causal relationship between essential hypertension and chronic high salt intake has not been established, recommendations at this time should be limted to the restriction of *excessive* salt intakes. According to current concepts, only a fraction of the population is genetically susceptible to developing essential hypertension by middle life. It is therefore unwarranted to impose restrictions that are difficult to follow on the entire population. However, restrictions of salt to the "advisable intake" (Chapter 11) is recommended for patients—including children—with a family history of hypertension, patients with a blood pressure in the upper range of normal, and obese people.

Potassium

Hyperpotassemia is rarely caused by dietary excess, because the normal kidney can excrete substantial quantities of potassium. Thus, hyperpotassemia is, in most instances, due to impaired renal excretion or a shift of potassium from the cell. Pseudohyperpotassemia, caused by the release of potassium from muscle tissue during prolonged use of a tourniquet for venipuncture, should be ruled out.

Clinical effects are due to the high extracellular potassium concentration, because the capacity of the cell to retain a comparable amount is limited. The resultant decrease of the ratio between intra- and extracellular potassium causes a reduction in membrane potential and abnormalities in cardiac rhythm and the rate of conduction. Initially, patients complain of paresthesias, and the neurological exam may show impaired vibratory and position sense. Hypotonia and hyporeflexia are common. The ECG shows tall, peaked T waves, a prolonged PR and shortened Q-T interval, decreased amplitude of the P wave, and widening of both the P and the QRS complex. The P wave ultimately disappears, and as the QRS complex merges with the T wave, a characteristic sine wave pattern results. The effects of hyperpotassemia are exaggerated by hypocalcemia and hyponatremia. Cardiac arrest is a major threat. The neurological manifestations eventually progress to include mental confusion and flaccid paralysis, which usually spares the cranial nerves.

Treatment becomes urgent when serum potassium rises to 7 mEq/l or when widening of the QRS complex develops. Reduction of total body potassium can be accomplished by reducing potassium intake and increasing its excretion in stool and urine. Dietary manipulations are useful only for the management of chronic conditions associated with potassium excess. Hyperpotassemia in the range of 7 mEq/l or more should be treated acutely through oral administration of a cation exchange resin (Kayexalate 1 g/kg) to enhance fecal potassium excretion or—in severe cases—peritoneal dialysis or hemodialysis. Infusion of 10–20% glucose solutions with insulin (0.1 U/kg or 1 U/2 g glucose) and of bicarbonate solutions (2–4 mEq/kg) force potassium back into the cell and thus help to reestablish a normal ratio between intra- and extracellular potassium concentration. Drugs with aldosterone-like activity are helpful only in cases where the secretion of this hormone is deficient.

Calcium

Dietary calcium excess rarely causes disease, because calcium absorption is limited in the absence of a comparable increase of vitamin D. Bone serves as the reservoir and serum calcium does not rise without vitamin D. Hypercalcemia is therefore only seen after an overdose or hypersensitivity to vitamin D, in disorders causing PTH excess, in metastatic bone disease, and with prolonged immobilization. (Table 12-5)

Table 12-5. Causes of Hypercalcemia

In infancy
Idiopathic hypercalcemia (D hypersensitivity)
Maternal hypoparathyroidism
Neonatal parathyroid hyperplasia, familial
Subcutaneous fat necrosis
At all ages
Hypervitaminosis D
Hypervitaminosis A (PTH stimulation)
Primary hyperparathyroidism
Transient ("relative") hyperparathyroidism following renal transplantation
Multiple endocrinopathy (autoimmune)
Benign familial hypercalcemia (autosomal dominant)
Thiazide diuretics
Metastatic bone disease
Prolonged immobilization

Phosphorus

Dietary phosphorus excess as the sole cause of disease has not been observed, although phorphorus is ubiquitous in the ordinary diet. Excess ingestion may result from laxative abuse, in which case the deposition as hydroxyapatite in bone causes hypocalcemia.

Magnesium

Hypermagnesemia has not been reported as a consequence of dietary excess but does occur following laxative abuse and when magnesium salts are given as antacids. Since the kidney is able to excrete excess magnesium rapidly, plasma elevations are not sustained and rarely reach toxic levels of above 4 mEq/l. Minor elevations occur in renal failure and in patients on dialysis. The combination of renal failure and high magnesium intake has caused symptomatic hypermagnesemia in a number of reported cases, with levels up to 7 mEq/l or more—which is the range where lethal cardiac complications occur. Hypermagnesemia has been reported in newborn infants whose mothers were given magnesium sulfate for toxemia (68).

Clinical manifestations are due to depression of the central nervous system and transmission at neuromuscular junctions. They consist of lethargy, muscular weakness, decreased tendon reflexes, dysarthria, and ataxia. Nausea and vomiting, a feeling of warmth, and flushing due to vasodilation appear to be specific, as they have been observed following rapid intravenous infusion of magnesium (69). Other manifestations, including weakness and ECG changes, reported in cases with renal failure, may have been caused by associated other abnormalities, such as hypercalcemia.

REFERENCES

1. Forbes GB: Prevalence of obesity in childhood, in Bray GA (ed): *Obesity in Perspective,* vol 2. US Dept of Health Education and Welfare, 1975.
2. Haase KE, Hosenfeld H: Zur Fettsucht im Kindesalter. Z. Kinderheilk. 7:11, 1950.
3. Bour H: Problèms généraux de obisité. *Social Demogr Med* 8:24, 1975.
4. Fabry P: Metabolic consequences of the pattern of food intake, in: *Handbook of Physiology.* Section 6: *Alimentary Canal.* Washington, DC, American Physiological Society, 1967, p 31.
5. Rosenstock IM: Psychological forces, motivation, and nutrition education. *Am J Public Health* 59:1992, 1969.
6. Decke E: Effects of taste on the eating behavior of obese and normal persons, in Schacster S (ed): *Emotion, Obesity, and Crime.* New York, Academic Press, 1971.
7. Nisbett RE: Determinants of food intake in human obesity. *Science* 159:1254, 1968.
8. Miller DS, Mumford R, Stock MJ: Gluttony: 2. Thermogenesis in overeating man. *Amer J Clin Nutr* 20:1223, 1967.
9. Kaplan ML, Leveille GA: Calorigenic response in obese and nonobese women. *Am J Clin Nutr* 29:1108, 1976.
10. Krieger I, Whitten CF: Energy metabolism in infants with growth failure due to maternal deprivation, undernutrition or causes unknown: Relationship between nitrogen balance, weight gain and postprandial excess heat production. *J Pediatr* 75:374, 1969.
11. Van Itallie TB, Campbell RG: Multidisciplinary approach to the problem of obesity. *J Am Diet Assoc* 61:385, 1972.
12. Mayer J: Regulation of energy intake and body weight: Glucostatic theory and lipostatic hypothesis. *Ann NY Acad Sci* 63:15, 1955.
13. Brobeck JR: Food intake as mechanism of temperature regulation. *Yale J Biol Med* 20:545, 1948.
14. Kennedy GC: Rose of depot fat in hypothalamic control of food intake in rat. *Proc Roy Soc Biol* 140:578, 1953.
15. Knittle JL, Hirsch J: Effect of early nutrition on the development of rat epididymal fat pads. *J Clin Invest* 47:201, 1968.
16. Boulton TJC, Dunlop M, Court JM: The growth and development of fat cells in infancy. *Pediatr Res* 12:908, 1978.
17. Chirico AM, Stunkard AJ: Physical activity and human obesity. *N Engl J Med* 263:935, 1960.
18. Stern JS, Johnson PR: Spontaneous activity in the Zucker obese rat. *Fed Proc* 33:677, 1974.
19. Garn SM, Clark DC: Trends in fatness and family line aspects of obesity: From the committee to advise the Ten-State Nutrition Survey. *Pediatrics* 56:443, 1975.
20. *Ten-State Nutrition Survey.* DHEW Publication (HSM) 72-8130. US Dept of Health, Education and Welfare, 1972.

21. Alexander MK: The postmorten estimation of total fat, muscle and bone. *Clin Sci* 26:193, 1964.

22. Soper RT, Mason EE, Printen KY, et al: Gastric bypass for morbid obesity in children and adolescents. *J Pediatr Surg* 10:51, 1975.

23. Rabinowitz D, Zierler KL: Forearm metabolism in obesity and its response to intra arterial insulin: Characterization of insulin resistance and evidence for adaptive hyper-insulinism. *J Clin Invest* 41:2173, 1962.

24. Wise JK, Hendler R, Felig P: Evaluation of alpha cell function by infusion of alanine in normal diabetic and obese subjects. *N Engl J Med* 288:487, 1973.

25. Parra A, Schultz RB, Graystone JE, et al: Correlative studies in obese children and adolescents concerning body composition and plasma insulin and growth hormone levels. *Pediatr Res* 5:605, 1971.

26. Scriba PC, Bauer M, Emmert D, Fateh-Hoghadon A, et al: Effects of obesity, total fasting and realimentation on T_4, T_3, RT_3, TBG, cortisol, thyrothropin, CBC, transferrin, alpha haptoglobin and C_3 in serum. *Acta Endocrinol* 91:629, 1979.

27. Vanden Brande JL, Du Caju MVL: Plasma somatomedin activity in children with growth disturbances, in S Raiti (ed): *Advances in Human Growth Hormone Research.* DHEW Publ (NIH) 75:612, Bethesda, Md, 1974, p 103.

28. Forbes GB: Lean body mass and fat in obese children. *Pediatrics* 34:308, 1964.

29. *Build and Blood Pressure Studies, 1957,* vol 1. Chicago, Society of Actuaries, 1959.

30. Kannel WB, Pearson G, McNamara PM: Obesity as a force of morbidity and mortality in adolescence, in Heald FP (ed): *Adolescent Nutrition and Growth.* New York, Appleton-Century-Crofts, 1969, p 51.

31. Mann GV: The influence of obesity on health (second of two parts): Coronary heart disease. *N Engl J Med* 291:226, 1974.

32. Kannel WB, Gordon T: Physiological and medical concomitants of obesity: The Framingham Study, in Bray GA (ed): *Obesity in America,* NIH Publication 79-359, 1979, p 125.

33. Garrison RY, Wilson PW, Castelli WP, et al: Obesity and lipoprotein cholesterol in Framingham offspring study. *Metabolism* 29:1053, 1980.

34. *Obesity and Health.* US Department of Health Education and Welfare, US Public Health Service, 1977, p 23.

35. Council on Foods and Nutrition, American Medical Association: I. A critique of low carbohydrate ketogenic weight reduction regimens: A review of Dr. Atkins' diet revolution. *JAMA* 224:1415, 1973.

36. Genuth SM, Castro JH, Vertes V: Weight reduction in obesity by outpatient semistarvation. *JAMA* 230:987, 1974.

37. Bistrian BR, Blackburn GL, Stanbury JB: Metabolic aspects of a protein-sparing modified fast in the dietary management of Prader-Willi obesity. *N Engl J Med* 296:774, 1977.

38. Linn R, Stuart SL: *The Last Chance Diet.* New York, Bantam Books Inc, 1976.

39. Isner JM, Sours HE, Paris Al, et al: Sudden, unexpected death in avid dieters using the liquid protein modified fast diet: Observations in 17 patients and the role of the prolonged QT interval. *Circulation* 60:1401, 1979.

40. *Facts About Obesity.* Washington, DC, National Institutes of Health, 1976.

41. Wheeler ME, Hess KW: Treatment of juvenile obesity by successive approximation control of eating. *J Behav Ther Exp Psychiatry* 7:235, 1976.

42. Kingsley RG, Shapiro J: A comparison of three behavioral programs for the control of obesity in children. *Behav Res Ther* 8:30, 1977.

43. Aragona J, Cassady J, Drabman RS: Treating overweight through parental training and contingency contracting. *J Appl Behav Anal* 8:269, 1975.

44. Epstein LH, Parker L, McCoy JF, et al: Descriptive analysis of eating regulation in obese and nonobese children. *J Appl Behav Anal* 7:402, 1976.
45. Bellack AS, Rozensky R, Schwartz J: A comparison of two forms of self-monitoring in a behavioral weight reduction program. *Behav Res Ther* 5:523, 1974.
46. Mason EE, Ito C: Gastric bypass. *Ann Surg* 170:329, 1969.
47. Soper RT, Mason EE, Printen KJ, et al: Gastric bypass for morbid obesity in children and adolescents. *J Pediatr Surg* 10:51, 1975.
48. Simeons ATW: Action of chorionic gonadotrophin in obese. *Lancet* 2:946, 1954.
49. Lebon P: Action of chorionic gonadotrophin in obese. *Lancet* 2:268, 1961.
50. Asher WL, Harper HW: Effect of human-chorionic gonadotrophin on weight loss, hunger, and feeling of well-being. *Am J Clin Nutr* 26:211, 1973.
51. Food and Drug Administration: *Federal Register* 39:42397 (Dec 5) 1974.
52. Wittenbom JR, Weber ESP, Brown M: Niacin in long-term treatment of schizophrenia. *Arch Gen Psychiatry* 28:308, 1973.
53. Counts SJ, Baylink DJ, Shen FH, et al: Vitamin D intoxication in an anephric child. *Ann Intern Med* 82:196, 1975.
54. Brumbaugh PF, Haussler MR: 1,25-Dihydroxy-vitamin D_3 receptor: Competitive binding of vitamin D analogs. *Life Sci* 13:1737, 1973.
55. Miller JZ, Nance WE, Norton JA, et al: Therapeutic effect of vitamin C: A co-twin control study of the effects of vitamin C. *Prog Clin Biol Res* 24:151, 1978.
56. Herbert A, Jacob E: Destruction of vitamin B_{12} by ascorbic acid. *JAMA* 230:241, 1974.
57. Report of Committee on Nutrition: Vitamin K compounds and the water-soluble analogues use in therapy and prophylaxis in pediatrics. *Pediatrics* 28:501, 1961.
58. Salmon MA, Wright T: Chronic copper poisoning presenting as pink disease. *Arch Dis Child* 42:108, 1971.
59. Walker Smith JA, Blomfield J: Wilson's disease or chronic copper poisoning? *Arch Dis Child* 48:476, 1973.
60. Hodge HC, Smith FA: Some public health aspects of water fluoridation, in Shaw JH (ed): *Floridation as a Public Health Measure.* Washington, DC, American Association for the Advancement of Science, 1954, p 76.
61. Dean HT: The investigation of physiological effects by the epidemiological method, in Moulton FR (ed): *Flourine and Dental Health,* Am Assoc Adv Sci Publ No 19. Washington DC, 1942, p 23.
62. Hadjimarkos D: Selenium and dental caries susceptibility. *J Nutr* 103:1634, 1973.
63. Finberg L, Kiley J, Luttrell CN: Mass-accidental salt poisoning in infancy. *JAMA* 184:187, 1963.
64. Allen FM: Treatment of kidney diseases and high blood pressure. Morristown, NJ, *The Physiatric Institute,* 1925.
65. Tobian L: The relationship of salt to hypertension. *Am J Clin Nutr* 32:2739, 1979.
66. Dahl LK: Salt in processed baby foods. *Am J Clin Nutr* 21:787, 1968.
67. Kagan BM, Felix N, Molander CW, et al: Body water changes in relation to nutrition of premature infants. *Ann NY Acad Sci* 110:830, 1963.
68. Lipsitz PJ: The clinical and biochemical effects of excess magnesium. *Pediatrics* 47:50, 1971.
69. Kelly HG, Cross HC, Turton MR, et al: Renal and cardiovascular effects induced by intravenous infusion of magnesium sulfate. *Can Med Assoc J* 82:866, 1960.

13
Nutritional Management of Inborn Errors of Metabolism

AMINO ACID METABOLISM
Phenylketonuria (PKU)
Manifestations, Diagnosis and Treatment
Urea Cycle Enzyme Deficiencies
Manifestations, Diagnosis and Treatment
Organic Acidemias (Ketotic Hyperglycinemias)
Manifestations, Diagnosis and Treatment
Maple Sugar Urine Disease (MSUD)
Manifestations, Diagnosis and Treatment
Cystinuria
Manifestations, Diagnosis and Treatment
Homocystinuria
Manifestations, Diagnosis and Treatment
Hereditary Tyrosinemia
Manifestations, Diagnosis and Treatment
Hartnup's Disease
Manifestations, Diagnosis and Treatment
Hyperornithinemia
Manifestations, Diagnosis and Treatment
Lysinuric Protein Intolerance (Hyperdibasicaminoaciduria)
Manifestations, Diagnosis and Treatment
Hyperlactatemia
Diagnosis and Treatment

CARBOHYDRATE METABOLISM
Diabetes Mellitus
Overview
Control of Hyperglycemia and Prognosis
Dietary Management
Procedure for Planning the Measured Diet

Most inborn errors of metabolism are caused by deficiency of an enzyme protein that either is missing or, more commonly, is nonfunctioning because of a structural mutation. Deficient function can also be caused by absence or abnormality of a cofactor (coenzyme) necessary for enzyme function. Enzyme substrate, which may be toxic, accumulates as a result of the deficiency. Alternately, lack of enzyme products may cause disease in cases where the product is vital to normal function of the organism.

Since 1908, when Sir Archibald Garrod (1) described the first inborn errors of metabolism, many new disorders have been recognized, largely due to the development of new diagnostic techniques. Paper chromatography was the method that led to the detection of the largest number of disorders. The approach has been used in mass screening programs, which subsequently produced invaluable information on the incidence of inborn errors and their significance as a cause of disease. Some of these disorders turned out to be far more common than they were thought to be originally, while others, once considered the cause of symptoms, are now recognized as benign. Mass screening also facilitated early detection of inborn errors, which is necessary for treatment to be successful.

A significant number of once hopeless cases can now be treated. Dietary manipulation is still the most commonly used and the most successful treatment modality. One objective is the decrease of enzyme substrate in disorders where its accumulation is believed to be toxic. This can be accomplished by reducing the intake of a nutrient that is the precursor of the substrate, providing the organism cannot synthesize the substrate. Galactosemia, fructose intolerance, and phenylketonuria are examples of diseases where the omission or decreased intake of a single nutrient leads to complete recovery. In other disorders, therapy is aimed at the substitution of the deficient enzyme product. Hypoglycemia, caused by a block in the gluconeogenic pathway, and glycogen storage disease type I are examples of diseases where substitution therapy is effective. Only a few disorders of lipid metabolism lend themselves to these treatment approaches. Enzyme replacement and organ transplants are more promising avenues of therapy for this group of disorders.

Basic knowledge concerning the toxicity of accumulating metabolites, mainly amino acids, was originally not available and is still incomplete in many instances. Experience in the treatment of inborn errors through dietary manipulation has improved understanding, but because of the rarity of these disorders, large gaps in knowledge persist. Anyone who attempts to treat inborn errors should be cognizant of the limitations in knowledge and must respect the potential dangers of dietary manipulations. Infant formulas from which one or more amino acids are omitted have been used successfully in the treatment of aminoacidopathies. However, excessive restriction of a nutrient that is necessary for growth is a risk of therapy, as evidenced by early experiences in the treatment of PKU, when complete restriction of phenylalanine caused mental deficit. It should be realized that minimum amino acid requirements in patients with an enzyme block are not equivalent to minimum normal requirements, and that recommendations are often based on single case experiences. Another pitfall relates to the tendency to place undue emphasis on maintaining normal plasma concentration of the metabolite in question although it is often not known whether this metabolite is indeed the offending one. An example is congenital lactic acidemia. Misinterpretation of treatment effects is probably the most common mistake made, one that leads to false hopes for the parents and imitation of the treatment by other physicians. The literature is replete with single case reports, which are necessary but should not be overinterpreted or judged hastily.

The emphasis in this chapter is on inborn errors that are known to cause disease and that are responsive to medical—mainly dietary—management or megavitamin therapy. Only a limited amount of biochemical background data, necessary for the understanding of clinical management, are presented.

AMINO ACID METABOLISM

Phenylketonuria (PKU)

Manifestations

Phenylketonuria (PKU) is the most common aminoacidopathy; incidence less than 1:14,000. The disorder is caused by a lack of activity of the enzyme phenylalanine hydroxylase, which leads to the accumulation of phenylalanine and several of its metabolites—phenylpyruvic, phenyllactic, and phenylacetic acid—as well as phenylacetyl glutamine. There is no certainty yet as to which of these metabolites is toxic to the human brain. Phenylalanine hydroxylase converts phenylalanine to tyrosine, which is consequently decreased. Low tyrosine levels are manifested by a characteristic depigmentation of skin, hair, and eyes. In addition, there is eczema and a musty odor.

Diagnosis

The most reliable diagnostic test is based on the demonstration of elevated phenylalanine levels in blood. A simple screening test, the Guthrie bacterial inhibition assay, has been automated for use in mass screening. It is used in most parts of the United States, Canada, and Europe. The sensitivity of the test is usually adjusted so that a level above 4 mg/dl is considered positive. In response to a survey, showing that 7% of infants with PKU had on the third day of life plasma values between 2 and 4 mg/dl (2), some states have lowered the upper limit of normal and designate levels in excess of 2 mg/dl positive. Unfortunately, this has increased the incidence of false-positive tests. The practicing physician should be aware of the implications of a presumptive "positive" test and of the fact that only 5 to 10% of "positive" infants prove to be classical cases of PKU. The three major disorders other than PKU that may give rise to a positive test are (neonatal) transient mild, hyperphenylalaninemia (HiPhe), persistent mild HiPhe, and transient neonatal tyrosinemia. Making a distinction between the first two is difficult and, for practical purposes of early clinical management, not necessary.

Plasma phenylalanine levels in transient mild HiPhe usually range between 2 and 12 mg/dl, and from 12 to 20 mg/dl in persistent mild PKU. The level considered diagnostic of classical PKU is above 20 mg/dl. Tyrosine is not diagnostic in mild neonatal HiPhe. Mild neonatal HiPhe and neonatal tyrosinemia may be due to immaturity or partial genetic deficiency of metabolizing enzymes—phenylalanine hydroxylase in mild neonatal HiPhe, and *p*-hydroxyphenyl pyruvic acid (*p*HPPA) dioxygenase in transient neonatal tyrosinemia. Manifestations are aggravated by a high protein intake. Treatment with vitamin C and reduction of protein intake will speed reversal of laboratory signs in transient neonatal tyrosinemia.

Approximately 1 to 2% of infants heretofore considered to have classical PKU do not respond to dietary therapy. Their primary defect is reduced synthesis of dihydrobiopterin (3) or tetrahydrobiopterin (4), which is a cofactor necessary for adequate activity of phenylalanine hydroxylase. These children have what was called "malignant" PKU because of progressive CNS dysfunction despite therapy. Failure to recognize, early on, these clinical differences in patients with "hyperphenylalaninemia" has undoubtedly contributed to publicity that PKU programs received originally.

Treatment

In view of the odds favoring a benign condition, parents should be reassured when plasma phenylalanine is below 20 mg/dl, yet encouraged to cooperate fully with follow-up monitoring. While the management of PKU is best conducted at a genetic metabolic center, the local physician can help greatly by assuring dietary compliance and cooperation with the necessary diagnostic procedures. Familiarity with the condition will avoid giving parents conflicting information.

Nutritional management requires restriction of phenylalanine to the required amounts for age, based on body weight (Table 13-1). This is accomplished by use of elemental formulas, made from a casein hydrolysate with very low or no phenylalanine. Lofenalac and Phenyl-Free, both from Mead Johnson & Co., are the products used in the United States. Management of infants is relatively easy in that they may receive as much of this formula (Lofenalac) as any other child, with (1–3 oz) of evaporated milk (double for regular milk) added in order to make up the total requirement for phenylalanine (Table 13-2 and 13-3). The two milks may be mixed together. Addition of protein in amounts that maintain normal phenylalanine levels is crucial, because a phenylalanine-deficient diet is not growth supporting. Provision of calories is important during illness in order to prevent the breakdown of tissues, which may raise phenylalanine concentrations to levels that are injurious to the health of the patient. Hospital admission for the sole purpose of intravenous glucose feeding thus may be required if food is consistently refused during an illness. Infants and children who take pureed or solid foods will get their phenylalanine supplement from these sources, but dietary management becomes more difficult. Parents should be taught how to incorporate the prescribed amount of phenylalanine through using books that list the exact content of commonly used portions of food (5). They are encouraged to let the child choose low phenylalanine foods without too much restriction—making sure, however, that the amount of phenylalanine per day remains within the limits of the prescription. They also should be directed

Table 13-1. Recommended Daily Amino Acid Intakes in Select Aminoacidopathies

	PKU	*Tyrosinemia*	*Homocystinuria Tyrosinemia*	*Maple Sugar Urine Disease*		
Age	*Phenylalanine (11) (mg/kg/day)*	*Tyrosine (mg/kg/day)*	*Methionine (11) (mg/kg/day)*	*Isoleucine*	*Valine (mg/kg/day)*	*Leucine*
0–2 mos.	60–70	60–80 (6)	42	80 (12)	85 (12)	>76 (12)
2–6 mos.	40–60	61–82 (7)	42	80 (12)	85 (12)	>76 (12)
6–12 mos.	30–50	42 (8)	20			
1–4 yrs.	20–30	25–85 (9)	10–23			
4–7 yrs.	15–25	8–50 (10)	10–18			
7–11 yrs.	15–25	25	10–13	30 (11)	45 (11)	33 (11)

Table 13-2. Nutrient Content of Special Formulas[a]

	Lofenalac		*Phenyl-Free*		*MSUD Diet Powder*		*Product 3200 AB*		*Product 3200 K*		*Product 3232 A*	
	per 100 g. powder	*per quart of formula*	*per 100 g. powder*	*per 16 fl. oz. of formula*	*per 100 g. powder*	*per quart of formula*	*per 100 g. powder*	*per quart of formula*	*per 100 g. powder*	*per quart of formula*	*per 100 g. powder*	*per quart of formula*
Kilocalories	460	640	406	400	476	640	460	640	518	640	524	659
Protein, equivalent, g.	15.0	20.8	20.3	20.0	8.2	11.0	15.0	20.8	15.8	19.5	25.0	21.0
Carbohydrate, g.	59.6	82.8	66.0	65.0	63.7	85.1	59.6	82.8	51.1	63.1	34.0	83.0
Fat, g.	18.0	25.5	6.8	6.7	20.1	27.4	18.0	25	28.0	34.6	32.5	27.0
Ash, g.	3.6	5.0	3.8	3.7	2.9	3.8	3.6	5.0	3.0	3.7	5.8	
Caloric Distribution:												
Protein, % of calories	13		20		7		13		12		19	13
Fat, % of calories	35		15		39		35		49		55	50
Carbohydrate, % of calories	52		65		54		52		39		26	37
Essential Amino Acids, g.	1,151	1,600	2,030	2,000	1,190	1,600	1,151	1,600	1,296	1,600	1,916	1,600
Histidine	0.39	0.54	0.47	0.46	0.25	0.34	0.40	0.56	0.38	0.47	0.70	0.58
Isoleucine	0.75	1.04	1.10	1.08	none	none	0.86	1.20	0.76	0.94	1.42	1.19
Leucine	1.41	1.94	1.73	1.70	none	none	1.76	2.45	1.31	1.62	2.32	1.94
Lysine	1.57	2.16	1.89	1.86	0.80	1.08	1.91	2.65	0.98	1.21	2.08	1.74
L-Methionine	0.45	0.62	0.63	0.62	0.25	0.34	0.56	0.78	0.18	0.22	0.68	0.57
Cystine	0.025	0.035	0.35	0.34	0.25	0.34	0.042	0.06	0.11	0.14	0.075	0.063
(Methionine + Cystine)	(0.48)	(0.66)	(0.98)	(0.96)	(0.50)	(0.68)	(0.60)	(0.84)	(0.29)	(0.36)	(0.76)	(0.63)
Phenylalanine	0.08	0.11	0	0	0.55	0.74	0.08	0.11	0.86	1.06	1.18	0.99
Tyrosine	0.81	1.11	0.94	0.93	0.65	0.87	<0.042	<0.06	0.55	0.68	0.45	0.38
(Phenylalanine + Tyrosine)	(0.88)	(1.22)	(0.94)	(0.93)	(1.20)	(1.61)	(<0.12)	(<0.17)	(1.41)	(1.74)	(1.63)	(1.37)
Threonine	0.77	1.06	0.94	0.93	0.55	0.74	0.65	0.90	0.59	0.73	1.08	0.90
Tryptophan	0.19	0.26	0.28	0.28	0.20	0.27	0.20	0.28	0.18	0.22	0.24	0.20
Valine	1.20	1.66	1.26	1.24	none	none	1.28	1.92	0.80	0.99	1.78	1.49
Non-Essential Amino Acids												
Arginine	0.34	0.47	0.69	0.68	0.50	0.67	0.39	0.54	1.08	1.33	0.85	0.71
Alanine	0.64	0.88	0	0	0.45	0.61	0.76	1.06	0.68	0.84	0.82	0.68
Aspartic acid	1.34	1.86	5.20	5.12	1.14	1.53	1.60	2.22	1.94	2.40	1.92	1.60
Glutamic acid	3.78	5.21	1.88	1.85	2.09	2.81	4.31	5.99	3.12	3.85	5.58	4.66
Glycine	0.35	0.48	3.35	3.30	0.60	0.81	0.40	0.56	0.67	0.83	0.55	0.46
Proline	1.13	1.55	0	0	0.90	1.21	1.13	1.52	0.77	0.95	2.55	2.13
Serine	1.02	1.41	0	0	0.60	0.81	1.09	1.52	0.81	1.00	1.30	1.09

[a] *Formula Preparation* (Mead Johnson); Lofenalac (66 cal/dl): add 858 ml water to 139 g powder (phenylketonuria); MSUD formula (66 cal/dl: add 858 ml water to 134.5 g powder (MSUD); Product 300 AB (66 cal/dl): add 858 ml water to 139 g powder (tyrosinemia); Product 300 K (66 cal/dl): add 850 ml water to 123.5 g powder (homocystinuria).

Table 13-3. Essential Amino Acid Requirement and Content of Commonly Used Milks and Formulas[a]

	Histidine	*Isoleucine*	*Leucine*	*Lysine*	*Methionine*	*Cystine*	*Phenylalanine*	*Tyrosine*	*Threonine*	*Tryptophan*	*Valine*
Requirement[b]											
Infant (mg/kg)[c]	16–34	17–126	76–226	90–200	20–36	50	47–94	—	45–87	13–40	65–115
School Child (g/day)	nonessential	1.0	1.0–1.5	1.2–1.6	0.4–0.8	—	0.4–0.8	—	0.8–1.0	0.06–0.12	0.6–0.9
Young Adult (g/day)	"	0.25–0.7	0.17–1.1	0.3–1.2	0.15–1.1	0.1–0.2	0.3–1.1	0.2–0.9	0.1–1.5	0.05–0.25	0.23–0.8
Milk Content (mg/100 kcal)											
Human milk	29	91	133	97	33	29	64	81	57	24	93
Cow's milk	144	345	530	420	133	48	261	271	248	74	371
Enfamil	66	119	222	184	58	20	109	89	102	39	142
Prosobee	78	159	273	203	70	33	173	141	125	44	159
Nutramigen	102	206	328	297	97	11	169	66	153	34	253
Pregestimil	81	166	278	233	84	45	129	70	135	42	205

[a] Values for formula products are derived from Mead Johnson analytical data.

[b] Values are extremes from multiple sources (Ref. 82).

[c] Ref. 27.

to specialty products with low phenylalanine content, such as pastas, starches, breads, potato mixes, and egg replacers. These are currently available through several companies.* In order to have a greater variety of regular foods supply a major portion of both, calories and permissible phenylalanine, older children with PKU may be given Phenyl-Free (100 g diluted with water up to 600 ml contains 66 kcal/100 ml, vitamins, minerals, and 20 g protein with all essential amino acids except phenylalanine).

Calculation of Amino Acid Intake

1. Determine daily allowance of the restricted amino acid, based on age and body weight from Table 13-1.
2. Determine average daily volume of formula that the infant is expected to take.
3. Calculate amount of the restricted amino acid that will be taken by the infant who is given the determined amount of special formula (Table 13-2).
4. Subtract value 3 from value 1 = amount of amino acid that must be supplied from other sources, including infant foods, regular milk, etc.
5. To calculate milk supplement (Table 13-3) in infants on

   phenylalanine restriction: Divide value calculated in step 4 by 1.8 = ml of regular milk supplement.

   methionine restriction: Divide value calculated in step 4 by 0.84 = ml of regular milk supplement.

   tyrosine and methionine restriction (tyrosinemia): see text.

   isoleucine, valine, and leucine restriction (MSUD): need for supplementation should be determined by plasma levels of branched chain amino acids.

   leucine restriction in isovaleric acidemia: Do not exceed normal mean requirements of 150 mg/kg/day; use formulas with low protein content.

When effective dietary treatment is started before 1 month of age and when good control of plasma phenylalanine levels is maintained, patients with classical PKU will grow and develop normally. Controversy exists over the approach to persistent, mild HiPhe. Since these patients have persistent partial enzyme deficiency they may develop intermittently significant elevations of plasma phenylalanine when their protein intake is high. It is thus not surprising that several reports have appeared showing that patients with a seemingly "benign" form of hyperphenylalaninemia or tyrosinemia (13) had slightly decreased IQ levels when tested in later

* General Mills Chemicals, Inc., Minneapolis, Minnesota. Chicago Dietetic Supply, Inc., LaGrange, Illinois. Ener-G-Foods, Inc., Seattle, Washington.

years. Intermittent monitoring of plasma phenylalanine levels after protein loading is advisable in these cases. Some of these patients may require some protein restriction.

Urea Cycle Enzyme Deficiencies

The urea cycle is the major pathway for the removal of ammonia. When carbamylphosphate is formed from ammonia, 1 nitrogen atom enters the urea cycle and is carried to citrulline, which picks up a second nitrogen from aspartate to form argininosuccinic acid (ASA), and then arginine, which splits off urea with its 2 nitrogen atoms. A block due to deficiency of any one of the five urea cycle enzymes causes accumulation of ammonia (Fig. 13-1).

Manifestations

The symptoms of patients with different urea cycle enzymopathies are similar and appear to be the result of hyperammonemia. They consist of feeding difficulties, occasional vomiting, hypotonia, apathy, irritability, tremors, and ultimately convulsions and coma. Manifestations may be severe, with onset soon after birth, or they may occur intermittently. A milder form with insidious onset of mental retardation appears to be the usual manifestation of hyperargininemia although spastic diplegia may develop. *Carbamylphosphate synthetase (CPS) deficiency* tends to be more severe. A wide spectrum of clinical manifestations is seen in *ornithine transcarbamylase (OTC) deficiency*, which is the only X-linked disorder of the

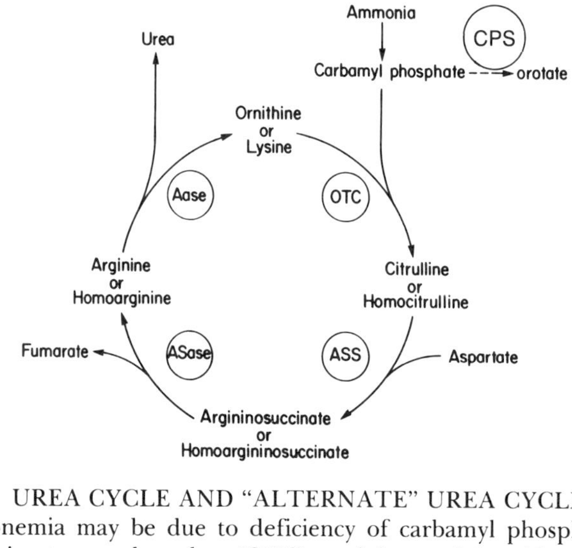

Figure 13-1. UREA CYCLE AND "ALTERNATE" UREA CYCLE
Hyperammonemia may be due to deficiency of carbamyl phosphate synthetase (CPS), ornithine transcarbamylase (OTC), argininosuccinic acid synthetase (ASS), argininosuccinic acid lyase (ASase), or arginase (Aase).

group. This disease is lethal in males, while heterozygous females have variable manifestations, ranging from mild protein intolerance with occasional vomiting or migraine after a high-protein meal to cyclic vomiting and attacks of coma and convulsions.

Diagnosis

Disorders other than the urea cycle enzymopathies that cause hyperammonemia in the newborn period must be excluded. They are transient neonatal hyperammonemia, lysinuric protein intolerance, propionic, methylmalonic and isovaleric acidemia and one form of hyperornithinemia (see below). Metabolic acidosis, associated with a large anion gap, is typical of the organic acidemias, while urea cycle enzymopathies have a normal pH or may be associated with respiratory alkalosis. Three of the urea cycle enzymopathies show in plasma or urine typical elevation of the respective amino acid, as indicated by the name. They are *ASAuria*, *citrullinemia* and *hyperargininemia*. Plasma and urine citrulline may be elevated in ASAuria but to a much lesser degree than in citrullinemia. In hyperargininemia, there is competition at the renal tubular transport site between dibasic amino acids and cystine, which results in a urinary amino acid pattern similar to cystinuria. Urinary orotic acid excretion is high in OTC deficiency because the substrate, carbamylphosphate, is diverted into the pyrimidine pathway, but amino acids of the urea cycle are not increased. CPS deficiency is characterized by hyperammonemia without elevation of either orotic acid or diagnostic amino acids. All hyperammonemias may show, periodically, nonspecific elevations of lysine, glutamine, and, in some cases, glycine and homocitrulline.

Transient neonatal hyperammonemia is not associated with specific amino acid elevation or a known enzyme abnormality. This makes it difficult to distinguish the disorder from OTC and CPS deficiency. Mild metabolic acidosis is common in neonatal hyperammonemia and requires exclusion of the organic acidemias through examination of the urine for organic acids. Early differentiation of the various causes of hyperammonemia in the newborn period is important because treatment varies. Whereas the transient neonatal form responds to nonspecific therapy, some urea cycle enzymopathies call for specific measures. Diagnosis of persistent hyperammonemia requires demonstration of the enzyme defect. Liver is currently the only tissue in which all five defects can be reliably demonstrated.

Treatment

Acute hyperammonemia in infancy requires immediate reduction of protein intake to 0.8 g/kg/day or complete withdrawal in infants unable to take oral feedings. Calories must be supplied, if necessary, by the intravenous route to prevent the need for gluconeogenesis and further accumulation of ammonia from endogenous protein sources. If prolonged nutritional maintenance by the intravenous route is required, an essential amino acid mixture (Nephramine, McGaw Laboratories) may be given to prevent protein catabolism, starting with 0.5 g/kg/day, and supplementing it gradually with oral protein. Peritoneal dialysis is most effective in removing accumulated ammonia in severe cases. Acute therapy of some urea cycle enzymopathies can be managed successfully with infusions of arginine and oral sodium benzoate and/or phenylacetate (see below).

Long-term treatment consisted in the past mainly of protein restriction (Table 13-4), but patients with severe enzyme deficiency did poorly on this regimen. Use of a protein-restricted diet supplemented with essential amino acids (Table 13-5) or nitrogen-free analogues (14) has been attempted and seemed to be promising, because the regimen can promote adequate growth during early infancy (15). Longer observation subsequently showed that this treatment does not prevent sudden occurrence of severe hyperammonemic coma, presumably precipitated by catabolic stress. Thus, a follow-up study indicated that most infants had died before 1 year of age (16). However, the approach should not be abandoned, since the degree of deficiency cannot be predicted in the individual case. A

Table 13-4. Low-Protein Formula Made with Protein-Free Base (Sample calculation for an infant weighing 4.8 kg)

1. Determine desired protein intake, based on body weight.
   Example: 1.2 g/kg = 5.8 g/day
2. Determine desired protein source.
   Example: The standard formula used by the patient contains 0.015 g protein/ml
   Amount of formula allowed = 5.8 ÷ 0.015 = 387 ml; equivalent to 260 kcal
3. Determine desired calorie intake, based on body weight.
   Example: 100 kcal/kg = 480 kcal/day.
4. Determine additional calories needed from protein-free base.
   Example: Use Product 80056 (Mead Johnson), 4.9 kcal/g
   Total calorie allotment (480) minus calories from formula (260) = 220 kcal to be derived from protein-free base.
   220 ÷ 4.9 = 45 g Product 80056 (Mead Johnson)
5. Determine calorie density.
   Example: 24 kcal/30 ml (ounce)
6. Determine total volume needed to make up a formula with above ingredients.
   Example: Total calories per day (480) ÷ 24 (ounces) = 20 (ounces) × 30 ml = 600 ml

Order: Infant Formula: 387 ml
Product 80056: 45 g
Add water to make 600 ml
Mix; feed 100 ml every 4 hours.

Table 13-5. Essential Amino Acid Formula Made from Nephramine

	Nephramine[b] (25 ml)	Enfamil (50 ml)	80056[c] (125 ml)	Total Amino Acids per dl	Total Amino Acids per 100 kcal[d]	Comparison[a] Snyderman [(mg/kg) =	Comparison[a] Batshaw (mg/100 kcal[d])]
Isoleucine, mg	140	39	—	89	131	150	83
Leucine, mg	220	74	—	147	216	190	150
Lysine, mg	160	60	—	110	162	130	127
Lysine acetate	225		—	112	165		
Methionine & cystine, mg	220	19	—				
	<5	6	—	119	175	56	37
Phenylalanine & tyrosine, mg	220	36	—			230	80
		30	—	143	210		
Threonine, mg	100	33	—	66	97	110	73
Tryptophane, mg	50	13	—	31	46	30	27
Valine, mg	160	47	—	104	153	130	70
Histidine, mg	62	11	—				
Calories, kcal	6	33	98	*TOTAL:*	68 kcal/dl		
Protein, g	1.3	0.75	—		1.0 g/dl		
Fat, g	—	1.85	4.5		3.2 g/dl		
Carbohydrate, g	—	3.5	14.2				

[a] SOURCE. ML Batshaw et al: *Johns Hopkins Med J* 148:34, 1981 (17). SE Snyderman et al: *Pediatrics* 56:65, 1975 (mixture no. 2) (14).

[b] Use of Nephramine with product 80056 allows better individual manipulation of calorie and amino acid intake than use of Aminaid (both by McGraw Laboratories).

[c] To 22 g powder, add water to make 125 ml.

[d] The intake of infants, expressed in mg/100 kcal, corresponds roughly to the same intake expressed in mg/kg.

starting dose for total protein intake, including essential amino acids or ketoanalogues, is 1 g/kg/day. Since this amount is not growth promoting in early infancy, higher intakes should be attempted gradually.

Recently, new treatment methods employing alternative pathways for nitrogen waste disposal by use of arginine, sodium benzoate, and phenylacetic acid were proposed and used with some success (17,18). Initial observations suggest that in many cases, mental retardation cannot be prevented even with this approach. However, this can be attributed to irreversible insult sustained during severe neonatal hyperammonemia. Consequently, early recognition and vigorous treatment hold promise of complete recovery. Chronic therapy requires close dietary supervision, dedication, and competent handling on the part of all caretakers.

Treatment with arginine is recommended for ASAuria and citrullinemia. It may be given orally as the free base, mixed with formula or milk, or intravenously on a short term basis as 10% arginine hydrochloride, 600 mg/kg/day, with sodium bicarbonate to prevent acidosis (17). Arginine, with 4 nitrogen atoms, enters the urea cycle and gives off 2 nitrogen atoms as urea. As it is carried through the cycle it picks up 1 nitrogen atom from ammonia and 1 from aspartate until it reaches the block. The accumulating argininosuccinic acid in ASAuria has 4 nitrogen atoms and is readily excreted in the kidney, which results in a net loss of 2 nitrogens. Treatment with arginine is theoretically less effective in citrullinemia, because citrulline is not excreted as readily as argininosuccinic acid and it removes only 1 waste nitrogen molecule. Success of this treatment should be monitored by measuring blood ammonia and plasma amino acids. Arginine and ornithine should be maintained below 200% of the upper normal limit. Plasma levels of ASA and citrulline may rise much higher, but, apparently, they have no adverse effects. Acceptance of these elevations is feasible only if they are indeed accompanied by significant excretion of nitrogen waste and maintenance of normal ammonia levels. Normal renal function is required.

The rationale for use of sodium benzoate and phenylacetate is based on its ability to induce conjugation with glycine and glutamine, respectively, to form hippurate and phenylacetyl glutamine, which are then excreted. Glycine and glutamine are expected to drain off waste nitrogen (18). Sodium benzoate may be given intravenously, 175 mg/kg/day, or orally, 250 mg/kg/day (17). Side effects consist of vomiting and irritability. They develop when the glycine pool decreases and hippuric acid is no longer formed, causing elevation in the level of free plasma benzoate.

The use of Lactulose has been advocated for treatment of hyperammonemia because it is believed to prevent passive diffusion of ammonia from the gut by acidifying the colonic content and converting ammonia into ammonium ions. Its usefulness is questionable, and it is not recommended for infants.

Organic Acidemias (Ketotic Hyperglycinemias)

This group of disorders was originally called ketotic hyperglycinemias, because episodes of ketoacidosis are common and elevation of plasma glycine levels was the only other detectable biochemical abnormality. They are now recognized to be due to several different metabolic defects, which lead to the accumulation of specific organic acids (Table 13-6) in addition to ketone bodies. The incidence is not known because newborn screening programs do not readily detect these disorders. Propionic acidemia and methylmalonic acidemia (MMAemia) appear to be the most common. Recognition is important because a significant number can be effectively treated, thus averting lasting CNS damage or death. MMAemia is one potentially curable organic acidemia that may be more common than is currently realized, because a recent report showed that screening of high-risk infants admitted to a metropolitan hospital with symptoms suggestive of the disease yielded 1 case of MMA per 26 tests (19). According to that series and an earlier literature survey (20), 30% respond to high doses of vitamin B_{12}. Another vitamin, biotin, is potentially curative in multiple carboxylase deficiency. (Chapter 10).

Manifestations

The degree of enzyme deficiency varies in these disorders. In particular, vitamin-responsive forms tend to be less severe, as indicated by experience with MMAemia. Consequently, clinical manifestations range from overwhelming disease in the newborn period, which progresses rapidly to coma and death, to a more chronic episodic illness with onset in the latter part of the first year and sometimes even later. An example of a benign course with onset of symptoms in late childhood is glutaric acidemia, (21). Organic acidemias cause intermittent episodes of ketoacidosis associated with lethargy and vomiting. The vomiting is particularily violent in isovaleric acidemia which is, in addition, marked by a characteristic odor of sweaty feet (22). Any one of these acute episodes can be life-threatening, even in the late onset, milder forms. Repeated episodes may cause irreversible CNS damage and mental retardation. The urine is positive for ketone bodies, and blood pH and CO_2 content are low, with a large anion gap. Occasionally, respiratory overcompensation develops, as evidenced by a slightly elevated pH, low pCO_2, ketosis, and a large anion gap. The central stimulation of respiration and metabolic rate (23), together with vomiting and acidosis, are features that these disorders share with salicylate poisoning. Leukopenia and thrombocytopenia have been described during ketoacidotic attacks of MMAemia, propionic acidemia, and isovaleric acidemia. Pancytopenia also occurs (24). A generalized rash is typical of multiple carboxylase deficiency. Hemolytic anemia occurs in pyroglutamic aciduria (83) manifested sometimes only by reticulocyte elevation.

Table 13-6. Disorders Associated with Organic Aciduria[a]

Disorder (Deficient Enzyme)	*Vitamin to Be Tested (Deficient Cofactor)*	*Precursor*[b] *(To Be Restricted)*	*Diagnostic Urinary Compound*[c]
Propionic Acidemia			
(Propionyl-CoA Carboxylase) (85)	*Biotin* (5–10 mg p.o.)	Isoleucine Threonine Methionine Cholesterol Odd chain FA	methylcitrate[d] 3-hydroxypropionate propionylglycine 3-hydroxyvalerate glycine
Methylmalonic Acidemia (20)			
(Methylmalonyl-CoA Mutase) (Methylmalonyl CoA Racemase) (86)	*Vitamin* B_{12} (1,000 μg) (Adenosylcobalamin) (Adenosyl and methylcobalamin)	All above plus valine and thymine	methylmalonate[d] and glycine; methylmalonate and homocystine
Multiple Carboxylase Deficiency (80)			
(Propionyl-CoA, 3-Methylcrotonyl-CoA and Pyruvate Carboxylase; probably due to deficient holocarboxylase synthetase).	*Biotin* (5–10 mg p.o.)	All above plus leucine and gluconeogenic amino acids	3-methylcrotonylglycine 3-hydroxypropionate 3-hydroxyisovalerate

Isovaleric Acidemia (22)			
(Isovaleryl CoA Dehydrogenase)	None	Leucine	isovalerylglycine[d] 3-hydroxyisovalerate
Glutaric Aciduria (81)			
(Glutaryl-CoA Dehydrogenase)	None	Multiple precursors	glutarate[d] glutaconate 3-hydroxyglutarate
Pyroglutamic Aciduria (83, 89)			
(Glutathione Synthetase, oxoprolinase)	None	Multiple precursors	pyroglutamic acid[d]
Beta-Ketothiolase Deficiency (84)			
(β-ketothiolase)	None known	Isoleucine	2-methylacetoacetate 2-methyl-3-hydroxybutyrate

[a] PKU and MSUD are also associated with organic aciduria but diagnosis does not require gas chromatographic analysis of urine for organic acids.

[b] Restriction of the precursor may be tried in vitamin unresponsive cases.

[c] Organic acids that are inconsistently excreted or present in small amounts are not listed.

[d] Organic acids which are present during remission and acute exacerbations.

Diagnosis (25)
A genetic organic aciduria should be suspected when no cause for ketoacidosis can be found and when protracted vomiting is not attributable to gastroenteritis, or when it is unassociated with alkalosis. Hyperglycinemia with glycinuria is not a reliable diagnostic feature, as it does not occur in all cases (Table 13-6). Mild to moderate hyperammonemia is common during acute episodes of ketoacidosis and should suggest the diagnosis, especially since urea cycle enzyme defects, as a rule, are not associated with ketoacidosis. Reye's syndrome enters the differential diagnosis because of the association of vomiting, hyperammonemia, and occasional elevation in plasma of short chain fatty acids, including propionate and isovalerate. A history of previous attacks and the absence of SGOT elevation speaks against Reye's syndrome. Massive elevation of urinary MMA levels is diagnostic of MMAemia if nutritional B_{12} deficiency can be ruled out, both by serum B_{12} determination and failure to respond to low doses of vitamin B_{12} (100 μg IM per week). Characteristic urinary organic acids are demonstrated by use of gas chromatography. The method is capable of detecting all pathognomonic organic acids (Table 13-6) and numerous other compounds. The test is available through metabolic laboratories, a fact that makes recognition of this group of disorders difficult. MMAemia is currently the only exception, as it can be diagnosed by use of a simple color test that can be made available in clinical laboratories (19). Confirmation of the diagnosis by enzyme analysis in fibroblasts or leukocytes is desirable, although it may not be necessary in typical cases of MMAemia and isovaleric acidemia, because the urinary excretion of massive amounts of MMA and isovalerylglycine, respectively, is diagnostic. Diagnosis of the B_{12}-responsive form of MMA is based on the clinical response to IM doses of 1000 μg. Correlation between clinical response and in vitro B_{12} responsiveness of the enzyme is poor.

Treatment
Trial therapy with pharmacological doses of vitamins (Table 13-6) should be tried in any case with a typical history and biochemical findings. In view of the relatively high incidence of B_{12}-responsive MMAemia, treatment may be tried in critically ill cases even before a firm diagnosis is made, providing diagnostic steps have been initiated (urine for organic acids and serum for B_{12} determination); 200 μg B_{12} may be added to the intravenous infusion, four times per day, or 1000 μg may be given daily IM. If no improvement occurs within 2 to 4 days, it must be assumed that the disorder is not vitamin responsive. This treatment must be accompanied by correction of the acidosis with bicarbonate and intravenous fluid therapy to facilitate excretion of the toxic metabolites. Biotin should be tried in cases with urinary propionate excretion or cases with symptoms of multiple carboxylase deficiency (Table 13-8). To reduce the catabolic

protein load, it is necessary to provide calories during acute episodes in the form of 10% intravenous glucose solution.

With improvement of the ketoacidosis, protein should be added gradually but must be limited to the lowest amount compatible with growth (i.e., 1.5 to 1.8 g/kg/day in the young infant and less with increasing age (0.8 to 1.0 g/kg). Dietary restriction of precursors is currently the only form of therapy available in vitamin-unresponsive forms, except isovaleric acidemia. When the affected organic acid originates from multiple sources (Table 13-6), precursor restriction is nearly impossible. This makes treatment of vitamin-unresponsive MMAemia and propionic acidemia difficult. Severe protein restriction, using only 0.5 to 1.0 g/kg/day, thus may be the only available form of therapy. Leucine restriction has been attempted with apparent success in a 17-day-old infant with isovaleric acidemia by using the formula for MSUD, to which isoleucine and valine were added (26). A formula marketed as a low-leucine product (Wyeth-S14) is not suitable for this purpose because the formula provides only 1.1 g/dl protein and accomplishes the "low" leucine concentration by diluting all amino acids to about 73% of the amount in standard infant formulas. Guidelines on amino acid requirements are not available, as it is difficult to evaluate the response to treatment in disorders that vary in severity from case to case. A new form of therapy was tried in a child with isovaleric acidemia (23,28) which seems to obviate the need for severe protein restriction. Glycine was given orally to induce conjugation of the acid with glycine to form isovaleryl glycine, which is nontoxic and is excreted in the urine. The patient was maintained on 80 to 100 mg/kg every 8 hours (1 teaspoon equals about 2 g). Glycine may be given as a rectal retention anema during episodes of vomiting. Folic acid supplementation is advisable in conjunction with glycine. Chronic alkali therapy is necessary in vitamin unresponsive cases. Bicarbonate (4–6 mEq/kg/d) is preferred; citrate is not tolerated.

Maple Sugar Urine Disease (MSUD)

Three different forms of the disease and one vitamin-responsive variety are known, all caused by deficient oxidative decarboxylation of α-ketoacids, which are the transamination product of the three branched chain amino acids (BCAA)—isoleucine, valine, and leucine. The combined incidence is 1:224,000 live-born infants, according to a recent survey of 9 million neonatal screening tests performed over 12 years (29). Distinction of the three forms is based on differences in the remaining degrative activity of the enzyme, which is usually below 2% of normal in the *severe* form of the disease. The *intermediate* variety, which represents about 25% of cases, is less severe clinically, and the enzyme activity varies from 2 to about 8% (30). This degree of involvement causes mental retardation if untreated.

The biochemical abnormalities of MSUD in plasma and urine are consistently present. By contrast, urine and blood may be normal in the *intermittent* form, but the patients develop on occasion attacks of vomiting, hypoglycemia, and CNS manifestations, similar to those seen in the classical form. BCAA and urinary α-ketoacids are increased during attacks. Enzyme activity is usually greater than 8% and less than 16% of normal (30). This form appears to be rare. Onset is usually during the first year of life, or as late as 8 years of age, when attacks are precipitated by illness. The disorder probably remains undiagnosed in many instances. A fourth variety of MSUD is responsive to thiamine.

Manifestations

In the classical form of the disease, onset is shortly after birth and consists of refusal to eat, vomiting associated with metabolic acidosis, and a peculiar odor that has been described as spicy-sweet and similar to maple sugar or burnt sugar. CNS manifestations are due to neurotoxicity of branched chain keto acids and consist of hypotonia or hypertonicity and opisthotonus, irritability, lethargy, respiratory difficulties, and, ultimately, convulsions and coma. The majority of cases succumb to their disease if untreated. Even with treatment few cases of the severe form escape CNS damage. Treatment holds promise of complete disease prevention if it is begun during the first week of life and able to maintain low plasma concentrations of branched chain α-keto acids. Permanent sequelae consist of retarded motor and intellectual development, abnormal EEG with a tendency to convulsions, and intermittent cerebellar ataxia.

Diagnosis

Newborn screening tests usually employ a simple bacterial inhibition assay, which detects plasma leucine concentrations in excess of 4 mg/dl, a level of sensitivity that should also detect the intermediate variety. Timely detection is necessary but may be impossible when specimens are collected as part of the routine of statewide PKU screening programs. It is therefore advisable in suspicious cases to perform a ferric chloride test, which gives a gray-blue or blue-green color and the equally simple 2,4-dinitrophenylhydrazine test, which forms a yellow precipitate in the presence of increased α-keto acids. Abnormalities detected with these screening tests should be followed by quantitative amino acid determination, which shows elevation of BCAA and alloisoleucine. In partial enzyme deficiency, quantitative amino acid analysis of blood may not show significant abnormality unless it is obtained 3 to 4 hours after a meal. Confirmation of the diagnosis requires measurement of the enzyme in white blood cells or fibroblasts. In atypical cases with high BCAA, deficiency of dihydrolipoyl dehydrogenase should be ruled out. This enzyme forms a cofactor that is necessary for the activity of branched chain ketoacid dehydrogenase and two other dehydrogenases. The disorder is rare, and manifestations are different from those of MSUD (31).

Treatment

Treatment of suspected cases should begin with the reduction of protein intake to minimum requirements, 0.8 to 1.2 mg/kg/day, and the provision of adequate calories to lower endogenous protein catabolism. This may require intravenous alimentation with 10% glucose and intralipid. If there is significant neurological involvement, peritoneal dialysis is indicated. Continued treatment requires limitation of BCAA through the use of MSUD-Formula (Mead Johnson). Close adherence to minimum recommended intakes, based on body weight (Table 13-2), is necessary to prevent the insidious development of mental retardation. This requires careful supervision by a dietitian and intelligent cooperation of the parents. Plasma levels of BCAA should be monitored frequently. The restrictive diet must be maintained throughout life. Trial therapy with thiamine is justified, 10–50 mg/day.

Cystinuria

Manifestations

This disorder is caused by an inherited transport defect of renal tubular and intestinal mucosal cells. The trait causes increased urinary excretion of cystine, lysine, arginine, and ornithine and decreased intestinal absorption of these four amino acids (type I). Inheritance is autosomal recessive. Based on differences in intestinal absorption, three types have been identified. Clinical significance of the disorder relates to the risk of forming renal stones. Failure to treat homozygotes on a chronic basis invariably leads to stone formation and renal failure. Heterozygotes of types II and III excrete moderate amounts of cystine and are at risk of forming stones if the amount of cystine excreted exceeds 1,000 μmoles/g creatinine (25).

Diagnosis

The disorder can be detected by use of a simple urine screening test based on the nitroprusside reaction. Recognition of the disorder is difficult in the newborn period, because normal infants also excrete cystine and lysine up to 6 months of age. Reevaluation of an infant with a positive screen and of the parents therefore should be conducted after 6 months. Diagnosis requires exclusion of hyperargininemia and hyperornithinemia through measurement of plasma amino acids. In these cases, overflow aminoaciduria causes competition at the transport site with excretion of cystine and possibly one or more of the other dibasic amino acids. Since citrulline may be increased in the urine of patients who are homozygous for cystinuria, citrullinemia must also be ruled out using plasma amino acid determination. Patients with hyperdibasic aminoaciduria excrete lysine, arginine, and ornithine and are not at risk of renal stone formation.

Treatment

Since fecal and urinary losses of the four amino acids are tolerated without adverse effects on growth, prevention of renal stone formation is the major goal of therapy. This can be achieved by keeping the urinary cystine concentration below saturation. One way to accomplish this is to decrease the amount of cystine that requires excretion. An alternate way consists of an increase in fluid intake to maintain a high urine volume. The reduction of cystine excretion by limiting dietary protein and methionine has met with variable success, especially in infants who require protein for growth. Fluid therapy apparently is often not successful because it requires large amounts of water and continuous administration throughout the 24-hour period. Dent (32) recommends that adults consume at least 4 and optimally up to 7 l of fluid per day, including 500 ml at bedtime and 500 ml at 2 A.M. Adequacy of fluid intake can be monitored by keeping specific gravity below 1,010. Finally, the solubility of cystine can be raised by alkalinization, using both dietary alkalinization (Table 13-7) and oral sodium bicarbonate therapy. To be effective, urine pH must be kept above 7.5 throughout the day. Penicillamine has been recommended but is not without risk. It lowers cystine excretion by forming penicillamine–cysteine mixed disulfide.

Homocystinuria

This disorder of sulfur amino acid excretion is a manifestation of four different enzyme abnormalities. Two abnormalities affect the degradation of homocysteine to cystathionine, a step that requires vitamin B_6. One of these two is a pyridoxine-responsive disorder seen in roughly 50% of cases. Marked hypermethioninemia is characteristic of both types. Two other, rare abnormalities affect cofactors involved in the remethylation of homocysteine to methionine—folate and vitamin B_{12} (Figure 10-2).

Manifestations

Symptoms of cystathionine synthase deficiency are characteristic. They affect the ocular, cardiovascular and skeletal systems, and the skin, causing mottling and malar flush. Arachnodactyly and dislocation of the lenses, usually bilateral, are the best known abnormalities. Other eye manifestations are myopia, retinal detachment, and secondary glaucoma. Skeletal defects include genu valgus, pes cavus or planus, pectus excavatum or carinatum, scoliosis, and contractures. The most serious manifestations are thromboembolic phenomena, which are responsible for a wide variety of neurological complications. This abnormality is due to increased platelet stickiness. It is not known whether a deficiency of cystine or cystathionine

Table 13-7. Effect of Foods on Urinary pH.

Acid-Producing	*Alkali-Producing*	*Neutral*
Bread	Milk	Butter
Cereals	Fruits	Candy, not chocolate
Cheese	Vegetables	Coffee
Corn	ESPECIALLY:	Cornstarch
Crackers	Almonds	Fats, cooking
Cranberries	Apricots, dried	Honey
Eggs	Beans, Lima, Navy	Lard
Lentils	Beet Greens	Salad Oils
Macaroni, Spaghetti, Noodles	Chard	Sugar
Meat, Fish, Poultry	Dandelion Greens	Tapioca
Pastries	Dates	Tea
Peanuts	Figs	
Plums	Molasses	
Prunes	Olives	
Rice	Peas, dried	
Walnuts	Parsnips	
	Raisins	
	Spinach	
	Watercress	
	Foods that contain Baking Powder or Baking Soda	

is responsible for the mental retardation that occurs in some cases. In contrast to cystathionine synthase deficiency, cases of homocystinuria due to defective remethylation had noncharacteristic clinical manifestations.

Diagnosis

The cyanide nitroprusside reaction is used in a simple urine screening test. A bacterial inhibition assay was incorporated in some mass screening programs that were originally started for the detection of PKU. This assay is considered positive if plasma methionine is above 2 mg/dl. However, the test fails to detect many pyridoxine-responsive cases, presumably because they are milder and the rise in methionine occurs slowly after birth. The nitroprusside test is often negative in affected newborns who may excrete relatively low amounts of homocystine. Consequently, many patients are diagnosed later in life on clinical grounds, mainly because arachnodactyly or eye changes arouse suspicion. Early recognition is important to prevent serious vascular accidents.

Treatment

Dietary treatment is aimed at reducing the elevation of methionine, which results in the increase of homocysteine in plasma and homocystinuria. Either may be the cause of toxicity, because experimental administration of homocysteine to rabbits (33) has produced some of the vascular features. Elevation of the levels of these amino acids could theoretically inhibit transport of other amino acids into the brain. Supplementing the diet with l-cystine has also been recommended (34), but it does not alter the deficiency of cystathionine which may be responsible for the mental retardation. Aside from these theoretical considerations, effectiveness of treatment also remains uncertain because the natural history of the disorder varies and follow-up of a sufficient number of cases is not available for this rare disorder.

A low protein–low methionine diet should be instituted as early as possible, because thrombotic complications occur already during the first year. Although controversy exists over whether adults should adhere to a strict regimen, this would seem advisable since the incidence of vascular disease from other causes increases with age and platelet stickiness can be expected to increase the risk. Adherence to a low-methionine diet (Table 13-2) is relatively easy in infants and small children, who receive most of their protein from milk because a low-methionine formula is now available (3200 K—Mead Johnson). This milk source should be used throughout life for cooking. Food exchange lists are available (35) that may be used for meal planning in adults. The diet excludes animal sources of protein, meat, fish, eggs, and dairy products. Other foods high in methionine, which are not essential and can be avoided, are corn, dried peas and beans, nuts, and spinach. Excessive intake of rice, potatoes, oatmeal, white and whole-wheat flour should also be avoided. Treatment with pyridoxine (300–500 mg/kg/d, by mouth) should always be tried first.

Hereditary Tyrosinemia

Although the disorder is common in a French-Canadian isolate, with an estimated carrier rate of 1 in 20 or 30, it is rare in other areas, where the incidence is probably not higher than 1:500,000. Nevertheless, knowledge of its manifestations is important to the pediatrician because hereditary tyrosinemia enters the differential diagnosis of two disorders that are more common, transient neonatal tyrosinemia (TNT) and hereditary fructose intolerance (HFI). Approximately 0.5 to 1.0% of all newborns and about 25% of premature infants develop elevations of plasma tyrosine. HFI has been estimated to occur in 1:30,000 to 75,000 live newborns, depending on the area. The primary enzyme defect is not known.

Manifestations

Hereditary tyrosinemia manifests itself in two forms: an acute, early onset variety that causes liver failure; and a chronic form with renal disease, clinical signs of Fanconi's syndrome, rickets, and nodular hepatic cirrhosis. Both forms have been reported within the same family. Acute attacks of porphyria may occur at any time in either the acute or chronic disease. It is not known whether all these manifestations are the result of tyrosine toxicity. Acute episodes of liver failure are heralded by vomiting and occasionally by diarrhea. The liver enlarges, and there may be a peculiar cabbagelike odor, attributed to methionine metabolites. Jaundice, splenomegaly, and ascites may develop rapidly, with laboratory signs indicative of massive parenchymal damage. SGOT values may rise above 1000, even in the absence of jaundice. Acute exacerbations are accompanied by multiple clotting factor defects, which tend to be resistant to routine treatment with fresh frozen plasma. Hemorrhagic complications consist of ecchymosis, epistaxis, melena, hematuria, and other internal hemorrhages that may result in sudden demise. The acute form may revert to the chronic disease, but sudden exacerbations with liver failure may occur at any time.

Plasma tyrosine is elevated in both the chronic and acute disease, while methionine shows significant elevations only during acute exacerbations. The tyrosine metabolites, *p*-hydroxyphenyl lactic (*p*HPLA), *p*-hydroxyphenyl pyruvic (*p*HPPA), and *p*-hydroxyphenyl acetic acid (*p*HPAA), are excreted in the urine. They are the cause of a positive reaction by the nitrosonaphthol test, which can be used for screening purposes. In the acute form, α-feto protein (AFP) is elevated in serum, and α-amino levulinic acid (ALA) may appear in the urine.

Diagnosis (25)

It is desirable to make the diagnosis soon after birth in infants at risk, but this is difficult because tyrosine is elevated in TNT. In this disorder, tyrosine peaks in the first or second week of life, but the elevation may persist for several more weeks or longer if the newborn is deficient in vitamin C. TNT is due to transient deficiency of *p*HPPA dioxygenase. Reversal of the tyrosinemia can be hastened by treatment with daily doses of 50 mg vitamin C. AFP is said to be considerably higher in newborns with tyrosinemia than in those with TNT (36).

The differential diagnosis includes HFI if the patient has been exposed to fructose. This disorder is an exact phenocopy of tyrosinemia, providing the amount of fructose ingested is large and persistent enough to have caused liver and/or renal damage. Diagnosis of HFI requires a liver biopsy for measurement of fructose-1-phosphate aldolase activity. However, both, the enzyme and fructose tolerance test may be abnormal during an acute attack of tyrosinemia because this disorder is known to be associated with multiple liver enzyme deficiencies which are nonspecific. Timely diagnosis is further complicated because liver biopsy for enzyme analysis is contraindicated if clotting abnormalities exist. It is therefore advisable to discontinue fructose first and observe the response. If there is improvement of liver functions, a tolerance test may be performed, followed by a liver biopsy for enzyme studies if the test is compatible with HFI. Enzyme studies are inconclusive in tyrosinemia. Nonmetabolic liver diseases may be confused with hereditary tyrosinemia when they are associated with plasma amino acid elevations, including tyrosine. However, in these cases, methionine is rarely elevated to the degree seen in hereditary tyrosinemia. An association with Fanconi's syndrome and renal rickets is not seen in nonmetabolic liver diseases, but requires exclusion of galactosemia, hereditary fructose intolerance, and cystinosis. Isolated tyrosinemia without liver disease requires exclusion of the *Richner–Hanhart Syndrome* (90).

Hereditary tyrosinemia has been attributed to a deficiency of *p*HPPA dioxygenase. However, multiple other deficiencies, including α-amino levulinic acid dehydratase, porphobilinogen synthase, and various enzymes of the transsulfuration pathway, are also present. Deficiency of fumarylacetoacetase was described recently (37). This defect leads to the accumulation of succinylacetoacetate and succinylacetone, two metabolites that inhibit prophobilinogen synthase (38). This secondary defect is probably responsible for the attacks of acute porphyria, which are occasionally observed in these patients.

Treatment

Limitation of tyrosine intake improves both liver and renal manifestations (7-10). Limitation of tyrosine and phenylalanine intake is accomplished through use of an elemental formula designed for treatment of tyrosinemia (3200 AB, Mead Johnson). Phenylalanine must be restricted because it is converted into tyrosine. However, since the methionine content of 3200 AB is unusually high, it may be advantageous to use a combination of 3200 AB and a low-methionine formula, 3200 K (Table 13-2). This recommendation is supported by observations of rats who developed a condition similar to tyrosinemia on a high intake of methionine (39). A patient with hereditary tyrosinemia, a direct descendant of the settler who brought the disease into Quebec, was treated successfully in this manner (21). During her first episode of liver failure, plasma methionine was 759.7 μmoles/l (*N:* 15.2 ± 4.8). She was treated exclusively for 1 year with low-methionine 3200 K (Mead Johnson). Methionine dropped to 50.0 within 6 weeks and remained in that range. The patient recovered clinically, although tyrosine remained elevated, 555 μmoles/l (*N:* 54.5 ± 12.9). She was subsequently given low-tyrosine 3200 AB and had another acute liver attack within 4 months. On a mixture of the two formulas, she has remained asymptomatic for 2 years.

Strict adherence to minimum recommended intakes of tyrosine is probably not essential if the liver disease is stable. Thus, infants may be given the special formula 3200 AB ad libidum, limiting only the total protein intake, which should be kept at 1.8 g/kg/day in infancy and at

RDA values thereafter. Foods to be excluded are meat, cheese, egg, and vegetables with a high tyrosine content, peas, beans, corn, spinach, broccoli, and turnips. Amino acids, SGOT, and clotting time should be monitored. Greater dietary restriction and limitation to the minimum recommended intakes of tyrosine, phenylalanine, and methionine are necessary if the outlined regimen does not maintain amino acids in a near normal range. During exacerbation of the liver disease, no fructose should be given, because the conversion of fructose into glucose constitutes a drain on ATP, which is limited when the methionine level is elevated. It may be advisable to avoid large quantities of fructose on a chronic basis.

Tyrosine restriction in Richner–Hanhart syndrome with 3200 AB is successful in that it reverses the eye and skin lesions.

Hartnup's Disease

This is another genetic disorder that affects both the intestinal and renal tubular transport of a group of amino acids that share a common transport site. They are the monoamine-monocarboxylic amino acids: alanine, serine, threonine, asparagine, glutamine, valine, leucine, isoleucine, phenylalanine, tyrosine, tryptophan, histidine, and citrulline.

Manifestations

Although a large number of amino acids are affected, significant deficiency does not develop except for tryptophan. Thus, there are no signs of generalized protein deficiency, although aminoaciduria is a persistent phenomenon. The manifestations of tryptophan deficiency are attributable to niacin deficiency and include dermatological signs precipitated by exposure to sunlight, diarrhea, and neurological and psychological changes. The defect is more apt to cause disease in infancy, probably because the infant relies to a large extent on tryptophan for the generation of NAD since milk has a relatively low niacin content.

Diagnosis

The specific aminoaciduria is characteristic, although on paper chromatographic tests, an increase of so many amino acids may suggest generalized aminoaciduria. However, quantitative analysis shows that two amino acid groups, which share a common transport site, are not affected. These are cystine, together with the dibasic amino acids, and the imino acids: proline and hydroxyproline with glycine. An oral tryptophan load is diagnostic of the intestinal transport defect when the rise in plasma tryptophan is low. Patients have variable increases of urinary indoleacetic acid and indican, which originate from intestinal bacterial metabolism of tryptophan. The disorder should be distinguished from isolated intestinal malabsorption of tryptophan, known as the "blue diaper syndrome," and from isolated tryptophanuria.

Treatment

Niacin supplementation 50–200 mg/day, is curative, a fact that proves that manifestations in Hartnup's disease are indeed comparable to those of pellagra and are caused by tryptophan deficiency.

Hyperornithinemia

Two different types of hyperornithinemia have been described. One type is associated with hyperammonemia and is probably due to a defect in mitochondrial ornithine transport that causes deficiency of the urea cycle. Clinical manifestations are similar to those of urea cycle enzyme deficiencies. Only three cases have been reported.

The second type is due to a metabolic defect in ornithine metabolism (ornithine-ketoacid transaminase) and is associated with gyrate atrophy of the choroid and retina. This disorder is not associated with hyperammonemia.

Manifestations

A majority of patients described in the literature have been adults. Although onset appears to be in childhood, early manifestations probably remain undected in many cases. Night blindness and loss of peripheral vision are the first complaints. With progressive disease there is development of cataracts, myopia and ultimately total blindness. Chorioretinal atrophy is distributed circumferentially around the fundus, extending in extreme cases up to the optic disk. The rapidity of disease progression varies greatly, possibly as a function of protein intake and hyperornithinemia. Objective records of the dysfunction can be obtained by measuring electroretinographic responses and dark adaptation. Delayed growth and development have been described. Speech appears to be more affected than motor development. The youngest observed case was 11 months old (21). Although asymptomatic, eye ground changes were already present, consisting of a thinned retina and granular appearance of the otherwise normal pigment in the area that becomes characteristically involved.

Diagnosis

Plasma ornithine levels show a 10–20 fold increase and there is overflow hyperornithinuria. The increase of ornithine in cerebral spinal fluid and the aequeous humor of the eye is of similar magnitude. Since ornithine competes for the renal tubular absorption site with cystine and the dibasic amino acids, an increased excretion of cystine, lysine and arginine may be found. Confirmation of the diagnosis requires demonstration of the enzyme defect in skin fibroblasts.

Treatment
A moderate decrease of plasma ornithine can be accomplished by limiting dietary protein, especially in patients who have been on high protein intakes. Since arginine is a precursor of ornithine and since arginine but not ornithine is a constituent of food protein, dietary restriction of both, protein and arginine has been attempted with some success (87). Some patients respond to treatment with high doses of vitamin B_6, 200–400 mg/day (88). Thus, a decrease of plasma ornithine to levels 2–3 times the upper limit of normal can be accomplished with little inconvenience to the patient. Improvement of electroretinographic abnormality may be observed in responsive patients already after a brief period of therapy. Treatment is life long. Early detection is important, because atrophy of the retina is irreversible.

Lysinuric Protein Intolerance (Hyperdibasicaminoaciduria).

Although rare, this disease gains importance to the pediatrician because it is associated with hyperammonemia. The disorder is due to a transport defect that affects intestinal absorption and renal tubular reabsorption of dibasic amino acids, lysine, arginine, and ornithine. There are indications that impaired urea cycle function is a direct result of intracellular arginine and ornithine depletion. The severity of the deficiency is probably related to both, decreased absorption and increased urinary losses of these amino acids. Intestinal loading with dibasic amino acids may precipitate diarrhea.

Manifestations
Affected infants thrive fairly well on breast milk. However, when they are switched to cow's milk, they tend to develop diarrhea and vomiting. Blood ammonia levels rise because of the higher protein content of cow's milk. They develop an aversion to protein-containing foods, which contributes to the failure to thrive. A variety of other manifestations, which may be unrelated to the metabolic defect, have been reported, including eye fundus pigmentation, lens opacities and hyperelasticity of the skin and joints. Manifestations, such as ataxia and convulsions, appear to be a direct result of hyperammonemia. Hepato-splenomegaly and muscle weakness also occur.

Diagnosis
Increased urinary excretion of the three dibasic amino acids is characteristic. Urinary orotic acid is also increased. An elevation of cystine may be present, but it is very mild compared to cystinuria. The finding of normal plasma amino acids rules out overflow aminoacidurias. An intravenous l-alanine load (500–600 mg/kg over 90 minutes) precipitates hyperammonemia, but addition of arginine or ornithine to the load prevents the rise (40). Citrulline may have the same effect.

Treatment
Substitution of the two deficient amino acids, arginine and ornithine, is the major objective of therapy. Although oral arginine and ornithine supplementation has been used with some success, their absorption may be insufficient. Treatment with citrulline should be tried in these cases, with and without lysine (41).

Hyperlactatemia

Hyperlactatemia, with or without acidosis, is a cardinal feature of several genetic metabolic diseases, including the enzyme deficiencies listed in Table 13-8. It has been described in a variety of movement disorders, such as cerebellar ataxia, and in periodic paralysis. It is also seen in infants with nonspecific neurological manifestations associated with hypotonia. These ill-defined disorders are sometimes referred to as congenital lactic acidosis. Onset may be soon after birth, in which case the clinical course is rapidly progressive, or the disease begins during the first few years of life and is slowly progressive, with intermittent or acute exacerbations. Mild intermittent lactate elevations are also a feature of two well-defined genetic syndromes that are probably caused by an enzyme defect: Leigh's subacute necrotizing encephalopathy (see genetic vitamin B_1 deficiency) and oculocraniosomatic neuromuscular disease or Kearns-Shy syndrome. Tolerance tests with specific nutrients are used in the diagnosis of many of these disorders (Table 13-8). Dietary or vitamin therapy are of help in some types and may be tried even before a diagnosis has been made through positive identification of an enzyme defect, because the response is used as guide in the identification of the enzyme defect. A working knowledge of this complex group of disorders is therefore helpful for the pediatrician who must attempt to gain time through trial therapy until a diagnosis can be made, a process that is usually difficult and time-consuming.

Diagnosis
Diagnosis rests upon the demonstration that hyperlactatemia is indeed caused by a primary disease process and is not an artifact of sample collection or due to transient hypoxemia. Whereas the normal range of plasma lactate is between 4 and 13 mg/dl, values up to 20 mg/dl are not unusual in venous blood samples of normal infants—even when blood is collected without a tourniquet—because crying, hyperventilation, breath holding, and muscle tension cannot be avoided. The lactate/pyruvate ratio helps to identify the cause of the hyperlactatemia. Whereas the normal ratio is low, infants have a ratio of up to 20 because of the often unavoidable artifact of sample collection. The ratio is markedly elevated in hypoxemia, ischemia, or circulatory failure. Severalfold lactate elevations and ratios above 20 occur in acute respiratory failure, following shock,

and with strenuous exercise. A metabolic defect that may be responsive to dietary therapy should be suspected if hypoxia and hyperventilation have been ruled out and there is (*1*) an elevation of pyruvate, (*2*) an elevation of alanine, or (*3*) a history of hypoglycemia. Table 13-8 lists the major manifestations of genetic metabolic diseases associated with hyperlactatemia. (The more common defects are discussed in detail in the appropriate section under aminoacidopathies and disorders of carbohydrate metabolism.)

Figure 13-2 shows the position of lactate in metabolic reactions that are central to the generation of energy substrate. Tolerance tests may provide clues to the possible cause of hyperlactatemia (Table 13-8), but they are not diagnostic and therefore require confirmation by enzyme analysis.

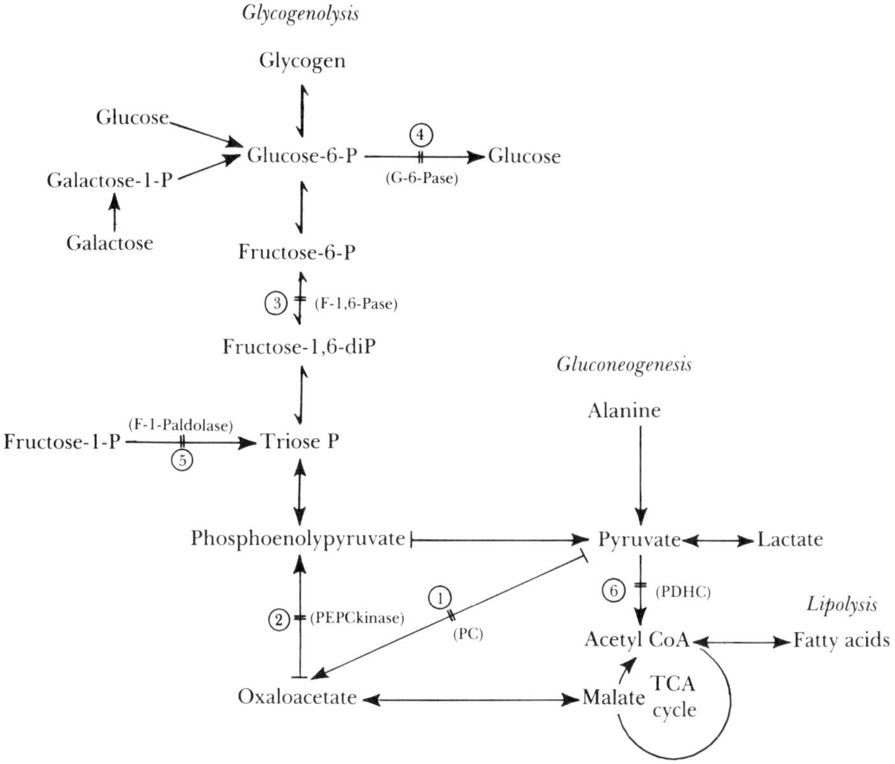

Figure 13-2. DIAGRAM OF THREE MAJOR PATHWAYS AFFECTED BY INBORN ERRORS, CAUSING HYPERLACTATEMIA
Six metabolic steps are indicated, which involve enzymes for which defects have been described that cause hyperlactatemia: (*1*) pyruvate carboxylase, (*2*) phosphoenolpyruvate carboxykinase, (*3*) fructose-1,6-diphosphatase, (*4*) glucose-6-phosphatase, (*5*) fructose-1-phosphatealdolase, and (*6*) pyruvate dehydrogenase complex.

Table 13-8. Diagnosis of Hyperlactatemia by Use of Nutrient-Related Tests

Defect	*Major Manifestation*	*Nutrient-Related Tests*
Gluconeogenic Enzyme Defect	Fasting hypoglycemia and acidosis	Fasting causes hypoglycemia and hyperlactatemia
Pyruvate carboxylase[a]	Fatty liver, enlarged	
Phosphoenolpyruvate carboxykinase	Fatty liver, enlarged	
Fructose-1,6-diphosphatase		Fructose and glycerol cause hypophosphatemia, and hyperlactatemia
Excessive Glycogenolysis		
Glycogen storage disease I (Glucose-6-phosphatase)	Hepatomegaly, nonicteric	Galactose causes hyperlactatemia and is not converted to glucose
Pyruvate Utilization Defect		
Pyruvate dehydrogenase complex (E_1, E_2, E_3) α-ketoglutarate dehydrogenase complex (E_3)	Psychomotor retardation and ataxia	Glucose causes hyperlactatemia; ketogenic diet may decrease hyperlactatemia
Deficient Lactate Excretion		
Hereditary Fructose Intolerance (Fructose-1-P aldolase)	Vomiting Hepatorenal disease	Fructose causes hypoglycemia and hypophosphatemia
Aminoacidopathies		
Organic acidemias[a]	Intermittent acidosis	Protein load causes exacerbation (see table 13-6)
Methylmalonic acidemia	Hyperglycinemia	
Propionic acidemia	Hyperglycinemia	
Isovaleric acidemia	Sweaty smell	
Multiple carboxylase deficiency	Alopecia and erythematous rash	

[a] See also Table 13-6.

Treatment

The metabolic pathways and the result of tolerance tests provide the rationale for dietary therapy. It is obvious that the nutrient that causes exacerabation upon challenge should be omitted from the diet. Thus, either fructose or galactose or both must be omitted in some disorders. The need for gluconeogenesis after a prolonged fast must be avoided in others. In glucose-6-phosphatase deficiency, frequent feeding of starchy foods prevents excessive glycolysis. A block in pyruvate utilization due to pyruvate dehydrogenase complex deficiency can be circumvented by using fat, about 66% of total calories, as substrate for the TCA cycle. Other dietary measures are discussed in more detail in the sections covering the respective diseases. A ketogenic diet (Table 7-1) may be tried in patients who respond to a glucose load with hyperlactatemia. However, lactate must be monitored accurately and repeatedly, both before and after the diet change. There is also justification for the use of thiamine, which is a cofactor for the pyruvate dehydrogenase complex, (50–100 mg), and of biotin (5–10 mg), the cofactor of pyruvate carboxylase. Improvement after pharmacological doses of thiamine has been reported in cases with pyruvate carboxylase deficiency, presumably because it "opened up" the pathway from pyruvate to acetyl-CoA as an alternate route.

CARBOHYDRATE METABOLISM

Diabetes Mellitus

Overview

Diabetes mellitus is a disorder of energy metabolism due to deficient insulin activity. In early onset disease, either insulin release is impaired or there is a complete shutdown of insulin production. By contrast, insulin is released, but appears to be ineffective in maturity onset diabetes. In either disorder there is hyperglycemia and "overflow" glucosuria. Ketoacidosis and coma develop in untreated cases. Insulin deprivation prevents transport of glucose into the cell, increases lipolysis, and promotes protein breakdown. Ketosis results when the rate of lipolysis exceeds the need for fatty acids.

Plasma insulin levels are low in juvenile onset diabetes and normal or high in maturity onset diabetes. The corresponding alternate names for these two entities are "insulin-dependent" (IDDM) and "nondependent" diabetes mellitus. The recent observation of children with congenital rubella, who develop diabetes by the time they reach puberty, suggests that viral infections are one cause of IDDM. An autoimmune mechanism is implicated by the demonstration of specific antibodies against islet cells in certain types of diabetes mellitus (42). A familial incidence, which has been recognized for some time, probably reflects a genetic disposition to develop immunodeficiency diseases. Recently, strong evidence has been presented indicating linkage of IDDM to gene loci of the histocompatibility (HL-A) system (43).

A high intake of sucrose and other carbohydrates was once considered a contributing factor in the development of diabetes. In the past, this has been disproven, both in population studies and among individuals within a given population. However, an association between obesity and the incidence of maturity onset diabetes has been confirmed. The mechanism responsible for the development of insulin insensitivity is not known. By contrast, IDDM is not diet related. Onset may be gradual in IDDM, but in the majority of cases it is sudden, often precipitated by an infection.

Ketoacidosis is a common complication in IDDM, whereas it is uncommon in maturity onset diabetes. After treatment of the initial attack, there may be some return of β-cell function in IDDM, associated with a decrease of insulin requirements. Inevitably, however, insulin dose must be stepped up again, especially with stress and during periods of rapid growth. Complications may develop as early as a decade after the onset of IDDM. These complications consist of hypertension, retinopathy, neuropathy, kidney disease, and myocardial infarcts.

Control of Hyperglycemia and Prognosis

Whether the late complications of IDDM are due to poor control of hyperglycemia and other metabolic consequences of diabetes mellitus or to independent genetic factors is not known and has been the subject of controversy. New data suggest that control of hyperglycemia is important in preventing these complications. One such piece of evidence is the finding of high sorbitol concentrations in the lens of the eyes and in peripheral nerves of experimental diabetic animals (44). Accumulation of this sugar alcohol appears to be related to increased glucose concentrations in extracellular fluid. It is of interest in this context that the late manifestations of diabetes affect tissues that do not require insulin for glucose entry into the cells and therefore may be injured by high concentrations of glucose.

Another important observation in favor of strict blood sugar control is the demonstration of excessive protein glycosylation secondary to hyperglycemia (45). A glycosylated hemoglobin derivative (Hg A_{Ic}) was shown to be a good indicator of blood sugar control. Since Hg A_{Ic} has greater affinity for oxygen than normal hemoglobin, tissue hypoxia could be the factor in diabetes mellitus that contributes to the development of microangiopathy. Evidence is thus strong that microangiopathy is a consequence of poor control. By contrast, atherosclerosis is influenced by many other risk factors that make it difficult to prove a relationship with the degree of diabetes control. Hyperlipidemia is one recognized risk factor of atherosclerosis that is present in diabetes mellitus when hyperglycemia is poorly controlled. Hyperlipidemia, in turn, causes platelet stickiness. Both blood lipids and platelet function have been implicated in the pathogenesis of atherosclerotic vascular disease. Actual proof that better control prevents complications is difficult to obtain in humans. Evidence from animal experiments is fairly conclusive, however, and there are new human data showing that the degree and duration of hyperglycemia are related to the incidence of neuropathy, microangiopathy, and retinopathy (46).

Dietary Management

The goal of therapy in children with diabetes mellitus has been defined as follows (47):

1. Control of symptoms caused by hyperglycemia (i.e., polyuria, polydipsia, and polyphagia)
2. Control of ketoacidosis and prevention of hypoglycemia due to insulin overdose
3. Normal somatic and emotional growth and sexual maturation and the leading of a normal life
4. Maintenance of a serum cholesterol level below 210 mg/dl, and an overnight fasting serum triglyceride level of less than 130 mg/dl
5. Achievement of a urine glucose concentration that is generally 1% or less, and a 24-hour urine glucose loss that is below 20 g/m^2 or 7% of the dietary carbohydrate intake

Achievement of these goals in IDDM requires insulin therapy, dietary management, education, and psychological guidance. Ideally, insulin should be injected on a continuous basis and at a changing rate, depending on instantaneous physiological need, as reflected by blood sugar levels. Since this is not yet feasible, patients on home management are given either single or multiple insulin injections. The preferred method is to give two injections, using both short- and intermediate-acting insulin, in hopes that the complementary action of the two will achieve fairly uniform blood sugar levels. Regular insulin begins to work in about 15 to 30 minutes, with maximum activity between 2 and 4 hours; whereas NPH insulin starts to act within 2 and 4 hours, achieves peak activity between 4 and 6 hours, and is no longer effective after 12 to 14 hours. The proportion of each kind of insulin to be used depends on the patient's activity level and eating habits. Since most activity occurs during the day, two-thirds of the total insulin dose should be given in the morning. The dose must be adjusted upward during periods of increased excercise, emotional stress, or infection and downward when food intake decreases.

Since insulin requirements and diet are interrelated, diabetic control obviously depends on both. The choice of diet and strictness of management have been the subject of controversy. Proponents of a free diet claim that the effectiveness of strict control has not been proven to prevent late complications, a claim which is no longer justified.

A "weighed diet" is the strictest form of management and appears unnecessary to this observer. The "unmeasured" (free) diet represents the opposite extreme. It may be used temporarily in children after the diagnosis of IDDM has been made, because the adjustment process is difficult enough without the burden of measuring all food. Young adolescents also tend to rebel against regimentation and will benefit from a more relaxed attitude. Moreover, during an initial period on the unmeasured diet, an opportunity exists to observe the course of the disease, the effectiveness of insulin in the individual case, and the pattern of glucosuria. Since the choice of foods is important, the young patient may have to be reeducated, and since a suitable diet for the diabetic is good dietary practice for healthy individuals as well, it is feasible and helpful to the patient if the entire family participates in the reeducation process.

Simple sugars should be avoided since they are rapidly absorbed and tend to flood the system, causing sudden peaks of hyperglycemia that are unopposed by endogenous insulin. The diet should be calorically adequate but not excessive. Adequacy is best monitored in children by following the growth curve. Animal fats, including butter, should be avoided because they are high in saturated fatty acids. Use of 2% milk is advised. Total intake should be divided into three meals and three between-meal snacks, and each should be offered at regular times. The amount eaten at each meal is allowed to vary with the child's appetite, in the expectation that it is controlled in the psychologically stable child by physiologic need. Assuming that this is the case, insulin requirements should remain fairly constant, providing illness does not adversely affect both the appetite and the need for insulin. Sweets such as candy, orange juice, and cola drinks are advised in the event of prodromal symptoms of hypoglycemia.

The "measured diet" is a compromise between the weighed diet and the unmeasured diet. It still requires considerable attention to detail and knowledge of foods. As young teenagers mature and learn to accept and manage the disease, they should slowly be switched over to this regimen. It is based on an exchange system where foods are divided into six groups (Table 13-9). Measured amounts of the respective foods in each food group have a similar value in calories, carbohydrate, protein, and fat composition, which allows exchange of different foods without tedious calculations. A new revised exchange list was published in 1976 by the American Diabetes Association and the American Dietetic Association.

Procedure for Planning the Measured Diet (Table 13-10)

1. Determine the calorie requirements for age and weight based on RDA (Table 1-2).
2. Choose calorie distribution per day; the following ranges have been recommended: 50 to 55% from carbohydrates, 12 to 20% from protein, and 30 to 35% from fat. Convert these figures into grams per day (see footnote, Table 13-10a).
3. Decide on the number of meals and snacks per day (six are recommended) and the percentage of the total carbohydrate allowance per day to be given at each. This should be guided by the time of day when either sugar is consistently spilled or when hypoglycemia tends to develop (Table 13-10a).
4. Select the number of allowed exchanges per day, which is determined by the calorie allotment per day (Table 13-11).
5. Distribute the exchanges containing carbohydrates (milk, fruit, vegtable,

Table 13-9. Exchange List for Meal Planning in Diabetes Mellitus

Bread Exchanges — *Carbohydrate, 15 g*	*Protein, 2 g*	*Calories, 70*	
Bread			
White (including French and Italian)	1 slice	English muffin, small	½
		Plain roll, bread	1
Whole wheat	1 slice	Frankfurter roll	½
Rye or pumpernickel	1 slice	Hamburger bun	½
Raisin	1 slice	Dried bread crumbs	3 tbs
Bagel, small	½	Tortilla, 6″	1
Cereal			
Bran Flakes	½ cup	Pasta (cooked), spaghetti, noodles, macaroni	½ cup
Other ready-to-eat, unsweetened cereal	¾ cup	Popcorn (popped, no fat added)	3 cups
Puffed cereal (unfrosted)	1 cup	Cornmeal (dry)	2 tbs
Cereal (cooked)	½ cup	Flour	2½ tbs
Grits (cooked)	½ cup	Wheat germ	¼ cup
Rice or barley (cooked)	½ cup		
Crackers			
Arrowroot	3	Pretzels, 3⅛″ long × ⅛″ dia	25
Graham, 2½″ sq	2	Rye wafers, 2″ × 3½″	3
Matzos, 4″ × 6″	½	Saltines	6
Oyster	20	Soda, 2½″ sq	4

Table 13-9. (Continued)

Bread Exchanges			
Carbohydrate, 15 g	*Protein, 2 g*	*Calories, 70*	
Dried Beans, Peas, and Lentils			
Beans, peas, lentils (dried and cooked)	$\frac{1}{2}$ cup	Baked beans, no pork (canned)	$\frac{1}{4}$ cup
Starchy Vegetables			
Corn	$\frac{1}{3}$ cup	Potato, white (whole)	1 small
Corn on cob	1 small	Potato, white (mashed)	$\frac{1}{2}$ cup
Lima beans	$\frac{1}{2}$ cup	Pumpkin	$\frac{3}{4}$ cup
Parsnips	$\frac{2}{3}$ cup	Winter squash, acorn or butternut	$\frac{1}{2}$ cup
Peas, green (canned or frozen)	$\frac{1}{2}$ cup	Yam or sweet potato	$\frac{1}{4}$ cup
Prepared Foods			
Biscuit, 2″ dia (omit one fat exchange)	1	Potatoes, french fried, 2″ to $3\frac{1}{2}$″ long (omit one fat exchange)	8
Corn Bread, 2″ × 2″ × 1″ (omit one fat exchange)	1	Potato or corn chips (omit two fat exchanges)	15
Corn muffin, 2″ dia (omit one fat exchange)	1	Pancake, 5″ × $\frac{1}{2}$″ (omit one fat exchange)	1
Crackers, round, butter type (omit one fat exchange)	5	Waffle, 5″ × $\frac{1}{2}$″ (omit one fat exchange)	1
Muffin, plain, small (omit one fat exchange)	1		

Milk Exchanges

Carbohydrate, 12 g *Protein, 8 g* *Fat, Trace* *Calories, 80*

Nonfat fortified milk	
Skimmed or nonfat milk	1 cup
Powdered milk (nonfat, dry, before adding liquid)	$\frac{1}{3}$ cup
Canned, evaporated, skimmed milk	$\frac{1}{2}$ cup
Buttermilk made from skimmed milk	1 cup
Yogurt (plain, unflavored), made from skimmed milk	1 cup
Low-fat fortified milk	
1% fat fortified milk (omit one-half fat exchange)	1 cup
2% fat fortified milk (omit one fat exchange)	1 cup
Yogurt (plain, unflavored), made from 2% fortified milk (omit one fat exchange)	1 cup
Whole milk (omit two fat exchanges)	
Whole milk	1 cup
Canned, evaporated whole milk	$\frac{1}{2}$ cup
Buttermilk made from whole milk	1 cup
Yogurt (plain, unflavored), made from whole milk	1 cup

Table 13-9. (Continued)

Vegetable Exchanges		
Carbohydrate, 5 g	*Protein, 2 g*	*Calories, 25*
(One exchange is $\frac{1}{2}$ cup)		
Asparagus	Greens	Rhubarb
Bean sprouts	Beet	Rutabaga
Beets	Chards	Sauerkraut
Broccoli	Collards	String beans, green or yellow
Brussels sprouts	Dandelion	Summer squash
Cabbage	Kale	Tomatoes
Carrots	Mustard	Tomato juice
Cauliflower	Spinach	Turnips
Celery	Turnip	Vegetable juice cocktail
Cucumbers	Mushrooms	Zucchini
Eggplant	Okra	
Green pepper	Onions	
The following raw vegetables may be used as desired		
Chicory	Escarole	Radishes
Chinese cabbage	Lettuce	Watercress
Endive	Parsley	

Fruit Exchanges			
	Carbohydrate, 10 g	*Calories, 40*	
Apple	1 small	Mango	$\frac{1}{2}$ small
Apple juice	$\frac{1}{3}$ cup	Melon	
Applesauce (unsweetened)	$\frac{1}{2}$ cup	Cantaloupe	$\frac{1}{4}$ small
Apricots, fresh	2 medium	Honeydew	$\frac{1}{8}$ medium
Apricots, dried	4 halves	Watermelon	1 cup
Banana	$\frac{1}{2}$ small	Nectarine	1 small
Berries		Orange	1 small
Blackberries	$\frac{1}{2}$ cup	Orange juice	$\frac{1}{2}$ cup
Blueberries	$\frac{1}{2}$ cup	Papaya	$\frac{3}{4}$ cup
Raspberries	$\frac{1}{2}$ cup	Peach	1 medium
Strawberries	$\frac{3}{4}$ cup	Pear	1 small
Cherries	10 large	Persimmon, native	1 medium
Cider	$\frac{1}{3}$ cup	Pineapple	$\frac{1}{2}$ cup
Dates	2	Pineapple juice	$\frac{1}{3}$ cup
Figs, fresh	1	Plums	2 medium
Figs, dried	1	Prunes	2 medium
Grapefruit	$\frac{1}{2}$	Prune juice	$\frac{1}{4}$ cup
Grapefruit juice	$\frac{1}{2}$ cup	Raisins	2 tbs
Grape juice	$\frac{1}{4}$ cup	Tangerine	1 medium

Table 13-9. (Continued)

Meat Exchanges

Protein, 7 g *Fat, 3 g* *Calories, 55*

Lean Meat

This list shows the kinds and amounts of lean meat and other protein-rich foods to use for one, low-fat meat exchange.

Beef	
Baby beef (very lean), chipped beef, chuck, flank steak, tenderloin, plate ribs, plate skirt steak, round (bottom, top), all cuts rump, spare ribs, tripe	1 oz
Lamb	
Leg, rib, sirloin, loin (roast and chops), shank, shoulder	1 oz
Pork	
Leg (whole rump, center shank); ham, smoked (center slices)	1 oz
Veal	
Leg, loin, rib, shank, shoulder, cutlets	1 oz
Poultry	
Meat without skin of chicken, turkey, cornish hen, guinea hen, pheasant	1 oz
Fish	
Any fresh or frozen	1 oz
Canned salmon, tuna, mackrel, crab and lobster	$\frac{1}{4}$ cup
Clams, oysters, scallops, shrimp	5 or 1 oz
Sardines, drained	3
Cheeses containing less than 5% butterfat	1 oz
Cottage cheese, dry and 2% butterfat	$\frac{1}{4}$ cup
Dried beans and peas (omit one bread exchange)	$\frac{1}{2}$ cup

Fat Exchanges			
Fat, 5 g		*Calories, 45*	
Margarine, soft, tub or stick	1 tsp	Margarine, regular, stick	1 tsp
Avacado, 4″ dia	$\frac{1}{8}$	Butter	1 tsp
Oil, corn, cottonseed, safflower, soy, sunflower	1 tsp	Bacon fat	1 tsp
		Bacon, crisp	1 strip
Oil, olive	1 tsp	Cream, light	2 tbs
Oil, peanut	1 tsp	Cream, sour	2 tbs
Olives	5 small	Cream, heavy	1 tbs
Almonds	10 whole	Cream cheese	1 tbs
Pecans, large	2 whole	French dressing	1 tbs
Peanuts		Italian dressing	1 tbs
Spanish	20 whole	Lard	1 tsp
Virginia	10 whole	Mayonnaise	1 tsp
Walnuts	6 small	Salad dressing, mayonnaise type[a]	2 tsp
Nuts, other	6 small	Salt pork, $\frac{3}{4}$″ cube	1

SOURCE: *Exchange List for Meal Planning.* New York: American Diabetes Association, and Chicago: American Dietetic Association, 1976.

Table 13-10a. Example of Meal Planning for a Patient with Diabetes Mellitus, requiring 2,000 kcal/day[a]

Exchange:					*Milk*[b]			*Fruit*		*Vegetable*			*Bread*			*Meat*			*Fat*
Nutrient/exchange: (g/exchange)					*Carbohydrate (CHO) (12)*	*Protein (8)*		*CHO (10)*		*CHO (5)*	*Protein (2)*		*CHO (15)*	*Protein (2)*		*Protein (7)*	*Fat (3)*		*Fat (5)*
Planned exchanges	*CHO*																		
	planned		*Actual*	*number per day*			*number per day*		*number per day*			*number per day*			*number per day*			*number per day*	
	(%)	*(g)*	*(g)*	*3*	*(g)*	*(g)*	*4*	*(g)*	*3*	*(g)*	*(g)*	*11*	*(g)*	*(g)*	*4*	*(g)*	*(g)*	*14*	*(g)*
Breakfast	20	50	52	1	12	8	1	10				2	30	4				3	15
Snack	10	25	25				1	10				1	15	2				1	5
Lunch	20	50	47	1	12	8			1	5	2	2	30	4	1	7	3	3	15
Snack	10	25	25				1	10				1	15	2				1	5
Dinner	30	75	77	1	12	8	1	10	2	10	4	3	45	6	2	14	6	4	20
Snack	10	25	30									2	30	4	1	7		2	10
Total (g)		250	256		36	24		40		15	6		165	22		28	9		70

[a] Plan: CHO: 50% = 1000 kcal = (1000:4) = 250 g
Protein: 15% = 300 kcal = (300:4) = 75 g
Fat: 35% = 700 kcal = (700:9) = 77 g

[b] 2% Milk.

Table 13-10b. Comparison of Planned and Actual Nutrient Distribution per Day and Meal

	Planned (g)	*Actual (g)*	*Actual*	*CHO*	*Protein*	*Fat*
CHO/day	250	256	Breakfast	52	12	15
Protein/day	75	80	Lunch	47	21	18
Fat/day	79	79	Dinner	77	32	26
			Snack	25	2	5
			Snack	25	2	5
			Snack	30	11	10

Table 13-11. Meal Plan for patients with Diabetes Mellitus, Based on Exchanges

	Number of Exchanges per Day								
Food	*1,100 calories*	*1,300 calories*	*1,400 calories*	*1,600 calories*	*2,000 calories*	*2,200 calories*	*2,500 calories*	*2,700 calories*	*3,000 calories*
Milk, skim	2	2	2	3	3	3	3	3	3
Fruit	2	3	3	3	4	4	4	5	5
Vegetable	1	1	2	3	3	3	3	3	3
Bread	6	7	7	8	11	12	15	16	18
Meat	2	2	3	3	3	4	5	6	7
Fat	7	9	9	10	14	15	19	17	19

SOURCE: *Exchange Lists for Meal Planning*. New York: American Diabetes Association, and Chicago: American Dietetic Association, 1976.

bread) over the six meals and snacks to provide approximately the percentage of carbohydrate planned for each (Table 13-10a).

6. Distribute the remaining exchanges; try not to provide more than 50% of the total protein allotment at any one single meal. Provide 10 to 20% of total protein in the late night snack.
7. Choose foods according to the patient's preference from the exchange list (48) (Table 13-9).
8. Calculate the actual grams of carbohydrate, protein, and fat provided by the menu, and compare them with the planned amount of each (Table 13-10b).

Hypoglycemias

Low blood sugar levels are seen in many divers disorders. Only some have nutritional implications, either because food is the cause of the hypoglycemia or because diet is an essential part of treatment. Moreover, the relation of hypoglycemia to food intake is important even in disorders that have no etiologic connection with nutrition. The foods that cause hypoglycemia in people with metabolic disorders are those containing galactose, fructose, glycerol, leucine, and specific amino acids. These disorders are the subject of this section, excluding galactosemia, hereditary fructose intolerance, organic acidemias, and aminoacidopathies, because they are discussed individually. Familiarity with all causes of hypoglycemia is essential for the diagnostic process. A brief outline of metabolic and endocrinologic disorders that can cause hypoglycemia is therefore presented.

Diagnostic Approach

The blood sugar level at which acute clinical manifestations occur varies in different disorders and among patients. By and large, symptoms of hypoglycemia may be expected when blood sugar drops below 40 mg/dl in infants and children, below 30 mg/dl in full term neonates, and below 20 mg/dl in low birth weight infants. Patients with glycogen storage disease may be asymptomatic at lower levels and are also less prone to develop brain damage as a result of hypoglycemic episodes. By contrast, other disorders, such as leucine-sensitive hypoglycemia, carry a risk of permanent neurological damage. A high degree of suspicion is necessary to establish a diagnosis, because many of the manifestations of hypoglycemia are nonspecific. They include apathy, headache, nausea, weakness, convulsions, giddiness, and confusion. Small infants are jittery and have tremors. Symptoms of hypoglycemia may be overshadowed by the manifestations of coexisting disease. Moreover, the fact that blood sugar levels are often no longer elevated when the patient is examined presents further difficulties. Pallor, hunger, sweating, and cold clammy skin are most suggestive of hypoglycemia. If the patient is examined after the acute symptoms have subsided, spinal fluid may be analyzed, because the glucose abnormality tends to persist longer in CSF than in blood. Since it may be difficult to ascertain the diagnosis of hypoglycemia, patients with a suggestive history should be given instructions on how to obtain a blood glucose determination in the event of another attack.

Diagnosis of the cause of hypoglycemia is the next step in the workup. Only a few causes can be ruled out by the physical exam (Table 13-12). Diagnosis rests mainly on a careful history, characteristic biochemical abnormalities during the acute attack (Table 13-13), and select provocative tests. Thus, it may be helpful to give the patient a written note with instructions to physicians in attendance at another acute attack, requesting frozen plasma for later use in specific diagnostic tests. The sequence of provocative tests should be individualized, based on the presumptive diagnosis derived from historical data.

History

Since the disease onset varies in different types of hypoglycemia, a history should ascertain the time at which the first suggestive manifestations of hypoglycemia occurred. Thus, leucine-sensitive hypoglycemia starts generally before 6 months of age, ketotic hypoglycemia between 1 and 6 years, and hypoglycemia due to insulin excess, either right after birth or after 3 years of age. The relation of the first episode to the introduction of new food items, such as fruits or lactose-containing formulas, is important, as well as the relation of hypoglycemic attacks to meals, illness, or other stress. The duration of the fast prior to an attack may be fairly characteristic. Attacks occur in reactive hypoglycemia 3 to 4 hours after a meal, in disorders of gluconeogenesis and in glycogen storage disease type III after a longer fast, and in glycogen storage disease type I already after 2–3 hours. The type of meal may provide a clue in leucine sensitivity and in fructose intolerance. Finally, the history should explore the possibility of alcohol or drug ingestion, including salicylates, propranolol, and specific hypoglycemic medications. Characteristic features of different disorders are listed on Table 13-12.

Laboratory Workup

After a physical examination, which rules out such causes as growth hormone deficiency, Beckwith syndrome, and glycogen storage, other disorders that have episodic hypoglycemia as the only manifestation must be excluded. It is generally necessary to first confirm the diagnosis of hypoglycemia and the relation to meals through serial blood sugar measurements, including preprandial measurements during the day, followed by a 12-hour fast at night. These tests should be done at 2- to 3-hour intervals, preferably by use of a heparin-filled venous line to avoid disturbing the patient since crying accelerates development of hypogly-

Table 13-12. Differential Diagnosis of Hypoglycemia

Cause	*Diagnostic Features*
Endocrine Disorders	
Growth hormone deficiency	Deficient growth hormone response to stimulation
Insulin excess	Increased insulin/glucose ratio; normal to low β-hydroxybutyrate and FFA
β-cell hyperplasia, adenoma	Onset at birth, or after 4 years
Beckwith syndrome	Macroglossia, omphalocele, gigantism
"Infant giant"	Gigantism at birth, microcephaly
Inborn Errors of Metabolism	
Glycogen storage (types I, III, and VI)	Large liver, ketoacidosis, increased lactate, β-hydroxybutyrate, triglycerides and FFA
Galactosemia	Urinary-reducing sugar (galactose), hepatorenal disease, cataracts, mental retardation
Hereditary fructose intolerance	Urinary-reducing sugar (fructose), vomiting, hepatorenal disease, elevated plasma tyrosine
Deficient gluconeogenesis	Fasting hypoglycemia with elevation of lactate, β-hydroxybutyrate, and alanine
(Pyruvate carboxylase)	
(PEPcarboxykinase)	Hepatomegaly
(Fructose-1,6-diphosphatase)	Fructose and glycerol cause hypoglycemia, hyperlactatemia, and hypophophatemia
Glycogen synthetase deficiency	Fasting hypoglycemia; galactose tolerance normal for glucose conversion but lactate rises
Maple sugar urine disease	Elevated plasma leucine, valine and isoleucine; fasting hypoglycemia with low alanine and lactate
Organic acidemias	Ketoacidosis; specific organic aciduria (see Table 13-6) plasma glycine and ammonia may be elevated.
Other Metabolic Disorders	
Ketotic hypoglycemia	Hypoglycemia induced by ketosis; onset 12 months to 6 years; abnormal glucagon test during ketosis; hypoglycemia associated with elevated β-hydroxybutyrate, FFA and triglycerides; normal lactate, low-normal alanine, low insulin, and elevated glucagon
Leucine sensitive hypoglycemia	Onset before 6 months; no ketosis; leucine load causes hypoglycemia and increase of plasma insulin; fasting hypoglycemia may occur.

Table 13-12. (Continued)

Cause	*Diagnostic Features*
Neonatal hypoglycemia	Transient, unless caused by disorders listed above; common in small or large for gestational age infants, in erythroblastosis, and infants born after perinatal stress, or to diabetic and toxemic mothers

cemia. Infants should be allowed water during the fast. Preliminary tests at the bedside with Dextrostix may have to be done more frequently during the prolonged fast, in order to protect the patient from sudden hypoglycemia. In the event of hypoglycemia, blood should be withdrawn first for biochemical tests (Table 13-13), followed by glucagon (30 μg/kg/M, up to 1.0 mg) and-ie no response-25% glucose. It is not necessary to continue a fast much beyond 12 hours, because many normal infants and children also develop hypoglycemia if fasting is continued beyond that time (49). A blood glucose value below 40 mg/dl after a 12-hour fast is pathologic (i.e., <2 SD below normal). The following blood tests should be performed during hypoglycemia: plasma insulin, glucagon lactate, pyruvate, β-hydroxybutyrate, free fatty acids, triglycerides, alanine, and cortisol. Alanine and lactate are elevated in disorders of gluconeogenesis, β-hydroxbutyrate and free fatty acids are elevated in ketotic hypoglycemia while lactate is normal. Low levels of β-hydroxybutyrate during hypoglycemia suggest hyperinsulinism, even if plasma insulin is not significantly raised (50). Tolerance tests should be limited to those most likely to provide a diagnosis, using a sequence of tests suggested by history and physical findings.

Table 13-13. Basic Laboratory Workup in Hypoglycemia

- Serial blood sugars (preprandial and during a 12-hour fast)
- Plasma insulin
- SGOT and SGPT
- Tests to be performed during hypoglycemia on blood
  - Insulin/glucose ratio
  - Glucagon
  - Lactate and pyruvate
  - Free fatty acids
  - β-hydroxybutyrate
  - Triglycerides
  - Amino acids (alanine, branched chain amino acids, glycine)
  - Cortisol

Nonspecific Acute Therapy

Known cases of hypoglycemia should be instructed on the treatment of an acute attack, especially on how to give glucose to an unconscious or convulsing patient. These patients may be given glucose concentrates under the tongue ("Glutose", Paddock). Intravenous therapy consists of 25% glucose, 1–2 ml/kg, given at a rate of 2 ml/minute.

Specific Therapy of Hypoglycemia in Metabolic Disorders

Hepatic Fructose-1,6-Diphosphatase Deficiency. The enzyme affected in this disorder is a key enzyme in gluconeogenesis (Fig. 13-2). Consequently, the gluconeogenic amino acid, alanine, and its immediate metabolic products, lactate and pyruvate are increased in blood. Uric acid elevation occurs secondarily to the hyperlactatemia. The defect causes hypoglycemia after a period of fasting or any event that results in hypercatabolic stress, including infections, fever, and exercise. Hypoglycemia developed in the first reported case after loading with fructose and glycerol, which cannot be converted to glucose (51). A high-fat meal may have a similar effect. Galactose is tolerated. As in hereditary fructose intolerance, serum phosphorus levels fall dramatically after loading with fructose or glycerol (1.0 g/kg, each, orally), because phosphorus is sequestered as fructose-1,6-diphosphatase. Hypoglycemia, which is due to inhibition of glycogen mobilization by intermediates of fructose metabolism, develops in hereditary fructose intolerance only after the fructose load. By contrast, fructose-1,6-diphosphatase deficiency causes hypoglycemia also after a prolonged fast because of deficient gluconeogenesis. The two disorders require differentiation by liver enzyme analysis since tolerance tests tend to be inconclusive.

Treatment consists of frequent feedings. The diet should be low in fat and free of fructose and sucrose. Total carbohydrate intake must be increased to about 55% of total calories in order to decrease fat intake to 30% or less. Prolonged fasting must be avoided.

Other Gluconeogenic Enzyme Defects. A few cases have been reported with a genetic deficiency of hepatic phosphoenolpyruvate carboxykinase and pyruvate carboxylase. They had fasting hypoglycemia, hyperlactatemia, and an elevated level of serum alanine, but fructose tolerance was normal.

Glycogen Synthetase Deficiency. This disorder results from a deficiency of glycogen formation and is characterized by fasting hypoglycemia. Glucagon (30 μg/kg), given after an overnight fast, produces an insufficient blood glucose response. Complete inactivity of this enzyme would seem incompatible with survival. The few reported cases that have been studied evidently survived because of some remaining in vivo activity, possibly by a reverse phosphorylase reaction. Consequently, glucagon may produce a blood glucose rise, especially after a shorter fast of several hours. Symptomatic hypoglycemia developed in the first reported case (52) when the night feeding was withheld at 7 months of age. Hypoglycemia was severe but not precipitous. The patient was microcephalic and mentally retarded, possibly as a result of repeated unrecognized hypoglycemia. In this disorder, galactose ingestion produces a blood glucose rise, which is accompanied by a rise of serum lactate (53), because the galactose that does not enter the circulation as free glucose cannot be stored as glycogen and floods the glycolytic pathway to form lactate (Fig. 13-2). A high-protein diet and late night feedings were of benefit in the reported cases.

Ketotic Hypoglycemia. Hypoglycemia may be associated with ketoacidosis in a variety of conditions, including organic acidemias, maple sugar urine disease, and gluconeogenic enzyme deficiencies. In addition to these disorders, there is another unique type of ketotic hypoglycemia, which is considered to be the most common hypoglycemia in childhood. To make the diagnosis, one must demonstrate that ketosis induces the drop in blood glucose. This disorder has similarities with starvation, as plasma ketones, free fatty acids, triglycerides, and glucagon are elevated while glucose, alanine, and insulin are low (54). Liver glycogen is depleted during ketosis. The depletion has been attributed to insufficient gluconeogenesis from alanine and unresponsiveness of the adrenal medulla. Absence of the expected rise of catecholamines prior to the development of hypoglycemia has been reported (55). The explanation that deficient gluconeogenesis is the cause of hypoglycemia in this disorder is supported by the ability of cortisol to prevent hypoglycemia if given just prior to the induction of ketosis.

The onset of ketotic hypoglycemia is usually during the second year of life, and the disorder persists for several years. Patients have sporadic episodes of hypoglycemia, commonly associated with convulsions and precipitated by a prolonged fast or illness. General health between attacks is good, and there is commonly a surprising lack of intellectual impairment, even after many severe hypoglycemic attacks.

Diagnosis is best established by use of a provocative ketogenic test (56,57). The patient must be adequately prepared prior to the test with a high-caloric diet for 3 days. After an overnight fast, baseline values for blood sugar, β-hydroxybutyrate, free fatty acids, triglycerides, alanine, insulin, and glucagon are obtained. The patient is then given a ketogenic diet consisting of 1,200 kcal/M^2 body surface area and containing 67% fat, 16% carbohydrate, and 17% protein calories. Blood sugar is measured every 4 hours, and serial urines are tested for ketones until they become positive. During this time patients are permitted normal activity. All biochemical tests are repeated when ketosis develops or when the blood sugar drops below 40 mg/dl. A glucagon test is performed at that time (30 μg/kg). In a typical case, no hyperglycemic response occurs, since the liver is depleted of glycogen. However, when the test is repeated after a 8- to 12-hour fast in the absence of ketosis, the response is normal.

Dietary management is aimed at avoiding prolonged fasting and a high fat intake. The patient should monitor the urine for ketones, especially at bedtime and on arising. If urine ketones are present, starchy foods and some sugar should be taken in the form of hard candy, orange juice, or Glucola. Glucagon is obviously not effective in the treatment of acute attacks. Cortisol may be tried in cases that are difficult to control by other means.

Leucine-Sensitive Hypoglycemia. Whereas normal children respond to leucine with a modest drop in blood sugar (58), patients with leucine sensitivity develop marked hypoglycemia. It has been estimated that the disorder makes up 30% of all childhood hypoglycemias. Onset is usually before 6 months of age. Attacks of hypoglycemia are provoked by a protein-rich meal, but they also tend to develop after a prolonged fast. The disorder shares characteristics with diseases causing insulin excess, including low levels of β-hydroxybutyrate. β-cell hyperplasia and hypertrophy have been reported in leucine-sensitive hypoglycemia (59). In both, onset is shortly after birth, and the prognosis is poor. Early onset and difficulty in preventing repeated attacks are probably responsible for the mental retardation that is common in the two disorders. The tendency to develop hypoglycemia in response to leucine may subside spontaneously at about 4 to 6 years of age (60).

Treatment of acute attacks consists of subcutaneous administration of glucagon, in addition to glucose concentrates, which may be given orally if possible. Long-term management consists of limiting the leucine intake to minimum requirements. This amounts, in essence, to a low-protein diet, although efforts should be made to select those protein foods with a lesser leucine content (Table 13-14). A formula, marketed as a low-leucine product (Wyeth S-14) accomplishes the "low leucine" content by diluting all amino acids to about 73% of the amount in standard formulas. The daily protein should be divided over four meals in order to decrease the leucine load at any one meal. Cortisol, which is sometimes used in hypoglycemia that is unresponsive to other measures, is probably not useful in this disorder, because the catabolic action of cortisol could raise the endogenous leucine load. Diazoxide has been tried with some success (8mg/kg/day, in 3 doses, up to a maximum of 20 mg/kg/d).

Glycogen Storage Disease (GSD)

The name *glycogen storage disease* (GSD) encompasses a group of at least 10 genetic disorders that are associated with quantitatively or qualitatively abnormal glycogen storage in one or more of the following tissues: liver, kidney, muscle, intestinal mucosa, WBC, or RBC. It is beyond the scope of this book to describe the disorders that are not responsive to dietary therapy. Thus, only GSD types I, III, and VI are presented, together with a discussion of the biochemistry and mechanism of these diseases to the extent necessary for an understanding of therapeutic principles (Fig. 13-2).

GSD Type I

A complex system of hormones and enzymes maintains glucose concentration in blood and tissues within a narrow range of normal. To accomplish this and supply energy when it is needed, glucose is stored in the form of glycogen, which allows rapid mobilization. Glucose-6-phosphate occupies a central position in glucose homeostasis because it is part of several pathways that lead to and from glycogen. Consequently, multiple disturbances are to be expected when the enzyme that releases glucose from glucose-6-phosphate is deficient. This enzyme, glucose-6-phosphatase (G-6-Pase), is deficient in glycogen storage disease type I.

When blood glucose declines, approximately 3 hours after a meal, phosphorylase is activated by glucagon and removes a glucose molecule from the branched glycogen molecule to produce glucose-1-phosphate. Glycogenolytic enzymes operate normally in GSD type I until the pathway reaches glucose-6-phosphate, from whence glucose cannot be liberated. As a result, hypoglycemia intensifies, only to stimulate phosphorylase further and flood the system with products of glycogenolysis. Instead of glucose formation, glucose-6-phosphate is degraded via the Embden-Meyerhof glycolytic pathway to acetyl-CoA and lactic acid. Since this amounts usually to more energy than is needed at the given time, lactic acid accumulates, and part of the glucose-6-phosphate is metabolized via the pentose shunt, resulting in TPNH, which stimulates fatty acid synthesis. Ketoacidosis is the inevitable result. Gluconeogenesis is ineffective in relieving the hypoglycemia, because this pathway also relies on G-6-Pase for the final release of glucose. If fructose and galactose are fed, they fail to relieve the hypoglycemia, because both fructose-1-phosphate and galactose-1-phosphate have to be converted first to glucose-6-phosphate. Hypoglycemia provokes hunger, but eating anything other than glucose only leads to an increase in glycogen and fat without reversal of the hypoglycemia. Liver enlargement is the result of both glycogen and fat accumulation.

The most prominent disease manifestation, which is present is GSD types I, III, and IV, is hepatomegaly. The liver is firm and smooth and extends downward to the iliac crest and beyond the midline to the splenic region. It is characteristically not associated with splenomegaly or jaundice. Since the patients are fat, they appear well nourished, but their muscles tend to be flabby. Older children with GSD type I are generally short. The face is plethoric, and the cheeks are chubby, which results in an appearance that has been compared with a "doll's face." Nosebleeds and easy bruising

Table 13-14. Leucine Content of Baby Foods

	mg/100 g	*mg/tbs*		*mg/100 g*	*mg/tbs*
Strained Meats			Applesauce and pineapple	7	tr
Beef	1,078	154	Apricots with tapioca	12	2
Beef/Beef hearts	996	139	Bananas with tapioca	17	2
Chicken	1,059	151	Peaches	17	2
Egg yolks	832	116	Pears	13	2
Egg yolk/ham	851	119	Pears and pineapple	17	2
Ham	1,170	167	Plums with tapioca	23	3
Lamb	1,235	176	Prunes with tapioca	37	5
Liver	1,375	196	Strained and Junior Vegetables		
Pork	1,145	164	Green beans	70	10
Turkey	1,116	159	Beets	37	5
Veal	1,077	154	Carrots	37	5
Junior Meats			Mixed Vegetables	43	6
Beef	1,197	171	Peas	243	34
Chicken	1,137	162	Creamed spinach	200	28
Ham	1,255	179	Squash	30	4
Lamb	1,251	179	Sweet potato	70	10
Pork	1,202	172	Strained and Junior Desserts		
Turkey	1,270	181	Fruit dessert	10	1
Veal	1,244	178	Custard pudding	233	33
Strained and Junior High Meat			Peach cobbler	20	3
Dinners			Dutch apple dessert	10	1
Beef with vegetables	451	64			
Chicken with vegetables	483	69			

Cottage cheese with pineapple	559	80
Ham with vegetables	511	73
Lamb with vegetables	644	90
Turkey with vegetables	426	61
Veal with vegetables	460	66
Strained and Junior Vegetables and Meats		
Beef and egg noodles	220	31
Cereal, egg yolks and bacon	189	26
Chicken noodle dinner	188	26
Cream of chicken soup	206	29
Macaroni, tomato, and beef	161	23
Turkey rice dinner	164	23
Vegetables and bacon	112	16
Vegetables and beef	130	18
Vegetables and chicken	140	20
Vegetables and ham	125	17
Vegetables and lamb	149	21
Vegetables and liver	191	27
Vegetables and turkey	139	19
Strained and Junior Fruits		
Applesauce	7	tr
Applesauce and apricots	13	2

Strained and Junior Cereal with Fruits (in jars)		
High protein cereal with applesauce and bananas	326	46
Mixed cereal with applesauce and bananas	86	12
Oatmeal with applesauce and bananas	65	9
Rice with applesauce and bananas	29	4
Dry Cereals		
Barley	767	18
High protein cereal	2,626	63
High protein cereal with peaches	1,913	46
Mixed cereal	939	23
Mixed cereal with bananas	925	22
Oatmeal	1,111	27
Oatmeal with bananas	991	24
Rice cereal	500	12
Rice cereal with strawberries	607	15
Miscellaneous	*mg/each*	
Animal cracker, Barnum	12	
Arrowroot biscuit	48	
Chicken sticks	124	
Meat sticks	122	
Turkey sticks	102	

SOURCE: Information on leucine content obtained from Gerber Products Company. For leucine content of commonly used foods, see: Church C, Church H: *Food Values of Portions Commonly Used.* 12th ed. Philadelphia, Lippincott, 1975.

are common and are attributable to loss of vascular integrity. Lipemia retinalis may be noticeable, and with time, xanthomas develop in children who maintain high lipid levels. Starting about 3 to 4 hours after a meal, if glucose is not provided, clinical manifestations of acidosis become apparent. These children breathe progressively faster, but often do not show signs of hypoglycemia even when blood sugar levels are very low.

Positive laboratory findings include a mild to moderately elevated SGOT, SGPT, and variable increases of serum lactate, pyruvate, triglycerides, cholesterol, and fatty acids. Uric acid elevation may be severe and persistent enough to cause gout in the older child. Kidney enlargement due to glycogen storage is readily noticeable on radiological examination of the abdomen, and the intravenous pyelogram shows elongation and compression of the renal pelvis and calyces. Bleeding time is prolonged, but platelet count and clotting time are normal. Tests measuring platelet adhesiveness frequently show decreased values, probably as a result of hyperlipidemia.

Providing the clinical picture is typical, the next diagnostic step is a liver biopsy for histological examination and enzyme analysis (must be collected on liquid nitrogen and stored at −70°F.) Several tolerance tests may be performed in questionable cases prior to biopsy. The glucagon test (30 to 100 μg/kg, maximum 1 mg) measures specifically the mobilization of glucose from liver glycogen. In patients with glycogen storage disease, plasma glucose level remains flat, or the rise is slow and does not exceed 50% of the baseline value. Plasma lactate, which does not rise in normal individuals, increases sharply. Since the test may be abnormal in GSD types III and VI and in nonspecific liver disease, it is advisable to follow a positive test with a tolerance test that evaluates the conversion of other hexoses to glucose-6-phosphate and glucose by use of either fructose (0.5 g/kg) or galactose (1.0 g/kg). These tolerance tests are positive for GSD type I if there is no rise in plasma glucose and elevation of lactate.

GSD Type III

The disorder GSD type III, which is caused by absence of amylo-1,6-glucosidase, has chemical similarities with GSD type I but tends to be milder. Plasma elevation of lactate is minimal and ketoacidosis is rare because patients are able to tolerate a longer fast. Biochemical abnormalities are absent in some cases even after a 12- to 18-hour fast. Liver enlargement is massive in all cases.

The glycogen molecule is multitiered and has more peripheral branches, the larger the molecule is. Phosphorylase cleaves off glucose molecules starting from the peripheral branch endings and working inward until a branch point is reached. This requires "debrancher" enzyme, amylo-1,6-glycosidase, in order to cleave glucose at its 1,6-linkage. This enzyme is deficient in GSD type III. Phosphorylase functions normally in response to glucagon stimulation and maintains normal plasma levels until fasting has exhausted all the glucose that is available from the most peripheral branches of the glycogen molecule. Since glycogenolysis stops at the branch points, hypoglycemia does not result in increased activity of the glycogenolytic pathway toward lactic acid and acetyl-CoA. Moreover, gluconeogenesis and conversion of galactose and fructose can proceed normally.

The glucagon test may reflect the specific biochemical defect if it is normal 4 to 6 hours after a meal, and abnormal after a longer fast when all glucose has been cleaved off the peripheral branches of the glycogen molecule and there is failure of glucose mobilization. Galactose and fructose tolerance tests are normal. Unfortunately, none of these function tests serve as a reliable diagnostic tool. Diagnosis requires analysis of the three enzymes that cause a similar clinical picture if they are deficient: G-6-Pase, phosphorylase, and debrancher enzyme. Although erythrocyte glycogen is elevated and the enzyme defect has been demonstrated in WBC and fibroblasts, routine use of these tissues for diagnosis is not advised, because the tissue of choice is the one that allows reliable testing of all three enzymes, namely liver.

GSD Type VI

Disorders of GSD type VI are caused by deficiency of liver phosphorylase or phosphorylasekinase. Complete absence of activity appears to be rare, and the degree of deficiency varies considerably from case to case. Consequently, biochemical abnormalities and clinical complications are usually less severe than in GSD type I. As little as 10% of normal enzyme activity appears to be sufficient for glucose homeostasis. Cases with more severe deficiency develop hypoglycemia 3–4 hours after a meal. Since endogenous glucagon is ineffective and does not flood the glycolytic pathway with metabolites, hyperlactatemia does not develop. Ketoacidosis, which is rare, may result when fat must supply the energy that cannot be supplied by glycogen. Patients have large livers and usually no evidence of significant hepatocellular dysfunction, although SGOT may be moderately increased. Their ability to withstand stress depends on the degree of enzyme deficiency.

Treatment

A major objective of treatment for all three types of GSD is the provision of glucose when it is needed. Since this varies in the three disorders and from case to case, it is necessary to individualize the treatment regimen, based on serial blood glucose determinations, both during the night and during daytime activities.

It is always necessary in GSD type I to provide frequent feedings throughout the 24-hour period, usually every 3 hours. Tolerance of a fast is generally much better in GSD types III and VI. Care should be taken in all three disorders to avoid excessive calorie intakes from any nutrient, because storage of unneeded energy only adds to the glycogen excess in the liver. Every feeding must contain a ready source of glucose from starch or glucose polymers. Both galactose and fructose must be avoided in GSD type I. Since gluconeogenesis from protein is possible in GSD types III and VI, it is advisable to give a mixture of glucose from starch and sugars plus some protein with every meal, in hopes that it will provide glucose through gluconeogenesis for an extended period after the meal. This is especially desirable for the bedtime snack.

Maintenance of 24-hour glucose homeostasis is a major task in GSD type I. Patients who require feedings every 3 hours benefit from nightly nasogastric drip infusion of glucose (61). Once the need has been demonstrated, it is best to start early in infancy, because young infants adjust more easily than toddlers to the nightly introduction of a nasogastric tube. Use of a permanent percutaneous intragastric tube has been tried successfully. Although this approach may seem radical, it has definite advantages for parents and patients who have difficulty with the nightly introduction of a tube. Moreover, this approach does not carry a risk of aspiration. It is also possible to infuse a concentrated (50%) glucose solution slowly into the oral cavity through a catheter that is attached nightly to the lower last molar by use of a permanent clip. However, this treatment increases the risk of severe caries. Continuous nightime feedings by intragastric drip should improve hyperlipidemia, lactate and uric acid elevations and may cause a decrease in liver size. Growth may also accelerate. Whether a patient improves or not depends on the degree of control that was accomplished prior to continuous nighttime feedings on a regimen consisting only of feedings every 3 hours.

During continuous nighttime intragastric feeding total 24-hour calorie intake must be kept within the normal range. The prescription of the feeding mixture should be calculated carefully to limit glucose to the absolute minimum necessary for the maintenance of normal blood sugar levels, because excess adds to the already abundant glycogen stores in the liver and increases the obesity which is characteristic of GSD type I. Composition and rate of infusion should be determined in the hospital by titration against blood sugar levels. These should be measured while the patient is asleep, thus imitating the energy output that will exist during the night at home. The mixture should not contain fat and need not contain protein. Since excess protein should be avoided, patients will appreciate the variety of a protein meal during the day. Once the amount of calories needed for nighttime feeding has been determined, the balance of the total requirements must be carefully proportioned to provide starch or glucose every 3 hours, both as a cracker between meals and a starchy food item as part of the three major meals. The remaining calories must provide enough protein for growth but not an excess. Fat is needed to the extent necessary to make food palatable. Since the formula must be free of galactose, fructose, and sucrose, only Pregestimil and Prosobee are suitable milk substitutes. Prosobee is preferred because the use of protein hydrolysate in Pregestimil is not necessary. If a high-caloric nutritional supplement is needed, Isocal may be used, since it is free of galactose and fructose. Beverages that contain rapidly dializable glucose polymers are Glucola, (33 g glucose/dl), Lemon Sour, and Grape Sour. Galactose restriction need not be as rigid as in galactosemia (Table 9-6).

Galactose Intolerance

Two genetic enzyme defects are known that have galactosemia as a major feature. They are galactokinase deficiency and galactose-1-phosphate uridyl transferase (transferase) deficiency. The incidence of galactokinase deficiency has been estimated to be 1:100,000 live births (62). Mass screening programs in the United States and Europe indicate that the incidence of transferase deficiency ranges, with few exceptions, between 1:40,000 and 70,000.

The first step after absorption of galactose from the gut requires phosphorylation to galactose-1-phosphate by the enzyme galactokinase. In the absence of this enzyme, galactose accumulates and is excreted in the urine. Elevated concentrations of galactose in the lens presumably lead to the formation of galactitol, a sugar alcohol that appears to be locally damaging. Transferase is required in the second step of galactose metabolism, which results in the formation of glucose-1-phosphate. If the enzyme is deficient, galactose-1-phosphate accumulates and inhibits galactokinase, thus causing galactosemia with urinary overflow of galactose. Galactose-1-phosphate is increased in tissues (RBC) and toxic to liver, kidney, and brain, apparently because oxygen uptake is impaired.

Galactose-1-Phosphate Uridyl Transferase Deficiency (Galactosemia)

A small nuclear cataract may be the first manifestation of galactosemia due to transferase deficiency in the offspring of a heterozygous mother who was not on a lactose-restricted diet during pregnancy. Since she appears unable to dispose of galactose as rapidly as normal people, increased concentrations of galactose apparently reach the fetus and cause damage to the lens before the third month of gestation, when lens formation takes place. The earliest manifestation of toxicity in the infant is aminoaciduria due to tubular damage, which can be detected as early as 3 to 5 days after galactose ingestion. Subsequently, there is failure to gain weight, vomiting, and diarrhea. Acute liver toxicity is reflected by jaundice and elevation of SGOT and SGPT levels. Liver cirrhosis develops if the insult is allowed to continue. Cataract formation progresses, and there may be irreversible brain damage. However, the ensuing mental retardation may not be a function of the degree of lactose exposure alone.

Diagnosis is based on recognition of reducing substances in the urine (Clinitest or Benedict's test). Mellituria is commonly associated with proteinuria and aminoaciduria. Specific tests for glucose (Clinistix, Testape, and Combistix) are negative. Qualitative tests of the type of sugar should be performed in either urine or blood. Elevated blood galactose levels are the basis for detection in states that include a bacterial inhibition assay (BIA) as part of their PKU screening program. Any child who has been exposed to galactose and has a positive BIA or evidence of galactosuria should be placed on a galactose-free diet until a firm diagnosis is established, based on red cell transferase activity. It is desirable to quantitate the transferase activity in heterozygous parents, since this confirms the diagnosis and helps to identify patients with the Duarte variant.

Hereditary fructose intolerance, acquired liver disease, biliary atresia, and sepsis should be considered in the differential diagnosis. Recent evidence suggests that sepsis and galactosemia may coexist, probably because galactose serves as a favorable substrate for the growth of certain organisms, mainly *E. coli*, which are a common cause of sepsis in newborns. Diagnosis is further complicated by the possibility that neonatal galactosuria may be a benign transient phenomenon, usually lasting no later than the sixth day in full term infants and the third week in premature infants. Finally, galactokinase deficiency should be ruled out in infants with a positive BIA or galactosuria.

Galactokinase Deficiency

The manifestations of galactokinase deficiency are less severe than in "classical" galactosemia due to transferase deficiency, as they do not include liver, kidney, and CNS disease. This observation shows that galactose-1-phosphate rather than galactose is responsible for these manifestations. On the other hand, galactose, which accumulates in galactokinase deficiency, appears to damage only the lens, causing the gradual development of cataracts. Beutler et al. (63) assayed the activity of galactokinase and transferase in 210 individuals with cataracts and found decreased activity in 94 cases. Two patients had total deficiency, and 92 had partial deficiency, compatible with heterozygosity. Onset of cataract development was before 1 year of age in all 94 cases, but no patient with onset after 1 year of age had deficient enzyme activity. The recognition of galactokinase deficiency thus has implications for heterozygous family members. Heterozygotes should limit galactose intake moderately, because gradual development of cataracts is a potential threat (64).

Recognition of the metabolic defect depends on demonstration of galactosuria or galactosemia in patients receiving galactose in the diet. A positive urine test for reducing substances coupled with a negative glucose oxidase reaction is indication to collect urine, while the patient is receiving milk, in order to identify the sugar. Transferase deficiency may be ruled out first, since this disorder is more common and the assay is more readily available. Infants with persistent galactosemia or galactosuria in whom transferase deficiency has been ruled out, as well as children with cataracts who excrete galactose upon loading but have no liver or kidney disease should be tested for galactokinase deficiency.

Treatment
Both disorders require galactose restriction. Prompt institution and strict adherence to a galactose free diet are most important in transferase deficiency. The finding of cataracts in patients with galactokinase deficiency suggests that these patients benefit from moderate restriction. In transferase deficiency, adherence to the diet should be lifelong, with minor relaxation after growth has ceased. Parents must be made aware of the deleterious effects on mental capacity if the diet is not followed. They should be instructed about the names of galactose-containing products and sugars, such as lactose, whey, milk solids, and so on. Filled milks contain some regular milk and should be avoided. Most nondairy creamers, on the other hand, are permitted. Some vegetables contain significant amounts of galactose. Infant formulas that are galactose free are Nutramigen and, currently, all soy products (Table 9-6).

Hereditary Fructose Intolerance (HFI)

Hereditary fructose intolerance (HFI) is a genetic disorder of fructose metabolism that appears to be at least as frequent as galactosemia, yet it is less well known. The disease gains importance to physicians caring for infants because it is potentially lethal, but disease expression can be prevented by relatively simple diet therapy, providing it is detected in time. Moreover, HFI enters into the differential diagnosis of several disorders that affect the liver and kidney, including tyrosinemia and galactosemia. There are indications that many cases of HFI that appear as overwhelming disease in early infancy are missed.

The disorder is due to genetic deficiency of fructose-1-phosphate aldolase in liver, renal cortex, and intestinal mucosa. Ingested fructose can be converted by fructokinase to fructose-1-phosphate but not further. Indirect evidence indicates that fructose-1-phosphate inhibits gluconeogenesis, as well as glycogen breakdown at the level of phosphorylase. As a result, severe hypoglycemia develops. Moreover, there is inhibition of fructokinase by the accumulating enzyme product, fructose-1-phosphate, which causes plasma fructose to rise. It is excreted in the urine, causing a positive test for reducing substances.

Manifestations
Onset follows the introduction of fructose to the diet, mainly in the form of fruits, sugar, and honey. The severity and the course of the disease appear to be a function of the frequency and amount of fructose ingested. A small infant may become shocky, convulse, and die after drinking a bottle of fruit juice. Repeated ingestion in early infancy causes liver disease

with high SGOT levels and jaundice. An unusually severe clotting defect is common in cases with liver involvement. Since it may be present before there is jaundice, it is easily missed and may cause unsuspected bleeding and death. Liver cirrhosis, hypoalbuminemia, and ascites ultimately develop. Acute hypoglycemic attacks may occur at any time and precipitate a catastrophic event with shock, hypoxemia, and irreversible brain damage. A more chronic form of the disorder affects mainly the kidney. Manifestations consist of those seen in Fanconi's syndrome: aminoaciduria, glucosuria, and phosphaturia resulting in hypophosphatemia. It is interesting that many patients develop an aversion to sweets, although they do not consciously link their symptoms with the dietary insult.

Diagnosis

Circumstances that bring the patient to the attention of the physician are such that the diagnosis can be easily missed. Routine urinalysis at the time of the first checkup after birth is negative when fruits have not been introduced. This is also the case if sudden onset of shock causes hospital admission and urine is collected after rehydration with intravenous fluids that usually do not contain fructose. Another set of circumstances that may delay recognition occurs when the disease starts with vomiting and failure to thrive. Since the commonly prescribed diet for vomiting does not contain fruits, diagnosis may be missed on the routine urine exam after hospital admission.

A positive test for reducing substances (Clini-Test), coupled with a negative test for glucose by the glucose oxidase method (Clinistix), suggests excretion of fructose, galactose, or lactose, each being symptomatic of a different disorder. In these cases, urine should be collected for qualitative sugar analysis providing the patient still has been receiving the offending sugar. A diagnosis of HFI is suggested by a history of vomiting, onset of symptoms concomitant with exposure to fructose, and evidence of either hepatic disease or both hepatic and renal tubular disease. This degree of clinical evidence is an indication for a fructose tolerance test under the supervision of a physician. It is the safest approach to the diagnosis, because unsupervised exposure to fructose for the purpose of urine collection can precipitate hypoglycemic shock.

Fructose may be administered orally (0.5 g/kg) or intravenously (3.0 g/M^2). In either case, an intravenous line must be open in case treatment of hypoglycemia becomes necessary. Plasma fructose must be monitored during the oral test to prove adequate absorption. The response of serum phosphorus and glucose to the fructose challenge is measured at 20, 40, 60, and 90 minutes in the intravenous test and at 30, 60, 90, 120, and 180 minutes in the oral test. Individuals with HFI and fructose-1,6-diphosphatase deficiency show a drop in serum phosphorus because of sequestration of phosphorus as hexose phosphates. A drop in plasma glucose generally follows the decline of serum phosphorus. A presumptive diagnosis, based on tolerance tests, requires immediate fructose restriction and confirmation by enzyme studies in liver biopsy specimen. This should not be done until recovery from hepatocellular damage is complete.

Differential diagnosis of hereditary tyrosinemia may be difficult, because it is a phenocopy of HFI. In either disease, liver involvement is associated with elevation of plasma tyrosine and methionine levels, and clotting factors V, VII, and X are markedly reduced. Significant improvement after elimination of fructose from the diet occurs only in HFI. The chronic form requires exclusion of hereditary tyrosinemia and cystinosis.

Treatment

A strict regimen of complete withdrawal of fructose in any form is required (i.e., fruit, fruit juices, sucrose [cane or beet sugar], honey, sorbitol, levulose, and invert sugar). Polysaccharides and disaccharides, which are permitted, are starch, glycogen, maltose, isomaltose, and lactose. Patients should be aware of these technical names and should be instructed to read labels. For example, *sorbitol* is contained in many dietetic products. Attention must be paid to proper use of intravenous fluids, which may contain *invert sugar* or *levulose*. Some vegetables and legumes contain fructose, including broccoli, cucumbers, gourds, avocado, rhubarb, beets, asparagus, peas, and lentils (Table 13-15). Most hypoallergenic formulas contain sucrose. Patients should be restricted for the rest of their lives, although some relaxation is permissible after growth has ceased.

LIPID METABOLISM

Diet, Serum Lipids, and Health

Atherosclerotic vascular disease is a major cause of death in the American population. An impaired carbohydrate tolerance, cigarette smoking, lack of physical activity, obesity, and a family history of heart disease are recognized "risk factors" (65). Severe hyperlipidemias due to genetic disease or disorders like glycogen storage disease also predispose to atherosclerosis. Since mild elevations in plasma cholesterol of up to 30% above normal may be the result of diets high in saturated fats (66,67), a possibility exists that diet alone can lead to atherosclerosis. The typical American diet is high in fat (40%) and has an unfavorable ratio of polyunsaturated to saturated fats (0.2). Consequently, the feasibility of altering the American diet has been the subject of intense controversy in the past.

It is not certain, despite much research, whether cholesterol-reducing diets are indeed effective in lowering the incidence of coronary heart disease. A correlation between diet and coronary heart disease has been demonstrated in population groups, but data on the association between

Table 13-15. Sucrose-Fructose-Free Diet[a]

Food Groups	*Foods to Avoid*	*Foods Allowed*
Milk and beverages	Milk drinks containing sugar or sweetened chocolate, condensed milk, all fruit drinks, beverages containing sugar, fruits, or fructose	Whole, low fat, skim, buttermilk, imitation milk, evaporated milk; plain yogurt
Breads and baked goods	Breads made with sugar, baked goods made with fruits or sugar	All others
Cereals	Sweetened cereals, frosted flakes, cereals with raisins and other fruits	Cooked cereals, puffed rice, shredded wheat, saltines
Desserts	All desserts containing sugar, honey, or fruits, pie, cookies, candy, puddings, jello, ice cream, sherbet	Dietetic jello, dietetic ice cream, dietetic puddings
Eggs	None	All
Fat	Mayonnaise, salad dressings made with sugar	Butter, margarine, oil, homemade mayonnaise or French dressings made without sugar
Fruits	All	None
Meat, fish, and cheese	Ham, bacon, and lunch meats that are sugar-cured	Beef, veal, lamb, pork, chicken, turkey, fish, cheese
Potatoes and starchy foods	Sweet potatoes, yams	White potato (not stored), macaroni, noodles, spaghetti, polished rice
Vegetables	All others	Endive, escarole, kale, lettuce, spinach, swiss chard, rhubarb
Miscellaneous	Catsup, chili sauce, and other sauces containing sugar, honey, maple syrup, jam, jellies, preserves, sucrose, levulose, sorbitol, invert sugar, cane sugar, beet sugar	Vegetable juices (no tomato), coffee, tea, salt, condiments, sugar substitute, dietetic beverages, glucose, galactose

[a] For patients with fructose intolerance. (Note: Sucrose is not tolerated because it is hydrolyzed to fructose and glucose.)

dietary habits, serum lipids and coronary heart disease in individuals within populations are conflicting. There are many reasons to explain these findings including genetic individuality. Since a variety of etiologic factors are operative, failure to demonstrate a statistically significant relation between diet and the incidence of myocardial and cerebral infarcts does not prove the lack of any effect. It is significant, in this context, that prevention trials in adults living in a controlled environment have shown a beneficial effect of diets low in cholesterol (365 mg/day) and high in linoleic acid (40%).

Pediatricians may be asked about the type of diet that will prevent arteriosclerosis. Concern over the need for a prudent diet from childhood on stems from autopsy findings in adolescents of fatty streaks in the walls of coronary arteries in up to 83% of cases, and of raised atherosclerotic plaques in 22% (68). These lesions contain lipids that are similar in composition to those in blood. Moreover, death from coronary heart disease can occur in childhood when cholesterol is excessively high due to familial hyperlipidemia. Therefore, questions concerning a prophylactic diet for children have gained importance. Since conclusive answers are not yet available, and since the risk of atherosclerosis is not the same in all individuals, it seems unwise and unnecessary at this time to impose dietary restrictions on all healthy children. This philosophy is supported by epidemiological evidence that such a diet could promote bile stone formation. However, there is no lack of consensus concerning the management of children at risk. They should be placed on a diet that maintains normal weight, is low in fat (30 to 35% of total calories), and has a polyunsaturated to saturated fatty acid ratio of 1.0.

Since significant elevations of serum lipids in children are not likely caused by diet alone, efforts to detect hyperlipidemia should be aimed at the recognition of risk factors and diseases that cause it, rather than at large-scale investigation of dietary habits. Diabetes, glycogen storage disease, nephrotic syndrome, morbid obesity, hypothyroidism, and obstructive liver disease are associated with hyperlipidemia as a secondary phenomenon. Recognition of these disorders is not difficult since they are associated with other diagnostic manifestations. By contrast, elevation of serum lipids is the only manifestation early in the course of the hereditary hyperlipidemias, and timely recognition is therefore difficult.

Since it is not yet practical to screen all children for hyperlipidemia, testing of serum cholesterol, triglycerides, and lipoproteins should be restricted to certain high-risk groups. These are children with a family history of early myocardial infarcts or hyperlipidemia. Children are best tested after 2 years of age. Values for cholesterol over 200 mg/dl and of triglycerides in excess of 150 mg/dl warrant repeat testing with emphasis on adherence to a 12-hour fast prior to the test. If several determinations are in the upper normal range or above, it is advisable to place these children on a diet (see following). A positive diagnosis of genetic hyperlipidemia requires family studies and determination of lipoproteins in addition to plasma lipids.

Biochemistry

In recent years new information on cholesterol metabolism and the role of plasma lipoprotein in the transport throughout the body has become available which has been summarized in numerous reports (60–71). The current interpretation of these data is briefly presented here, since it forms the basis for an understanding of hyperlipidemias and their management.

Cholesterol can be found in every cell of the body as a major constituent of membranes. It makes up almost 50% of myelin and is a precursor of bile acids, adrenal and reproductive hormones, and vitamin D. It is synthesized at a sufficient rate to meet the body's need and is consequently not a dietary essential. Since it is also a constituent of animal tissues, it is present in meat, egg, fish, and milk products, but occurs only in small amounts in plant tissues. Vegetable fats contain no cholesterol.

Plasma cholesterol concentration is maintained remarkably steady through the action of a number of homeostatic mechanisms, including absorption. Although the percentage of absorption increases when dietary cholesterol is low, the absolute amount absorbed can be maintained at a low level through dietary measures. The availability of bile acids and of the hydrolytic products of dietary fats in the intestine is a major factor limiting absorption. Consequently, dietary fats aid the absorption of cholesterol and—since cholesterol is converted to bile acids—it seems to promote its own absorption indirectly. However, the total amount of available cholesterol is controlled through feedback inhibition of endogenous cholesterol synthesis in the liver. Diet is a major factor influencing cholesterol metabolism, since a high calorie intake increases cholesterogenesis and fats increase cholesterol absorption.

Following excretion into the gut, about 98% of bile acids are reabsorbed to be returned to the liver. Nevertheless, bile is a major pathway for the removal of cholesterol from the body. If a large amount is recycled, further bile production from cholesterol is inhibited. The primary bile acids produced from cholesterol are cholic and chenodeoxycholic acid, which are conjugated with glycine or taurine to yield bile salts.

Transport in blood or lymph requires a special carrier mechanism, because cholesterol is insoluble in aqueous solutions. Plasma lipoproteins serve this function. They are made up of specific apoproteins, phospholipids, and free cholesterol. A nonpolar core is capable of picking up cholesterol esters and triglycerides. Several classes of lipoproteins, which are based on increasing density, have been identified: chylomicron, very-low- (VLDL), low- (LDL), and high-density lipoproteins (HDL). The lipid-rich core of chylomicron consists mainly of triglycerides. Dietary and recycled cholesterol is carried together with triglycerides in chylomicron and VLDL via the thoracic duct to the blood stream. About 15% of total plasma cholesterol (35mg/dl) is bound to VLDL (71). When these particles enter the blood stream, they undergo several alterations. Mainly triglycerides are removed by action of lipoprotein lipase, leaving a remnant that picks up cholesterol esters, either from HDL or by esterification of free cholesterol on its surface. The responsible enzyme is lecitin-cholesterol transferase (LCAT) (72,73). Through a mechanism that is not fully understood, this process transforms VLDL into LDL. Cholesterol bound to LDL accounts for about 65% of total plasma cholesterol (145 mg/dl). LDL cholesterol is then taken up in various tissues by receptors on the surface of cells.

Excess cholesterol on the cell surface must be returned to the liver, where it may be converted to bile acids or excreted into plasma. HDL appears to play a very important role in this uptake of cholesterol, which protects the individual from excess accumulaton. The manner in which HDL seems to prevent cholesterol accumulation is not fully understood. It is possible that this is accomplished by HDL through direct blockage of cholesterol uptake by the cell, rather than removal from the cell after the fact. HDL carries about 20% of total cholesterol (45 mg/dl). The amount of HDL produced is influenced mainly by genetic and endocrine factors and relatively little by diet. Thus, women have higher values than men. Physical activity and alcohol ingestion increase circulating HDL. Cholesterol levels are a function of both genetic and environmental factors, including diet. The polyunsaturated to saturated fatty acid ratio is the most important of the dietary factors. Diet influences plasma cholesterol mainly by varying the excretion of steroids in the stool (73). Normal values for cholesterol and triglycerides have been established for American children (74) (Table 13-16).

Table 13-16. Plasma Lipid Concentrations in "Normal"[a] Americans

Age	*Cholesterol*		*Triglyceride*	
(years)	*(mean)*	*(upper 10%)*	*(mean, SD)*	*(upper 5%)*
6 (–12)	182	220	71 ± 36	140
(12–) 18	<182		108 ± 45	
Adults: 30–39	205	240		150
40–49	225	265		160
50–59	245	280		190

SOURCE: Values for children from Lauer RM et al: *J Pediatr* 86:697, 1975; for adults, from Fredrickson DS, Levy RI: *Metabolic Basis of Inherited Disease.* New York, McGraw-Hill, 1972, pp 545–614.

[a] Normal levels in the U.S. population are not to be considered safe levels.

Genetic Conditions Affecting Lipid Metabolism and Health

There are four genetic conditions that affect lipid metabolism and influence the incidence of peripheral vascular disease. Three major forms, which are easily distinguished on the basis of plasma lipid determinations, cause premature coronary heart disease; while one form, hyper-α-lipoproteinemia, protects the individual from atherosclerotic disease.

Primary Hyperlipidemias

The original classification of Fredrickson et al. (75), based on plasma lipoprotein patterns, has been simplified. Three major types are recognized in the pediatric literature. They are *hypercholesterolemia* (Fredrickson type IIa), *combined hyperlipidemia* (Fredrickson type IIb), and *hypertriglyceridemia* (Fredrickson type IV). LDL is increased and VLDL is normal in hypercholesterolemia; plasma cholesterol ranges usually from 250 to 500 mg/dl. LDL as well as VLDL are increased in combined hyperlipidemia, with cholesterol above 250 and triglycerides above 200 mg/dl. Only VLDL is increased in hypertriglyceridemia, and plasma triglycerides range from 200 to 500 mg/dl. The lipoprotein abnormalities reflect their function, since VLDL carries predominantly triglycerides and LDL carries cholesterol. *Familial hyperlipoproteinemia* (Fredrickson, type I) is a very rare disorder, with onset in childhood, that does not cause atherosclerotic vascular disease. Triglycerides, carried by chylomicrons, are markedly increased in this disorder and cause the plasma to appear milky, even after a fast. The biochemical defect of the three hyperlipidemias is not known. An enzyme, a carrier protein, or a membrane receptor may be involved. Lipoprotein lipase is apparently deficient in type I hyperlipoproteinemia.

Familial expression of these diseases is vertical. Approximately 50% of first-degree relatives are affected. Although this is compatible with an autosomal dominant mode of inheritance, it is possible that hypercholesterolemia is transmitted by a highly penetrant autosomal allele, with disease expression in heterozygous individuals. A homozygous form of hypercholesterolemia has been recognized where homozygotes have double the plasma concentrations of heterozygotes. Homozygotes rarely reach adulthood. The possibility of polygenic inheritance in some forms of hyperlipidemia should be considered.

Clinical manifestations are similar in the three major forms of hyperlipidemia. It has been claimed that these disorders are the cause of myocardial infarcts in almost 50% of cases who have their first attack before 50 years of age. Xanthomas are common and involve most frequently the eyelids (xanthelasma) and cornea (arcus corneae). Other favorite sites are tendons, mainly achilles tendon and the extensor tendons of the hand and fingers, and the areas over the elbows, knees, and buttocks. Xanthomas may be tuberous or flat (planar). They are skin colored or have an orange hue. Only hypercholesterolemia and hyperlipidemia type I are fully expressed in the pediatric age group. The best age for detection of hypercholesterolemia is not known. Current methods do not allow recognition in cord blood. Values in neonates are variable because they increase about twofold after birth and are influenced by the diet, with higher levels in breast-fed infants than in infants on cow's milk.

Treatment

The interrelationship between nutrient intake and plasma lipids and lipoproteins has been studied in schoolchildren of the Princeton school district (76,77). The finding of an inverse relationship between the polyunsaturated to saturated fatty acid ratio and plasma cholesterol-LDL supports earlier and generally accepted guidelines recommending a ratio of 1.0 to 1.5. In addition, an inverse relationship was found between total dietary carbohydrate and sugar content to plasma cholesterol-LDL. The cholesterol-lowering effect of a high-carbohydrate diet was offset by the finding of rising triglyceride concentrations with increasing calorie, carbohydrate, and sucrose intake. The value of traditional therapy of hypertriglyceridemia in adults, consisting of weight reduction and carbohydrate restriction, is being supported by these findings.

A low-fat diet with a polyunsaturated to saturated fatty ratio of 1.0 can be maintained by following a number of simple directives: (*1*) use of vegetable fats (except coconut oil) for cooking and of margarine made with corn oil as a spread; (*2*) limitation of meats rich in fat, mainly beef and pork, and substitution with fish and foul; (*3*) use of skim milk for adolescents and 2% milk for infants and small children; and (*4*) restriction of eggs to two or three per week.

The cholesterol-lowering effect of even the strictest diet is, unfortunately, not very effective in familial hypercholesterolemia since cholesterol is synthesized by the organism. The biochemical defect appears to have a far stronger effect than can be offset by diet. It is therefore almost always necessary to supplement a diet with drug therapy. A resin called cholestyramine, which binds bile acids and prevents their absorption, is the currently preferred drug for lowering plasma cholesterol. Although the drug interrupts the enterohepatic recirculation of bile acids and results in a net loss of steroids, this is apparently offset by a compensatory increase in cholesterol synthesis by the liver. Consequently, the cholesterol-lowering effect may not add more than 10% to the effect of diet alone. The drug has the additional disadvantage of unpleasant side effects, including bloating, constipation, and nausea. Moreover, it is not convenient to take. It comes in 4-g packets that must be mixed with a tall glass of juice or water and taken before meals, at least three times a day. Compliance is generally poor in children. Another cholesterol-lowering drug is D-thyroxine. Its mode of action is not fully understood. Since the drug has hypermetabolic action, it should be used with caution. The dose is 1 mg/

day, initially, and may be raised to 8 mg/day in adolescents. Individuals with familial hypertriglyceridemia may benefit from clofibrate (1 g, twice a day). The mode of action of this drug is also not known with certainty. Side effects include nausea, myositis, hair loss, agranulocytosis, and abnormalities of liver function. Patients taking the drug should be monitored periodically through blood count and liver function tests.

Familial Hyper-α-Lipoproteinemia

The name *familial hyper-α-lipoproteinemia* refers to a genetic condition characterized by an increase of α-lipoprotein, which is the term originally used for HDL. It has been estimated (78) that about half of all children with mild hypercholesterolemia of less than 250 mg/dl have normal values for LDL and above-average values for HDL. The phenomenon was studied in 18 kindred by Glueck et al. (79), who demonstrated vertical appearance of high cholesterol-HDL values in a total of 10 kindreds. Hyper-α-lipoproteinemia was identified by cholesterol-HDL levels above the 90th percentile (i.e., 70 mg/dl). It is necessary in such cases to rule out a secondary effect of alcohol ingestion or estrogen administration. Because of the known anti-risk effect of HDL, recognition of this condition in patients presenting with hypercholesterolemia is important. Joint determination of plasma lipids and HDL is advised in cases with hypercholesterolemia. This condition does not carry the risk of hypercholesterolemia, (type IIa).

REFERENCES

1. Garrod AE: Croonian lectures. *Lancet* II:1, 1908.
2. Holtzman NA, Meek AG, Mellits ED: Neonatal screening for phenylketonuria. *JAMA* 229:667, 1974.
3. Schaub J, Dauming S, Curtis H, et al: Tetrahydrobiopterin therapy of a typical phenylketonuria due to defective dihydrobiopetrin biosynthesis. *Arch Dis Child* 53:674, 1978.
4. Milstien S, Holtzman NA, O'Flynn ME, et al: Hyperphenylalaninemia due to the dihydropteridine reductase deficiency. *J Pediatr* 89:763, 1976.
5. Bowes A, Church CF: *Food Values of Portions Commonly Used*, ed 11. Philadelphia, Lippincott, 1972.
6. Bodegard G, Gentz J, Lindblad B, et al: Hereditary Tyrosinemia III on the differential diagnosis and the lack of effect of early dietary treatment. *Acta Paediatr Scand* 58:37, 1969.
7. Harries JT, Seakins JWT, Ersser RS, et al: Recovery after dietary treatment of an infant with features of Tyrosinosis. *Arch Dis Child* 44:258, 1969.
8. Fairney A, Francis D, Ersser RS, et al: Diagnosis and treatment of Tyrosinosis. *Arch Dis Child* 43:540, 1968.

9. Gentz J, Lindblad B, Lindstedt S, et al: Dietary treatment in Tyrosinemia (Tyrosinosis) with a note on the possible recognition of the carrier state. *Am J Dis Child* 113:31, 1967.

10. Halvorsen S: Dietary treatment of Tyrosinosis. *Am J Dis Child* 113:38, 1967.

11. Acosta P, Elsas L: *Dietary Management of Inherited Metabolic Disease: Phenylketonuria, Galactosemia, Tyrosinemia, Maple Sugar Urine Disease*. Atlanta, Ga, ACELMU, 1976.

12. Holt LE: *Protein and Amino Acid Requirements in Early Life*. New York, New York University Press, 1960.

13. Mamunes P, Prince PE, Thornton NH, et al: Intellectual deficits after transient tyrosinemia in the term neonate. *Pediatrics* 57:675, 1976.

14. Snyderman SE, Sansaricq C, Phansalkar SV, et al: The therapy of hyperammonemia due to ornithine transcarbamylase deficiency in a male neonate. *Pediatrics* 56:65, 1975.

15. McReynolds JM, Mantagos S, Brusilow SW, et al: Treatment of complete ornithine-transcarbamylase deficiency with nitrogen free analogues of essential amino acids. *J Pediatr* 93:421, 1978.

16. Brusilow SW, Batshaw ML, Walser M: Use of ketoacids in inborn errors of urea synthesis, in Winick M (ed): *Nutritional Management of Genetic Disorders*. New York, John Wiley and Sons, 1979, p. 65.

17. Batshaw ML, Painter MJ, Sproul GT, et al: Therapy of urea cycle enzymopathies: Three case studies. *Johns Hopkins Med J* 148:34, 1981.

18. Brusilow SW, Tinker J, Batshaw ML: Amino acid acylation: A mechanism for nitrogen excretion in inborn errors of urea synthesis. *Science* 207:659, 1980.

19. Krieger I, Nigro M, Taqi Q: Screening for metabolic disease in a metropolitan hospital. *Am J Dis Child*, to be published.

20. Hsia EY, Lilljeqvist AC, Rosenberg LE: Vitamin B_{12}-dependent methylmalonicaciduria: Amino acid toxicity, long chain ketonuria, and protective effect of vitamin B_{12}. *Pediatrics* 46:497, 1970.

21. Krieger I: Personal experience.

22. Tanaka K, Budd MA, Efron ML, et al: Isovaleric acidemia: A new genetic defect of leucine metabolism. *Proc Natl Acad Sci USA* 56:236, 1966.

23. Krieger I, Tanaka K: Therapeutic effects of glycine in isovaleric acidemia. *Pediatr Res* 10:25, 1976.

24. Inoue S, Krieger I, Sarnaik A, et al: Inhibition of bone marrow stem cell growth in vitro by methylmalonic acid: A mechanism of pancytopenia in a patient with methylmalonic acidemia. *Pediatr Res* 15:95, 1981.

25. Bremer HJ, Duram J, Kamerling JP, et al: *Disturbances of Amino Acid Metabolism*. Baltimore, Munich, Urban and Schwarzenberg, 1981, p 344.

26. Levy HL, Erickson AM, Lott IT, et al: Isovaleric acidemia: Results of family study and dietary treatment. *Pediatrics* 52:83, 1973.

27. Snyderman SE, Raitman EL, Boyer A, et al: Essential amino acid requirements of infants. *Am J Dis Child* 102:35, 1961.

28. Cohn RM, Yudkoff M, Rothman R, et al: Isovaleric acidemia: Use of glycine therapy in neonates. *N Engl J Med* 299:996, 1978.

29. Naylor EW, Guthrie R: Newborn screening for maple syrup urine disease (branched-chain ketoaciduria). *Pediatrics* 61:262, 1978.

30. Dancis J: Variants of maple sugar urine disease, in Nyhan WL (ed): *Heritable Disorders of Amino Acid Metabolism*. New York, John Wiley and Sons Inc, 1974, p 32.

31. Robinson BH, Taylor J, Sherwood WG: Deficiency of dihydrolipoyl dehydrogenase (a component of the pyruvate and α-ketoglutarate dehydrogenase complexe). Course of congenital chronic lactic acidosis in infancy. *Pediatr Res*, 11:118, 1977.

32. Dent CE, Friedman M, Green H, et al: Treatment of cystinuria. *Br Med J* 1:403, 1965.

33. McCully KS, Ragsdale BD: Production of arteriosclerosis by homocysteinemia. *Am J Pathol* 61:1, 1970.

34. Perry TL: Treatment of homocystinuria with low methionine diet and supplemented by l-cystine, in Carson NA, Raine DN (eds): *Inherited Disorders of Sulfur Metabolism*. London, Livingstone, 1971, p 245.

35. Roland DA: Nutritional care for children with inborn errors of metabolism, in Krause MV, Mahan LK (eds): *Food, Nutrition and Diet Therapy*. Philadelphia, London, Toronto, WB Saunders Company, 1979, p 777.

36. Bĕlanger L, Bélanger M, Larochell E: Existence α'alpha-1-foèto protéine circulante chez 8 patients souffrant de tyrosinémia héréditaire. *Union Med Can* 101:877, 1972.

37. Fallström SP, Lindblad B, Lindstedt S, et al: Hereditary tyrosinemia fumaryl aceto acetase deficiency. *Pediatr Res* 13:78, 1979.

38. Lindblad B, Lindstedt S, Steen G: On the enzymic defects in hereditary tyrosinemia. *Proc Natl Acad Sci USA* 74:4641, 1977.

39. Perry TL, Hansen S, MacGongall L: Methionine induction of experimental tyrosinemia. *J Ment Defic Res* 11:246, 1967.

40. Perheentupa J, Visakorpi JK: Protein intolerance with deficient transport of basic amino acids, another inborn error of metabolism. *Lancet* II:813, 1965.

41. Awrich AE, Stackhouse WJ, Cantrell JE et al: Hyperdibasicaminoaciduria, hyperammonemia, and growth retardation: treatment with arginine, lysine and citrulline.

42. Bottazzo GF, Florin-Christensen A, Doniach D: Islet-cell antibodies in diabetes mellitus with autoimmune polyendocrine deficiencies. *Lancet* 2:1279, 1974.

43. Nerup J, Platz P, Anderson OO, et al: HL-A antigens and diabetes mellitus. *Lancet* 2:864, 1974.

44. Gabbay KH: Hyperglycemia, polyol metabolism, and complications of diabetes mellitus. *Annu Rev Med* 26:521, 1975.

45. Koenig RJ, Peterson CM, Jones RL, et al: Correlation of glucose regulation and hemoglobin A_{1c} in diabetes mellitus. *N Engl J Med* 295:417, 1976.

46. Pirart J: Diabetes mellitus and its degenerative complications: A prospective study of 4,400 patients observed between 1947 and 1973. *Diabetes Care I* (pt I):168 (pt II):252, 1978.

47. Drash A: The control of diabetes mellitus: Is it achievable? Is it desirable? *J Pediatr* 88:1074, 1976.

48. *Exchange Lists for Meal Planning*. New York, American Diabetes Association; Chicago, American Dietetic Association, 1976.

49. Chaussain JL: Glycemic response to 24-hour fast in normal children and children with ketotic hypoglycemia. *J Pediatr* 82:438, 1973.

50. Stanley CA, Baker L: Hyperinsulinism in infancy: Diagnosis by demonstration of abnormal response to fasting hypoglycemia. *Pediatrics* 57:702, 1976.

51. Baker L, Winegrad AI: Fasting hypoglycemia and metabolic acidosis associated with deficiency of hepatic fructose-1, 6-diphosphatase activity. *Lancet* 2:13, 1970.

52. Lewis GM, Spencer-Peet J, Stewart KM: Infantile hypoglycemia due to inherited deficiency of glycogen synthetase in liver. *Arch Dis Child* 38:40, 1963.

53. Dykes JRW, Spencer-Peet J: Hepatic glycogen synthetase deficiency: Futher studies on a family. *Arch Dis Child* 47:558, 1972.

54. Haymond MW, Karl IE, Pagliara AS: Ketotic hypoglycemia: An amino acid substrate-limited disorder. *J Clin Endocrinol Metab* 38:521, 1974.

55. Koffler H, Schubert WK, Hug G: Sporadic hypoglycemia: Abnormal epinephrine response to the ketogenic diet or to insulin. *J Pediatr* 78:448, 1971.

56. Kogut MD, Blascovics M, Donnel GN: Idiopathic hypoglycemia: A study of twenty-six children. *J Pediatr* 74:853, 1969.

57. Colle E, Ulstrom RA: Ketotic hypoglycemia. *J Pediatr* 64:632, 1964.

58. DiGeorge AM, Auerbach UH, Mabry CC: Leucine-induced hypoglycemia: III. The blood glucose depressant action of leucine in normal individuals. *J Pediatr* 63:295, 1963.

59. Misugi K, Misugi N, Sotos J, et al: The pancreatic islet of infants with severe hypoglycemia. *Arch Pathol* 89:208, 1970.

60. Cochrane WA: Studies in the relationship of amino acids to infantile hypoglycemia. *Am J Dis Child* 99:476, 1960.

61. Greene ML, Slonim AE, O'Neill JA, et al: Continuous nocturnal intragastric feeding for management of type I glycogen-storage disease. *N Engl J Med* 294:423, 1976.

62. Cook JGH, Don NA, Mann TP: Hereditary galactokinase deficiency. *Arch Dis Child* 46:465, 1971.

63. Beutler E, Matsumoto F, Kuhl W, et al: Galactokinase deficiency as a cause of cataracts. *N Engl J Med* 288:1203, 1973.

64. Monteleone JA, Beutler E, Monteleone PL, et al: Cataracts, galactosuria, and hypergalactosemia due to galactokinase deficiency in a child. *Am J Med* 50:403, 1971.

65. Kannel WB, Castelli WP, Gordon T, et al: Serum cholesterol, lipoproteins, and the risk of coronary heart disease: The Framingham Study. *Ann Intern Med* 74:1, 1971.

66. Connor WE, Hodges RE, Bleiler RE: The serum lipids in men receiving high cholesterol and cholesterol-free diets. *J Clin Invest* 40:894, 1961.

67. Hegsted DM, McGrandy RB, Myers ML, et al: Quantitative effects of dietary fat on serum cholesterol in man. *Am J Clin Nutr* 17:281, 1965.

68. Strong JP, McGill HC Jr: The pediatric aspects of atherosclerosis. *J Atheroscler Res* 9:251, 1969.

69. Sabine JR: *Cholesterol*. New York, Marcel Dekker Inc, 1977.

70. Grundy SM: Cholesterol metabolism in man. *West J Med* 128:13, 1978.

71. Thompson P, Bortz WM II: Significance of high-density lipoprotein cholesterol. *J Am Geriatr Soc* 26:440, 1978.

72. Glomset JA, Verdery RB: Role of LCAT in cholesterol metabolism. *Expos Annu Biochim Med* 33:137, 1977.

73. Grundy SM: *Lipid Pharmacology*, vol 2, Paoletti R, Glueck CJ (eds). New York, Academic Press, 1976, p 127.

74. Lauer RM, Connor WE, Leaverton PE, et al: Coronary heart disease risk factors in school children: The Muscatine Study. *J Pediatr* 86:697, 1975.

75. Fredrickson DS, Goldstein JL, Brown MS: Familial hyperlipoproteinemia, in Stanbury JB, Wyngaarden JB, Fredrickson DS (eds): *The Metabolic Basis of Inherited Disease*. New York, McGraw-Hill Co, 1978, p 604.

76. Morrison JA, Larsen R, Glatfelter L, et al: Interrelationships between nutrient intake and plasma lipids and lipoproteins in school children aged 6 to 19: The Princeton School District Study. *Pediatrics* 65:727, 1980.

77. Morrison JA, DeGroot I, Edwards BK, et al: Plasma cholesterol and triglyceride levels in 6775 school children, ages 6–17. *Metabolism* 26:1199, 1977.

78. Neill CA, Ose L, Kwiterovich PO Jr: Hyperlipidemia: Clinical clues in the first two decades of life. *Johns Hopkins Med J* 140:171, 1977.

79. Glueck CJ, Fallat RW, Millett F, et al: Familial hyper alpha lipoproteinemia: Studies in 18 kindreds. *Metabolism* 24:1234, 1975.

80. Weyler W, Sweetman L, Maggio DC, et al: Deficiency of propionyl-CoA carboxylase and methyl crotonyl-CoA carboxylase in a patient with methyl crotonyl glycinuria. *Clin Chim Acta* 76:321, 1977.

81. Gregersen N, Brandt NY: Ketotic episodes in glutaryl-CoA dehydrogenase deficiency (glutaric aciduria). *Pediatr Res* 13:977, 1979.

82. Irwin MI, Hegsted DM: A conspectus of research on amino acid requirements of man. *J Nutr* 101:539, 1971.

83. Spielberg SP, Kramer LI, Goodman SI et al: 5-oxoprolinuria: Biochemical observations and case report. *J Pediatr* 91:237, 1977.

84. Hillman RE, Keating JP: Beta-ketothiolase deficiency as a cause of the "Ketotic Hyperglycinemia Syndrome". *Pediatrics* 53:221, 1974.

85. Hsia YE, Scully KJ, Rosenberg LE: Defective propionate carboxylation in ketotic hyperglycinemia. *Lancet* I:757, 1969.

86. Rosenberg LE, Scriver CR: Disorders of Amino Acid Metabolism; in: Bondy PK and Rosenberg LE (eds) Metabolic Control of Disease, WB Saunders Co. 1980.

87. Valle D, Walser M, Brusilow SW et al: Gyrate atrophy of the choroid and retina. Amino acid metabolism and correction of hyperornithinemia with an arginine deficient diet. *J Clin Invest* 65:371, 1980.

88. Shih VE, Berson EI, Gargiulo M: Reduction of hyperornithinemia with a low protein diet, low arginine diet and pyridoxine in patients with a deficiency of ornithine-ketoacid transaminase (OKT) activity and gyrate atrophy of the choroid and retina *Clin Chim Acta* 113:243, 1981.

89. Larsson A, Mattsson B, Wauters EA et al: 5-oxoprolinuria due to hereditary 5-oxoprolinase deficiency in two brothers—A new inborn error of the gamma-glutamyl cycle. *Acta Paediatr Scand* 70:301, 1981.

90. Fellman JH, Vanbellinghen PJ, Jones RT et al: Soluble and mitochondrial forms of tyrosine amino transferase relationship to human tyrosinemia. *Biochemistry* 8:615, 1969.

Index